Pathological Bodies

THE BERKELEY SERIES IN BRITISH STUDIES

Mark Bevir and James Vernon, University of California, Berkeley, editors

1. *The Peculiarities of Liberal Modernity in Imperial Britain,* edited by Simon Gunn and James Vernon
2. *Dilemmas of Decline: British Intellectuals and World Politics, 1945–1975,* by Ian Hall
3. *The Savage Visit: New World People and Popular Imperial Culture in Britain, 1710–1795,* by Kate Fullagar
4. *The Afterlife of Empire,* by Jordanna Bailkin
5. *Smyrna's Ashes: Humanitarianism, Genocide, and the Birth of the Middle East,* by Michelle Tusan
6. *Pathological Bodies: Medicine and Political Culture,* by Corinna Wagner

Pathological Bodies
Medicine and Political Culture

CORINNA WAGNER

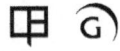

Global, Area, and International Archive
University of California Press
BERKELEY   LOS ANGELES   LONDON

The Global, Area, and International Archive (GAIA) is an initiative of the Institute of International Studies, University of California, Berkeley, in partnership with the University of California Press, the California Digital Library, and international research programs across the University of California system.

University of California Press, one of the most distinguished university presses in the United States, enriches lives around the world by advancing scholarship in the humanities, social sciences, and natural sciences. Its activities are supported by the UC Press Foundation and by philanthropic contributions from individuals and institutions. For more information, visit www.ucpress.edu.

University of California Press
Berkeley and Los Angeles, California

University of California Press, Ltd.
London, England

© 2013 by The Regents of the University of California

Library of Congress Cataloging-in-Publication Data

A catalog record for this book is available from the Library of Congress

ISBN: 978-1938169-08-3

22 21 20 19 18 17 16 15 14 13
10 9 8 7 6 5 4 3 2 1

For radical dandies, past and present

Contents

List of Illustrations ix

Acknowledgments xi

Introduction: Constitutions Both Corporeal and Political 1

PART I. REVOLUTIONARY PATHOLOGIES

1. The Case of Marie Antoinette: Revolutionary Politics and the Biologically Suspect Woman 17

2. Monstrous Mothers, Constitutional Amazons, and the Medicalization of the Breast 50

PART II. RADICAL PATHOLOGIES

3. Murder to Dissect: Godwin, Wollstonecraft, and the Pathology of Indifference 81

4. Hygiene, Contamination, and Tom Paine's Toenails 129

PART III. ROYAL PATHOLOGIES

5. Gout vs. *Goût:* Taste, Community, and the Monarchy 167

6. Hottentot Buttocks, "Strange Chinese Shapes," and George IV's Oriental Appetites 198

Coda: Medicine, Politics, and the Production of the Modern Body 231

Notes 239

Bibliography 273

Index 293

Illustrations

1.1 Anon., *Bravo, Bravo! la Reine se penetre de la Patrie* (1791) — 22
2.1. Thomas Rowlandson, *Political Affection* (1784) — 61
2.2. Anon., *Duchess of D—— in the Character of a Mother* (1784) — 62
2.3. Anon., *L'aristocrate; la democrate* (1790) — 65
2.4. James Gillray, *Un petit Soupèr a la Parisiènne* (1792) — 66
2.5. George Cruikshank, *The Belle-Alliance* (1819) — 67
2.6. Daniel Edwards, *Presidential Bust of Hillary Rodham Clinton* (2006) — 78
3.1. William Dent, *A Right Hon. Democrat Dissected* (1793) — 82
3.2. Anon., *A Dissection* (1797) — 83
3.3. James Gillray, *A Sphere, Projecting against a Plane* (1792) — 84
3.4. Pregnant woman with fetus showing, from Estienne, *De dissectione partium corporis humani libri tres* (1545) — 93
3.5. Standing and seated pregnant women, from d'Agoty, *Anatomie des parties de la generation de l'homme et de la femme* (1773) — 95
3.6. Abdominal viscera, from Hunter, *The Anatomy of the Human Gravid Uterus Exhibited in Figures* (1774) — 96
3.7. "The child in the womb, in its natural situation," from Hunter, *The Anatomy of the Human Gravid Uterus Exhibited in Figures* (1774) — 97
3.8. Thomas Rowlandson, *The Resurrection* (1782) — 99
4.1. James Gillray, *Tom Paine's Nightly Pest* (1792) — 148

4.2. James Gillray, *Fashion before Ease* (1793)   153
5.1. [William Heath], *A Pleasant Draught for Louis* (1814)   168
5.2. George Cruikshank, *A Levee Day* (1814)   169
5.3. James Gillray, *Temperance Enjoying a Frugal Meal* (1792)   177
5.4. James Gillray, *A Voluptuary under the Horrors of Digestion* (1792)   182
6.1. George Cruikshank, "The Folly at Brighton," from Hone, *The Joss and His Folly* (1820)   206
6.2. George Cruikshank, "A living teapot stands," from Hone, *The Joss and His Folly* (1820)   207
6.3. George Cruikshank, *The Court at Brighton a la Chinese!!* (1816)   208
6.4. Louis François Charon, *Les curieux en extase* (1815)   210
6.5. James Gillray, *Anti-saccharrites* (1792)   223
6.6. Isaac Cruikshank, *The Gradual Abolition off* [sic] *the Slave Trade* (1792)   224

Acknowledgments

As is usual with these projects, I have accumulated a long list of debts. Many people have become unfortunate victims of my fascination with all things bodily and all subjects medical. At dinner parties and receptions, I have waxed lyrical on intestinal parasites, skin disorders, gout, tumors, hysteria, hypochondria, and eighteenth-century techniques of kidney stone removal. The list of people who have been wonderfully patient interlocutors on these and other subjects include Victoria Bates, Andy Brown, Karen Edwards, Philipp Erchinger, Sally Flint, Regenia Gagnier, Sam Goodman, Helen Hanson, Matt Hayler, Gerald "Mac" Maclean, Alex Murray, Sam North, Angelique Richardson, Sharon Ruston, Jane Spencer, Darren Wagner, Paul Williams, Peggy Yoon, and Tricia Zakreski.

I must supplement this list with equally long-suffering discussants on a range of political subjects, from "rights, power, discourse" to coffeehouse culture. Thanks to Robert Lamb, Jon Mee, Alison O'Byrne, Frank O'Gorman, Steve Poole, and Jim Watt. I am most grateful to John Barrell, who was unstintingly sharp as a PhD supervisor and colleague. He won't remember, but years ago he asked me a tough question. I had suffered something of a crisis of faith and was producing some absolutely rubbish work. After reading one particularly dire piece, he sighed, turned to me, and asked, "Where is the excitement?" That question continues to stand me in good stead.

I also want to say something about other kinds of bodies: I have benefitted enormously from institutions, funding councils, associations, societies, and centers. Over the last ten years, I have been supported financially by the University of York Postgraduate Award Scheme, the Social Sciences and Humanities Research Council of Canada, the Arts and Humanities Research Council, the British Society for Eighteenth-Century Studies (BSECS), and the University of Exeter.

I have learned a great deal at Society for the Social History of Medicine conferences, Wellcome Trust events, and Morbid Anatomy's Congress for Curious Peoples symposia. This book has also benefited enormously from collaborative bodies at the University of Exeter, including the Centre for Medical Humanities (directed by the tireless and incredibly generous Mark Jackson), the Centre for Victorian Studies, and the Eighteenth-Century Research Group. I am very pleased, too, to be part of a wonderful collaboration between the University of Exeter (headed by Regenia Gagnier and John Dupré of Egenis) and Vanderbilt University (headed by Jay Clayton of the Curb Center for Art, Enterprise and Public Policy and Ellen Wright Clayton of the Center for Biomedical Ethics and Society). For consistently reminding me of the importance of collegiality, I want to thank the executive committee members of BSECS, including Michael Burden, Daniel Cook, Penny Corfield, Jeremy Gregory, Frank O'Gorman, Charlotte Roberts, and Debbie Welham.

I have spent wonderful hours in special collections in the libraries at the University of Glasgow, the University of York, the University of Cambridge, and the University of Oxford. I especially appreciate the staff, services, and collections of the British Library and the brilliant Wellcome Library. I look forward to many more happy years spent in your bowels.

The production of this book has been a real pleasure. For their enthusiasm and intelligence, thanks go to Mark Bevir and James Vernon, editors of the Berkeley Series in British Studies, and to Nathan O'Brien at the University of California Press. Julie Van Pelt had an amazing eye for detail, and Jane Spencer and two anonymous readers were insightful and encouraging. At just the right moment in this project, George Rousseau clearly articulated what I was doing and what was original about it. My sincere thanks.

On a more personal note, I am grateful to Edith, Harvey, Sheldon, and Jason Wagner for weeks of summer hospitality during the completion of this project. Finally, thank you, Andy Brown, for reminding me that, like Dorothy Parker, I care a very great deal "for fun and such." You are a gem.

Introduction: Constitutions Both Corporeal and Political

I begin this book by examining three passages. Although very different, all three express related ideas about "constitutions," both bodily and political.

My first selection is from a 1744 letter by one of the most famous anatomists and obstetricians of the eighteenth century, William Hunter. Then a medical student, Hunter counsels his ailing brother, James, who had recently given up his medical studies in London to convalesce at the family home in Scotland:

> If it is true that diseases are the strugles of nature endeavouring to extirpate the enemys of a Constitution, yours must now be very sound; for after so many attempts upon her Government, and the last so resolute a one, it is but reasonable to think that her excellency nature will now banish or destroy every malcontent, in short cut off the memory of Sedition. I wish you all pleasures in your Whey-drinking.[1]

William Hunter's political allegorizing of his brother's health expresses a long-standing association of the human body with the body politic. As revolution and rebellion assail the nation's constitution, so does disease attack and alter the body's structures and functions. Historically, the use of the body as political metaphor stretches back to the classical era and to Plato's *polis*; the use of political metaphor to make sense of the body has a similarly long history.

In the century before Hunter, writers commonly mediated lessons of anatomy and physiology with political referents. In his 1615 *Microcosmographia: The Body of Man*, the Suffolk anatomist and physician Helkiah Crooke compared the structure of government and the organic nature of civil society with the functioning of the hierarchized organs of the body. He provided a material framework for political debates about the relationship between governors and governed, and cast the material body as part of the social and political world. Crooke proposed that knowledge of the functioning of the brain would illustrate how princes could rule effectively, while the nourishing function of the liver might help them appreciate "bounty and liberality."[2] In the years following publication of his treatise, the relationship between politics and culture, medicine and morality, would become even more closely intertwined. In civil war pamphlets and in Restoration treatises, debates about political legitimacy and monarchical succession were often expressed in corporeal terms.

As this extremely brief foray into earlier periods should indicate, Hunter's comments tap into a long-standing politicomedical discourse. Yet, his language also reflects historically specific—and rather weighty—discursive transformations. Hunter anticipates the rise of what historians have identified as the age of both political and medical revolution (the philosopher Ian Hacking terms this one of medicine's "great periods of imperial expansion").[3] Hunter's letter expresses an amalgamation of political and medical ideas that, in the next century, would engender profound changes in both fields. His synopsis of the body's war against illness indicates a growing parity between medical and political attitudes about order and disorder. He also hints at the dominant aim of modern medical science: to return the body to its "natural" state by expelling the unnatural or contranatural elements that afflicted it. Enlightenment medicine was a contest to expunge from the patient's constitution any "seditious" elements that were subversive in nature. Hunter would seem to agree with Jean-Jacques Rousseau's conceptualization of illness as resulting from straying "from the path of nature."[4] The surgeon-to-be's advocacy of the prescribed whey cure may indicate a faith in medical knowledge that Rousseau would not share, but the mutual belief that the ailing body should be returned to its natural, or right and proper, state is significant. The way to do so, paradoxically, was to employ all the tools of medical progress and its developing technologies.

Scientific experimentation and innovative procedures would advance knowledge about the body, and the physician would acquire ever greater expertise about the human constitution. However, he (invariably "he") would always act as *agent* of "her excellency nature." This same paradox lies at the heart of ideas about political reform: progress and improvement were cultural buzzwords in this era of revolutions, but political change was bound by, and in the service of, nature. The conflation of political and medical language became all the more significant at the end of the century, in large part as a response to the French Revolution. In the 1790s, the language about excising sedition and banishing the enemies of the British constitution was pivotal in debates about serious constitutional questions. The greatest effects on British political culture would be felt when reactionaries, spurred on by the violent excesses committed across the channel, employed medical discourse to initiate moral and political reform. The resulting effects on wider culture, as I will show in this book, were profound.

. . .

Compare William Hunter's use of the term *constitution* with this second passage, from Edmund Burke's critically influential *Reflections on the Revolution in France* (1790):

> We have given to our frame of polity the image of a relation in blood; binding up the constitution of our country with our dearest domestic ties; adopting our fundamental laws into the bosom of our family affections; keeping inseparable, and cherishing with the warmth of all their combined and mutually reflected charities, our state, our hearths, our sepulchres, and our altars.[5]

Frequently quoted in analyses of the British response to the French Revolution, Burke's articulation of the interconnectedness of familial, communal, and national ties would quickly become a structuring paradigm of public and private life. While this passage has been fairly well mined for its statements about an emerging political conservatism and an increasingly symbiotic relationship between political and domestic interests, I want to draw attention to the "materiality" of Burke's bodily language. Words such as *frame, constitution, bosom,* and *blood* carry powerful political connotations as much as they are physiological referents. Burke's visceral language grounds his political philosophy in the natural order of things, against the abstract philosophies of radicals and revolutionaries. He poses the rhetorical question, "What is the use of discussing a man's abstract right to food and medicine?" To which he answers, "I shall always advise to call in the aid of the farmer and the physician, rather than the professor of metaphysics."[6] This is to clearly situate himself against abstract theories, which in spite of their immateriality, still managed to give monstrous birth to the Revolution.

In Burke's passage, the state functions very much like the human body, with its own anatomy, physiology, and pathologies. The nation and the nation's families can develop "normally" or they can atrophy; they can become diseased or grow strong and healthy. The people owe their constitution to past generations, just as familial bloodlines transmit physical vigor alongside moral values such as affection, honor, and loyalty. Unlike the revolutionary French, Britons were grateful for their inheritance and had not succumbed to revolutionary fever. They had not yet been "embowelled" of their "natural entrails," since they still felt "inbred sentiments" and had respect for "manly morals."[7] Manliness, as we will see in the following chapters, is in the process of being redefined here, in accordance with new ideas about the body and in the context of growing emphases on domesticity. Burke may use a material language to make his point about substance over abstraction; yet, conversely, he also pits a metaphysical representation of the English constitution against the all too earthly character of French politics. In the *Reflections*, as Timothy Morton rightly points out, "the benign body of the English state must seem so mystical: if it is too material, it will fall into the category of nature-to-be-dominated."[8] Like Marie Antoinette herself, the constitution must appear as a star in the firmament, out of reach of all too human hands. If the constitution were to be stripped of its aura, it would become like the French monarchy, "a delicious repast" for all too material "appetites."[9] Burke's famous description of the storming of Versailles, which left the royal residence "polluted by massacre, and strewed with scattered limbs and mutilated carcases," presents an image of the human literally reduced to a sum of its parts.[10] In this political atmosphere, the value of human life is drastically reduced, as Burke's slyly provocative use of the word *polluted* indicates. Tapping into related fears about dirt, contamination, and the spread of disease, Burke suggests that like dangerous epidemics, political theories spread through a population equally as fast. The result is similarly devastating.

• • •

While Burke's famous text established many of the key terms of the revolution debate of the 1790s, a very different kind of political text appeared in the years immediately following its publication. In 1792, the radical libertine Charles Pigott produced the first of his *Jockey Club* series, a three-part collection of scurrilous anecdotes about the great and the good of British society. Pigott linked the ravaged bodies of morally debauched aristocrats with what he saw as the equally ravaged British constitution. My third and final passage about constitutions is from one of Pigott's many scandalous anecdotes—this one about the Whig Duke of Norfolk, known for his love of drink, his aversion to soap, and his fondness for distinctly inappropriate mistresses:

> This *constitutional* Peer evinces his enthusiasm for the constitution, by an inverse mode of proceeding; by the most daring unconstitutional acts; by a continual interference at elections for Members of parliament, contrary to the first leading principles of the constitution he professes to reverence. Let us, however, be just, and setting the darling constitution aside, develop the real motive of his Grace's zeal and ardour on these occasions: . . . it gives him an excellent opportunity of indulging [habits] . . . at no other expense to himself, than the expence of his own purse and *constitution*, which suffers at least equally with the constitution of his country.[11]

Pigott himself uses italics to emphasize *constitution* and *constitutional*, and it is worth noting that variations of this word appear no less than *seven* times in this short passage. Pigott does not want his readers to miss the inseparable links between the duke's alcoholism, his shattered constitution, and his political corruption. This passage demonstrates clearly how, in the 1790s, an individual's private life had everything to do with his or her political role. That the duke's excesses and depravities destroyed his own health indicates his unworthiness for public office and demonstrates the risk he poses to the body politic. Pigott may have been on the side of libertinism, but his focus on private life signaled a change in the tenor of political debate. Personal habits and morality had become the center of the discussion.

Pigott's scurrilous anecdotes demonstrate how biographical genres—memoirs, confessions, eyewitness accounts, letters, tales of scandal, and newspaper gossip columns—became politically inflected in this era. Memoirs targeted the lives of radicals, scandal entered royal bedrooms, and eyewitness accounts described the lives of republicans, revolutionaries, and "new philosophers." In his Habermasian-inflected study of autobiographical writing in the eighteenth century, John Brewer describes how "the private realm" became "coextensive with civil society."[12] In the 1790s, private life took on new significance in light of violent revolutionary excess across the channel and the resultant conservative atmosphere in Britain. Government repression in the form of the Treason Trials, prosecutions for seditious words and libel, the suspension of habeas corpus in 1794, the introduction of the "Two Acts" in 1795 (which limited civil liberties in an effort to crush radicalism), and the spread of moral associations (the collective backbone of "the reform or ruin movement") all contributed to making visible and to politicizing those actions and deeds that had previously been protected from the public gaze. As John Barrell details, politics entered spaces that, according to an earlier paradigm of privacy, had been "outside" the realm of politics: the dressing room, the cottage, and places of conviviality and free exchange.[13]

A series of paradoxes emerges around the realignment of the categories of public and private in this period. For one thing, efforts to separate these spheres and to define modern civil society also effected the conflation of public and private. In *Secret History of Domesticity*, Michael McKeon demonstrates how, with the onset of modernity, public interest derived "from a multitude of private ones."[14] In a chapter on the relationship of family to state, he describes how eighteenth-century views of marriage—a public, political, and religious act—increasingly focused on intimate experience and individual interiority. Then, at the end of the century, the French Revolution further complicated the public-private relationship by making private life the business of the state and the focus of public opinion in new—and insidious—ways. In Britain, the idea that an individual's character and personal life were the best indicators of political trustworthiness became a foundational principle of modern political culture.[15] Another paradox emerges with the "invention of intimacy" that occurred earlier in the century: the sharing of intimate information contributed to what Brewer describes as the onset of "a seamless and transparent publicness" that emerged at the end of the century.[16] Indeed, *transparency* is a word that is used often in discussions of the history and politics of revolution, yet its importance has not been highlighted enough in British cultural history. The emphasis on visibility and clarity pervades medical writing, political discourse, and literature, all of which focus on the interior self and previously private practices. An unprecedented amount of attention was focused on one's habits, one's sex life, and one's ailments. During these times of political expediency, when the very existence of civil society seemed to be at stake, it became incumbent on every Briton to ensure that their politicians were living upstanding, healthy lives.

MEDICINE AND THE MIGRATION OF IDEAS

What precisely is the relationship between these three passages and their various uses of the term *constitution*? What does the politicizing of private life that we find in Burke and Pigott have to do with William Hunter's letter? The longer answers will come in the following chapters, but I can offer a short reply here: these passages demonstrate how medicine, politics, and morality began to share a common language in the eighteenth century. Developments in anatomy and physiology produced new theories about human vitality and organic function, about sexuality and reproduction, cleanliness and contamination, and about diet, drink, and disease. In the late eighteenth and early nineteenth centuries, these new theories circulated not only in popular medical manuals, where we would expect to find them, but also in all forms of political expression, including broadsides, philosophical treatises, pornography, tracts relating scandal, biography, confession, anti-Jacobin novels, plays, poetry, and graphic art. These diverse texts shared a vocabulary rich in anatomical terms and medicalized normative categories, such as *natural, universal, proper, clean,* and *moral,* as well as their oppositional cognates *unnatural, unsanitary,* and *immoral.*

The historical connections between medicine and politics are important and have had lasting influences, yet they have been overlooked. We have not sufficiently reflected upon how these medical categories have shaped political culture, often having detrimental consequences, as we will see. This book addresses this gap by tracing the ways that knowledge about the functioning of the body, new methods of diagnoses, innovative treatments, and changing ideas about the prevention of disease migrated into political culture. In effect, my aim is to map out a *tripartite* relationship between the political, the private, and the medical. Further, I argue that a normal/pathological paradigm—borrowed from medicine—was used to identify certain individuals as "naturally" or biologically unsuitable for politics.

In terms of methodology, this project addresses the lacuna that still exists between medical history, on the one hand, and literary and cultural history on the other. Important work by scholars in both these fields has done much to uncover the various interfaces between medicine, art, society, and culture. In particular, Roy Porter, Ludmilla Jordanova, W. F. Bynum, George Rousseau, and a successive generation of scholars have done much to forge links (or to reforge the links that existed in previous centuries) between science and the arts—or between the "two cultures," to use C. P. Snow's well-used adage.[17] The interdisciplinary terrain is in many ways no longer a terra incognita, as it was in those days when, as George Rousseau recalls, "the copula of science and the humanities constantly loomed in our daily conversations, even if we were unaware of its contexts."[18] Yet, as he also points out, there is still much work to be done. I am guided by his observations and those of Nikolas Rose who, following Michel Foucault, argues that we should pay close attention to, rather than disregard, "the *heterogeneity* of the events with which 'medicine' has been engaged" and should identify "the diversity of interventions carried out in the name of health" as well as "the diversity of ways of relating the language of medicine to the language of politics."[19] Rose's statements were first made in 1994, yet much about the varied ways that medicine—and all that falls under the aegis of medicine—has inflected politics remains relatively uncharted territory. In particular, this book more fully provokes and explores his comment about how language links the political and the medical.

As befits such diversity, and because this is a cultural study about the migration of medical into political discourse, the range of textual materials gathered here is accordingly varied: I refer to political pamphlets, philosophical treatises, poetry, novels, caricatures, literary reviews, newspapers, letters, biographies, and memoirs. These texts come in both "high" and "low" forms, from the most academic, research-oriented, and expensively produced treatises, such as William Hunter's lavishly illustrated *Anatomy of the Human Gravid Uterus* (1774), to such popular manuals as, for instance, William Buchan's *Domestic Medicine* (1769). As scholars have cautioned, medical knowledge in the eighteenth century should not be conceived of as a "top-down" affair, since knowledge circulated widely and in all directions.[20] In this era, medical information intermingled with other forms of writing: the findings of anatomical studies were deciphered by popular writers, while surgeons transmitted knowledge to the wider public through a range of popular medical books and pamphlets. Medical historian Mary Fissell also cautions against presuming a certain socioeconomic background for readers of medical treatises.[21] She points out that in early-modern England, cheaply printed manuals were popular among people of all social classes, and this is even more the case in the post-Enlightenment world. Medical books had a wide audience that often transcended class and gender divisions. Correspondence and other forms of textual evidence indicate that medicine was accessed fairly democratically by citizens, who consulted a range of materials, including household manuals, advice books, satirical prints, journals, newspapers, and popular treatises. As such, it is possible to draw at least some tentative conclusions about how widely pervasive were attitudes regarding health and disease, pollution and vitality. Regardless of genre and the socioeconomic background of readers, medical literature shares a vocabulary of well-being, personal responsibility, improvement, and reform.

The breadth of my materials implies a strong interdisciplinary impetus. This, it seems to me, is requisite given that the fairly firm disciplinary boundaries that segregate the academy did not exist in the same way in earlier periods. In addition, medical ideas circulated as much in the visual as in the textual. In histories of the body, we do not always credit images, particularly "lower" forms of graphic art, with as much significance as written materials. I hope to demonstrate how medical knowledge, and the vocabulary of physiologists and surgeons, migrated into visual forms of expression as much as into literary forms. I will excavate the ways that scientific ideas, "facts," and "findings" became part of larger, overarching narratives. Narrative has always been a structuring device, a means of processing knowledge and making sense of new ideas, not only in literature and visual culture, but also in medicine, law, and the hard sciences. Narratives and their component parts—metaphor, metonymy, synecdoche, imagery, rhetorical devices, figurative language—transcend disciplinary boundaries. Narrative is part of the historicist, genealogical approach I employ here, in that I seek to uncover the connections between political actions and the medical beliefs and desires that generated them.[22]

In this book, I use that particularly treasured tool of literary scholars, close textual analysis, to excavate latent meanings in graphic satire, medical treatises, and political scandal. My goal is to expose the workings of what Ludmilla Jordanova has helpfully termed "bridging concepts." These are key terms, such as *temperament, sensibility,* and *constitution,* that forge links between biology, politics, and morality. These terms gain cultural purchase through their reiteration in literature, art, politics, medicine, and everyday conversation.[23] We have already seen how the term *constitution* migrated between discourses and was redefined and redeployed in different contexts. The other bridging concepts that appear often in this book are *contamination, excess, susceptibility, rationality, reason,* and most often, *nature,* or *natural.* Under the auspices of these flexible terms (flexible because they are both technically medical and more widely cultural words), the political and scientific merged. Importantly, bridging concepts are laden with cultural value. They are regulative: they are the means by which the properly loyal and politically trustworthy British body is defined.

Clearly, this study owes something to Foucault's work on the emergence of modern medical techniques, the fashioning of bodies, the identification of "normal" and deviant sexual practices, and the various ways that power and disciplinary mechanisms operate. After Foucault, we understand that in the modern era, disciplinary mechanisms have operated in increasingly nuanced ways on what he terms "docile bodies."[24] Discipline is not simply wielded by an agent on another individual; instead, discipline and power operate as a dispersed network of strategies. However, in the following case studies, it may seem that political writers, both revolutionary and counterrevolutionary, do act as agents, promoting certain medicomoral values and wielding discipline. Indeed, we will see how medicopolitical discourse *does* certain things: it disqualifies female bodies, it pathologizes rebellious radicals, and it censors luxuriating elites. This discourse is aimed, too, at the docile bodies of the public. This last statement may seem particularly at odds with Foucault's arguments. The following pages will reconcile this seeming contradiction more fully, but I would also offer a few points here.

This book echoes some Foucauldian themes but not others. At certain points, Foucault appears: the following chapters owe much to his important work on dietetics, the use of pleasure, the medicalization of appetite, the birth of the clinic, the medical gaze, and especially governmentality, or the conduct of conduct. But this study should also be seen as an attempt to broaden the concept of governmentality, by moving away from a strict fidelity to Foucault. As I have already emphasized, this study pays close attention to discourse, but it does not "treat meanings as things that exist as part of systems of signs quite apart from the actors who make them." In his study of the ways we might rethink historicist, genealogical approaches to the concept of governmentality, Mark Bevir rightly points out that work on governmentality "can lose sight of the fact that people create meanings and practices."[25] Clearly, we can never fully define "the public," nor can we identify its precise role in the circulation of medicopolitical discourse. Part of the reason we cannot is precisely because, as Foucault indicates, discipline is subtle and insidious, and it operates in all directions. Yet, neither can we ignore the actors—and their beliefs, motives, goals, fears, interests, and narratives—in a study that seeks to uncover how certain of our beliefs about the normal and the pathological have developed. Nor can we disregard the role of the public in a study that scrutinizes those beliefs, with the aim of denaturalizing them. As we will see in the coming chapters, medicopolitical discourse was powerfully disciplinary; there were clear political and cultural consequences to its circulation. But while this discourse did not *belong* to anyone, intentional agents used language in political and moral struggles. The following case studies will demonstrate how medically inflected narratives built up around bridging concepts were debated, negotiated, and dispersed throughout society.

CASE STUDIES

The first two chapters demonstrate how biology was used to define appropriate social and political roles for women. Chapter 1 explores how political pornographers as well as serious political writers exploited contemporary knowledge about such medical conditions as uterine furor (or nymphomania), hermaphroditism, and onanism (or masturbation) to insist on the exclusion of women from politics. I begin with the case of Marie Antoinette: although a fair amount has been written about her, I consider how her body was *anatomized* in print and represented as pathological. Both French and British audiences were told that she suffered from a range of medical conditions that included a diseased womb, drooping breasts, and a grossly enlarged clitoris (an alleged symptom of hermaphroditism). These diagnoses legitimized her exclusion from the public sphere and played a role in her death. More important for this study, these verbal and visual representations of the French queen were exported to Britain and refashioned in support of arguments—made on biological grounds—against female succession and the participation of women in the world of politics more generally.

Chapter 2 continues this theme but focuses specifically on the ways that motherhood and the practice of breast-feeding became a locus of moral-medical debate. Political philosophers and physicians alike argued that breast-feeding was a natural, healthy act that expressed higher virtues and counteracted political and social disaffection. I argue that these problematical arguments, founded in emerging ideas about gendered biological difference, circumscribed women's roles. Together, these first two chapters show how woman's so-called maternal "nature" and her inherently unstable sexual "nature" were used to make ideological arguments about her inability to withstand the demands of public life.

Chapter 3 focuses on the case of the philosopher William Godwin and his wife, the feminist writer Mary Wollstonecraft. It is fairly well known that Godwin's candid confessions about her life, made in *Memoirs of the Author of "A Vindication of the Rights of Woman,"* deeply harmed the couple's political and personal reputations. In this chapter, however, I focus on the perceived ethical problems surrounding Godwin's detailing of the medical particulars of her death from puerperal, or childbed, fever. To scores of observers, his willingness to discuss her bodily symptoms (particularly in the rational language of a physician) provided a compelling example of why his political philosophy—which emphasized utility above all other considerations in decisions concerning government, justice, and human relations—was immoral and untenable. Godwin was castigated for acting the anatomist: he displayed a clinical disinterestedness in matters of the heart but an enthusiasm for a rationalist politics that violated human sanctity. In fact, earlier fears about anatomy (before the 1830s debates surrounding the Anatomy Act) form an important, and little considered, cultural context to the anti-utilitarian movement. In the last few decades of the eighteenth century, new medical theories about pregnancy, childbirth, and women's constitutions provided material for conservatives like the Cornish poet and clergyman Richard Polwhele, who argued that Wollstonecraft's death in childbirth reminded the world that women's bodies, which were prey to a completely different set of afflictions than those of men, proved women's unsuitability for philosophy, politics, and medicine.

In chapter 4, I argue that scandalizing the private lives and pathologizing the bodies of British radicals became an efficient means of silencing their political arguments. Focusing on Thomas Paine as my case study, I show how, as the rather loose standards of eighteenth-century hygiene and sanitation gave way to the more fastidious nineteenth-century emphasis on cleanliness, biographers made much of Paine's allegedly questionable personal hygiene. In a culture that had recently become intent on defining the boundaries between contagion and cleanliness, and on drawing ever closer analogies between dirt and disorder, Paine appeared threateningly contagious—a representation that had direct and dire consequences for the status of political radicalism and for rights-based political arguments.

Chapter 5 demonstrates how attitudes about temperance, middle-class moderation, taste, and gourmandizing had much to do with the refashioning of monarchical roles and the transfer of political power from the throne to the House of Commons. George IV became a figure whose excessive drinking and eating, and his resultant obesity and gout, were construed as symptomatic of the kind of aristocratic excess that threatened national cohesion and *sensus communis* (the set of cultural sensibilities shared by communities and nations). Drawing on treatises on gout, guides on diet, and the new gastronomical manuals promoting rational eating over excess, writers and artists linked George's habits of consumption to his suspect morals and his political incapacity. In an age that increasingly aligned taste with eating practices and also urged personal restraint and self-discipline, George's body—its corpulence, its goutiness, its intemperance—demonstrated that immoderation had catastrophic effects on the body politic.

Chapter 6 delves deeper into the propaganda leveled at George IV, but the focus here is on how new ideas about nutrition, local food economies, empire, and vegetarianism connected to anxieties about cross-cultural contamination through the exchange of goods and colonial diseases. Vegetarianism was one of many modern practices that sought to extend life, promote human sociability, and increase happiness by improving eating habits and routines. Physicians, moralists, poets, and political philosophers argued that the history of consumption paralleled the history of humanity's decline or progress; as such, political leaders had a responsibility to eat "locally," to avoid obesity, and to shun "artificial" food like Oriental cuisine.

My intention is to use these case studies to demonstrate how frequently medicine, politics, and morality were discursively and thus ideologically yoked. Representations of disease and vigor, monstrosity and normalcy, growth and decay had profound and lasting effects on political culture, social relations, and personal identity. Ultimately, I want to draw attention to how immune, or at least how desensitized, we have been (and continue to be) to the political exploitation of words like *natural* and *normal*. Each of the public figures who comprises a case study—male or female, monarch or subject, conservative or liberal, royal or republican—was used to enforce a division between normal and pathological bodies, between morally acceptable and unacceptable acts; and more to my point, to distinguish between appropriate and inappropriate political participants.

This remains the situation today. Certainly the lives and bodies of public figures are also exploited to challenge normative, gendered standards of behavior and to confront ideas about normal embodiment. But most often, I would argue, they are used to prescribe or to reinscribe rather narrow standards. How closely a public figure measures up to established models of appropriateness continues to be directly related to his or her perceived worthiness as a political actor. Crucially, as this book will demonstrate, the sexual behaviors, the habits and practices, and the bodies of average readers are measured by the same normative standards. As we judge, so are we judged.

PART I

Revolutionary Pathologies

1 The Case of Marie Antoinette

*Revolutionary Politics and the
Biologically Suspect Woman*

> The first and principal Cause of this *Furor* is a preternatural Irritation in the Parts of Generation; whence violent Impressions are made on the Brain.
> JOHN ASTRUC, "Of the Furor Uterinus,"
> in *A Treatise on All the Diseases Incident to Women* (1743)

> The Body Politic should be governed by the same rules that apply to the Body Physical.
> MARQUIS DE SADE, *Justine* (1791)

Through a barrage of verbal and visual images, political propagandists and pornographers transformed Marie Antoinette into one of the most vilified figures of the French Revolution. Earlier in the eighteenth century, publications of "libelles" and "private lives" had targeted courtiers and *salonnières*, but after 1789 the intensity and sheer number of pamphlets about royal private lives were unprecedented.[1] Cultural historians Sarah Maza, Chantal Thomas, Lynn Hunt and others have detailed how political pornographers cast the queen as an adulteress, a traitor, a lesbian, a sodomite, and an incestuous and murderous mother.[2] These scholars have ably demonstrated the cultural and political uses made of Marie Antoinette in revolutionary France. In *The Wicked Queen*, for instance, Chantal Thomas makes the point that antimonarchists so thoroughly gained control of the queen's image that the "real" woman was effaced by the monstrous queen of the pamphlets. She became an effigy at which a discontented populace could direct their fury over inflated food prices and political corruption.

More important, Thomas uncovers the ways that sexual norms were promoted alongside political values in this type of scandal. The queen and her alleged sexual crimes were presented as evidence not only of the corruption of the court and the ancien régime but also of woman's "nature." Her alleged behind-the-scenes machinations were used to hypostatize the political untrustworthiness of woman. In politico-pornographic writing, the French Jacobins drew on images of Marie Antoinette's body to buttress Enlightenment philosophies that advocated a gendered division of roles, in support of the new republic. The queen's trial in the press and in front of the revolutionary tribunal was, as Adriana Craciun aptly describes it, a virtual "morality play on the evil impact of women on the body politic"; a circumstance that effectively produced the "institutionalized elimination of women from the public political sphere."[3] In place of the old monarchical system, revolutionaries built a fraternal and distinctly masculine republican state that was, as Iain McCalman puts it, "contractual, virtuous, transparent and free of feminine contamination."[4]

Less attention has been paid, however, to the way British writers borrowed from their Continental neighbors to support a similar move to categorize women's bodies as "pathological." Indeed, the events surrounding the French queen's fall from power and her death were heavily reported, discussed, and debated in the British press. British propagandists fused representations of the queen's body with new medical knowledge to support their own arguments for the exclusion of women from politics. This attempt to circumscribe women's public role was largely accomplished through a discourse of biological incommensurability—the idea that there were essential physical differences between men and women, which determined gendered differences in character and ability and, thus, appropriate roles. A greater emphasis on bodily differences between men and women relied on a number of medical definitions, and political interpretations, of "women's nature."

In addition, the "depoliticizing" of women occurred through a genre of writing that has not generally been recognized as medical discourse. Political pornography, which exploded onto the print cultural scene in late eighteenth-century France, is grounded much more in contemporary medical research than has been typically acknowledged. The often anonymous authors of these lewd and inflammatory pamphlets went beyond exposing the queen's immorality. They also linked that immorality to deviance and to sexual perversity, which according to contemporary medical doctrine, originated in female physiology. Employing a gendered, medicopolitical discourse about "natural" biological functioning and gender-specific diseases, they used allegedly pathological public women as exemplars to demonstrate the limits of the female body and to support their arguments about the dangers of women in the political sphere. The attitudes that underpinned eighteenth-century medical theories about sexual function and dysfunction greatly shaped and continues to shape modern attitudes about gender, biology, and politics.

THE BIOLOGY OF INCOMMENSURABILITY

Any discussion of ideas about sex, gender, and the body must begin with Thomas Laqueur's groundbreaking claim that in the eighteenth century, beliefs about natural bodily processes and gender-specific pathologies were supported by what he terms the "biology of incommensurability." This medical paradigm was established by "writers of all sorts," who promoted what they viewed as "fundamental differences between male and female sexuality, and thus between man and woman," that were founded "on discoverable biological distinctions."[5] This was not always the case. In *Making Sex*, Laqueur takes a long view of medical history—from the Greeks to Freud—to trace an epistemic shift from the "one-sex" to the "two-sex" model of the body. Before the age of Enlightenment, males and females were thought to inhabit an essentially similar body (the one-sex body). Female and male sexual organs were thought to be generally homologous, and bodily secretions like blood, breast milk, and ejaculate were believed to be made of similar substances. Indeed, there are interesting connections between Laqueur's thesis and the observations of eighteenth-century writers on sexuality, who likewise identify a shift in medical beliefs about the sexed body.

For instance, in a 1741 treatise on hermaphroditism, physician and fellow of the Royal College of Surgeons James Parsons observes how previous generations of physicians drew "a great Analogy between the Male and Female Genitals." Both Greek and Arabic physicians asserted that male and female reproductive organs "differ in nothing but their Situation, that is, they compare the Cervix and Vagina Uteri to the Penis, and the Fundus to the Scrotum, only they are inverted or rather not protruded." In other words, Parsons explains to his modern audience, they believed "every Woman is a Man" except that she did not have the "heat" to "drive the inside of the Uterus, &c. outward."[6] As we will see later in this chapter, Parsons rejects the one-sex model and, along with it, ideas about the fluidity of sex and gender. In fact, he makes the argument that, historically, the belief in the one-sex model caused doctors to mistakenly read sexually anomalous bodies as hermaphroditic and led them to accept that, on occasion, it was possible for women to change sex, that is, for their bodies to grow male organs and to exhibit male characteristics.

Laqueur cautions us not to see the one-sex model as implying social, political, or cultural equality, but to see it as suggesting a lack of organic difference that then entails male superiority and female inferiority. As he puts it, "The relationship of men to women, like that of apples to oranges, was not given as one of equality or inequality but rather of difference."[7] However, a two-sex model emerged in the eighteenth century that categorized males and females as fundamentally different in kind, and these allegedly inherent biological differences were used to justify gender inequalities. We should not miss how profoundly political this medical paradigm became; in the words of Paul Youngquist, the "new biology of incommensurability sexed the flesh to new political ends."[8] Many of the medical writers I refer to in this chapter used this view of the gendered body and its functions as basis for their political arguments. Those arguments could be summed up as domestic roles for women and public ones for men.

Nowhere is this clearer than in Jean-Jacques Rousseau's merging of the political and the medical in his insistence on the biological incommensurability of men and women. In his renowned account of the nature of "man" in *Émile*, he recognizes a few resemblances between the sexes but generally emphasizes perceived differences, as determined by nature. He writes: "General differences present themselves to the comparative anatomist and even to the superficial observer; they seem not to be a matter of sex; yet they are really sex differences. . . . How far such differences may extend we cannot tell."[9]

Comparative anatomy, grounded as it is in reason, observation, and common sense, forms the bedrock of Rousseau's political judgments. The immutable physical "differences" between men and women must influence "moral nature," he argues.[10] Foundational principles of moral relations can be drawn from the "diversity" between the sexes that anatomists and physicians have identified. The first rule, which he articulates clearly in *Émile*, is that true to their natures, men must be "active and strong," while women are expected to be naturally "weak and passive."[11] From this supposedly biological principle, it follows that woman should please man, while man was born to wield power. This is not, Rousseau argues, "the law of love, but it is the law of nature, which is older than love itself."[12] Nature is biology, and biology determines gendered social roles. It follows, then, that women who violate these laws—by attempting to obtain power through their involvement in public affairs, by acting in a sexually aggressive way, or by altering their bodies in mannish ways—are gross violations of nature. As we will see, such violations became defined as deeply immoral acts in the age of revolution.

ANTIMONARCHICAL PROPAGANDA AND UTERINE FUROR

In the 1790s, a raft of pornographic pamphleteers and engravers portrayed France's foremost family in unprecedented ways. In an anonymously authored pamphlet titled *The Royal Dildo* (1789), readers encounter an incestuous queen who demanded, in crude and sexually violent language, that her father and children perform the most illicit acts on her body.[13] Like a disease, she corrupts the nation's religious, social, and political institutions, as she does her own home. Her desires taint the royal bloodline by producing bastard sons fathered by a number of men: in *The Austrian Woman on the Rampage; or, The Royal Orgy* (1789), her brother-in-law is the real progenitor of the dauphin; in *The Royal Bordello* (1789), she admits to one group of her lovers that her sons were fathered by her handmaid's lovers and by Cardinal de Rohan, who was implicated in the affair of the diamond necklace, which damaged the reputation of the royal household.[14]

In this pornography, one of the most politically damaging aspects of the queen's monstrosity is her pathological body. Propagandists insisted that the queen was prey to physiological disorders that materially demonstrated her biological weakness and thus her natural unsuitability for the rigors of politics. As the title of the pamphlet *The Uterine Furors of Marie-Antoinette* (1791) indicates, the queen was accused of being ruled by a disordered uterus that drove her to seek out sexual gratification at every turn. Revealingly, in *The Royal Dildo*, it is not *she* who is described as sexually lascivious; rather, it is her "cunt" that is so "amorous" it would "fuck its own father" and would take on an army of "delectable children" in search of sexual satisfaction.[15] In other words, her insatiable desires and immoral actions do not originate in her *character* or in conscious choice; rather, they emerge from deep within her pathological body. It is as if the woman's body has a mind of its own that overrides judgment, reason, or moral understanding. This theme is continued in a 1791 pornographic print in which the queen receives a line-up of soldiers (figure 1.1). As the audience, we watch with the three waiting men, becoming voyeurs in the monarchical bedroom. Everyone joins in the refrain, "Bravo, bravo! The queen is penetrated by the state."

The images of uterine furor in these "lower" forms of political writing are startlingly similar to representations of the then newly identified

22 / Revolutionary Pathologies

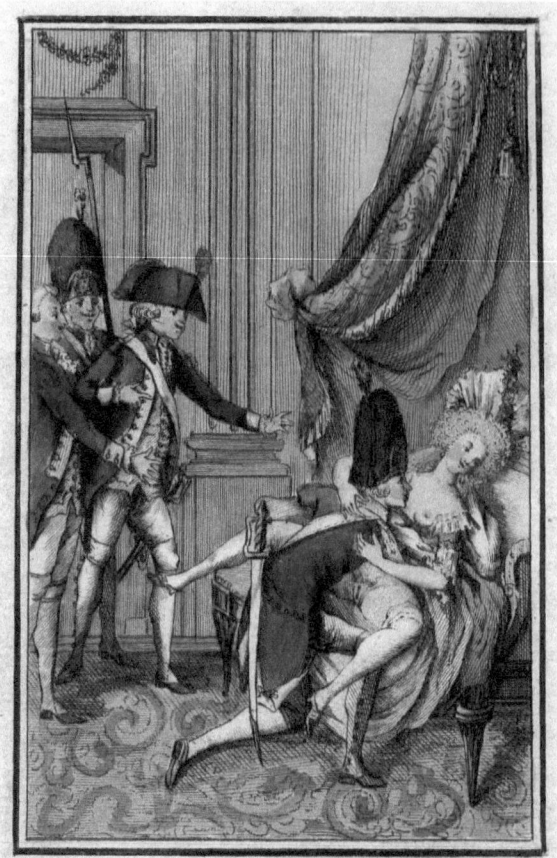

Figure 1.1 Anon., *Bravo, Bravo! la Reine se penetre de la Patrie* (1791 © Trustees of the British Museum, London)

disease of nymphomania. The French physician M.D.T. de Bienville's detailing of this disorder was translated for English audiences in 1775 by Edward Sloane Wilmot. Nymphomania became a particularly politicized disease in the 1790s and one of many diseases the queen was accused of having. Significantly, it was a notoriously shadowy, opaque disease: if the origins and effects of "normal" female sexual drives were somewhat obscure, then the unquenchable, dysfunctional, and multidirectional desires of the nymphomaniac were all the more so. Eighteenth-century medical texts tend to describe earlier forms of this condition as originating in the uterus, harking back to classical notions of the travelling womb, but in *Nymphomania; or, A Dissertation Concerning the Furor*

Uterinus, Bienville describes a disease that proceeded from the nerves of the uterus but was stimulated by the imagination.[16] Paradoxically, he also suggests that the cause of *furor* could be purely biological: an enlarged, elongated and penile clitoris would explain the sexual aggressiveness of certain women. Clearly, Bienville struggles to define the relationship between mind and body here. Yet, however shadowy the origin of the *furor*, it originated from somewhere within an inherently flawed and organically weak female body. According to Bienville, "the weakness of the sex" was due to woman's "organical construction." The "nature of the fibres, and muscles" of women and their sexual organs were clearly "more liable to inflammations than the organs of men."[17] This language reveals something of the paradoxical representation of woman's sexual "nature" in the eighteenth century. At times, woman was represented as sexually aggressive and untrustworthy, while at other times passionless and passive.

At any rate, for Bienville, secret thoughts, bodily compulsions, and monstrous behaviors were part of female nature, expressed by his consistent use of such terms as *elude* and *evade*. Contagion was an undetectable poison and its victims and agents were "monsters in human shape" (a phrase, interestingly, that was used often to describe Marie Antoinette). According to Bienville, nymphomaniacal women "perpetually dishonour themselves in secret by habitual pollutions" and "openly solicit" men "in the most criminal, and abandoned language."[18] These furious women "have not the power to conceal" their internal turmoil and therefore become increasingly bold until "they betray each shocking secret of their lascivious minds by proposals."[19] Bienville's nymphomaniacs, who solicit their lovers with graphic language, are models for the pornographer's Marie Antoinette, who likewise demands that countless sex acts be performed on her body by a phalanx of lovers. Like other nymphomaniacal women, she attempts to operate in secret but inevitably bears the marks of her disease and betrays herself to the world.

This sense of biological shadowiness and the untrustworthiness of hidden desires were particularly problematic symptoms in the newly transformed republican nation. Historian Lynn Hunt describes how the emphasis on public vigilance in 1790s' France emerged out of "the revolutionary belief in the possibility and desirability of 'transparency' between citizen and citizen, between the citizens and their government, between the individual and the general will."[20] "Transparency," she writes elsewhere, "was the perfect fit between public and private; transparency was a body that told no lies and kept no secrets."[21] The importance of ideas of coherence, visibility, and comprehensibility in all spheres of life in this period should not be underestimated. Openness was the highest virtue in civic and familial life—an idea that infused political discourse and structured human relations.

In *Discipline and Punish*, Michel Foucault emphasizes the role of public opinion in a rapidly modernizing nation. He argues that the revolutionary idea of justice was founded on a transparency that could only be maintained through public vigilance. Revolutionaries were intent to "prevent even the possibility of wrongdoing, by immersing people in a field of total visibility where the opinion, observation and discourse of others would restrain them from harmful acts."[22] Foucault emphasizes the subtle workings of power in this newly opened field of visibility: the ability to dispense discipline is dis-individualized and not overtly coercive. These observations on the politics of visibility provide important context to similar emphases in medicine. The eighteenth century was one of medical intervention, as he explains, in which "human behaviour and the human body were brought into an increasingly dense and important network of medicalization that allowed fewer and fewer things to escape."[23]

This thesis is supported by the evidence gathered here. Yet, something of a paradox emerges in this analysis: no matter how dis-individuated the disciplinary impulse might be, the public clearly participates in the process of making political judgments, of defining acceptable behavior, and of determining what are normal bodies. A vigilant public, who had greater access to the workings of government and to a large extent, each other's lives, was often described in this era as the principle means of obtaining a fully transparent society. A watchful corps of citizens defied the artificiality that characterized the ancien régime and opposed the secrecy, intrigue, and insincere manners of the court. Political pornography opened doors to reveal bedroom scenes and perverse domestic tableaux, so that the public could see the queen forcing champagne on the king, urging him to use his "power" tyrannically, and seducing him to "squander all the money" of "good Parisians."[24] The public could *see* the queen ensconced in her royal bedchambers, using her sexuality to corrupt ministers and to influence the king. Immersing her in such a field of visibility was a very pronounced step toward transforming France into a transparent nation. But the public had to be recruited into this disciplinary enterprise; ironically, that same public had no control over a normalizing process that was also operating on it.

The representation of the queen as a sexual predator coincides with the opposite representation of her husband. In fact, medical writers on the subject of nymphomania suggested that cold and weak, masturbating, impotent, or homosexual husbands were partially responsible for their wives' conditions. The symptoms associated with *furor uterinus* were amplified, Bienville argues, when women were "united either to an husband of so feeble a temperament, as to exact continence in his pleasures, or to a cold mate, but little sensible of the delights of enjoyment."[25] This was precisely the charge leveled at Louis XVI. He was represented as personally and politically impotent; his failures as a husband, father, and king contributed to his wife's licentiousness. In a scurrilous poem, *The Love Life of Charlie and Toinette* (1779), one pamphleteer recalls how Louis had not even the will or ability to father his own children:

> It is well known that that poor Gent,
> Condemned three or four times
> By the salubrious Faculty [of Medicine],
> For total impotence,
> Cannot satisfy Antoinette.
> Thoroughly convicted of this calamity,
> Since his matchstick
> Is about as thick as a bit of straw,
> And always limp and curled up,
> His Cock's only good for his pocket.[26]

There are several things to take from this passage. The king could only have been examined and "sentenced" by the respectable faculty of medicine in the wake of post-Enlightenment medicalization. The king is not simply "unmanned" by his wife; he is also unmanned by medical professionals, whose diagnosis erodes his political legitimacy all that much more. He is out of place in a modern, democratizing world in which elected representatives and professionals—not kings—now run the nation. Such an undressing of the king does more than desacralize him: he is rendered as politically powerless as he is sexually impotent. The fetal position adopted by his limp and "curled up" penis reflects his political vulnerability and his bodily abjectness. He is pathologized against emerging medical definitions of normalcy.

However, in spite of his lack, Louis is not the real villain of the piece. A perverse sort of sympathy existed for a king who, though spineless, submissive, impotent, and dim-witted, was horribly exploited by his manipulative and power-hungry wife. The difference in their reputations is confirmed by how relatively quickly Louis's image was rehabilitated in Britain immediately before and after his death. His execution was an event that, as John Barrell details at some length, provided British antirevolutionaries with a critical opportunity to refashion the king into the protagonist of a "domestic tragedy."[27] In sharp contrast to scandalous representations of Louis as ineffectual and effeminate, British loyalists portrayed him as a sympathetic father, a gentle, loving husband, and a compassionate brother.[28] In his private life, he was a model of domesticity and in his public capacity, a martyr. Engravings, coins, and pamphlets recalled the king's last "affecting" meeting with his family on the eve of his execution. By 1795, a journalist for the virulently antirevolutionary newspaper the *Tomahawk* could scoff at scandalmongers who had assumed it would be as easy to slander the reputation and memory of Louis as it had been his wife.[29] The attempt to convince Britons that he was a "beastly" and "blind husband" had failed, for in his final days it had become apparent that he "was a man whose *private life* would, in the days of superstition, have consecrated him a saint, and whose virtues and unmerited fate would have entitled him to the Crown of a Martyr."[30] These representations of the king's family tragedy were employed to polarize British public opinion in support of king and country.

An impetus behind the recovery of Louis's public character invariably stemmed from sympathy for his plight as the husband of a nymphomaniacal woman whose sexual and political aggression had been his political undoing. His impotence was excused because his disorder was *caused* by his wife's sexual dysfunction. He may have *contributed* to her nymphomania, but she had enervated and incapacitated him. As such, the attempts to erase from public memory the scandals surrounding the queen were much less successful. The dissenting scientist and philosopher Joseph Priestley termed her "a Medusa" and the radical orator John Thelwall described her as "an object of disgust" and a figure of "monstrous vices."[31] In his 1791 *Letters on the Revolution of France*, the friend of liberty and radical journalist Thomas Christie expressed his delight that the Revolution was a "severe" but "salutary lesson" for a queen who must be convinced "that the character of a virtuous wife, and an affectionate mother, confers purer joys than . . . the dissipated pleasures of an intriguing ambitious *virago*."[32] This same message was repeated consistently in the years following her death.

There are important connections between the medical projects of physicians like Bienville, the French pornographers who attacked Marie Antoinette, and the British propagandists who used the private lives of French monarchs to make salutary lessons. These three groups infiltrated private life in different ways, but more than that, they penetrated into women's bodies and scrutinized them in the name of science, progress, good order, and transparency. "Visualization," as art historian Barbara Stafford reminds us, was absolutely "central to the processes of enlightening."[33] The hysterical woman was a failure of the socializing, civilizing, and rationalizing process precisely because her biological urges had not been identified, addressed, treated, and disciplined. The revolutionary tribunals and courts attempted to render private life and personal loyalties transparent; similarly, medical treatises sought to clarify the biological functions of women. Once opened to the probing eye of science, unruly women would be exposed for what they really were: individuals driven by dysfunctional and *unseen* urges, which originated from deep within their bodies.

For Bienville, nymphomaniacs could be young virgins with too much liberty, widows suddenly deprived of marital sex, aristocratic women who had indulged too much in luxury and debauchery, or married women who had impotent or uninterested husbands (as was reportedly the case for Marie Antoinette and Louis XVI). What these women all had in common is that they did not live conventional, virtuous, restrained lives; they did not have "normal" marriages or family circles in which they found domestic contentment. In fact, Bienville goes some way to reconcile the oppositional views about the nature of women's sexuality by suggesting that women were naturally passive and had weak bodies, but could become sexual aggressors, if the necessary restraints to their activities were lifted. Women were naturally dominated by maternal feelings more than sexual feelings, but when their lives were not properly managed or their bodies were not kept in a state of calm equilibrium, then all hell broke loose. Their natural passivity was turned into an unnatural form of sexual deviance.

His conclusions as to treatment of nymphomania follow from these physiological and anatomical observations. Women needed to be watched, monitored, and thus preserved "from that impending wreck to which the sex are, by reason of their imbecility, exposed."[34] Since imagination was a factor, management of nymphomaniacal women was aimed at both mind and body. One way of keeping control over the furious woman was to keep her away from physical or mental stimulants. They must avoid luxurious foodstuffs, including chocolate, "rich sauce," "stimulating" meats, wines and spirits—a fairly common eighteenth-century prescription, found for instance in *The Lady's Dispensatory* of 1739, which identifies "high Feeding" and "provocative Medicines" as contributors to the "hysterical symptoms" associated with *furor uterinus*. Women's diets, the author cautions, should be limited, "thin and cooling."[35] In his 1786 *Principles of Midwifery; or, Puerperal Medicine*, Dr. John Aiken echoes his predecessors, insisting that "every suspected exciting cause" should be removed from the nymphomaniac's life.[36] Along with these dietary therapies, doctors advised women to stay close in the bosom of their families, to avoid the company of men, to restrain their dangerously roving imaginations, and to keep from conversations that may excite them.

These types of cures, which circumscribed women's activities and confined them to the domestic sphere, anticipated further emphases on restraint in the nineteenth century. Scholars have suggested that the rise of evangelicalism and the emergence of urban industrial capitalism in the late eighteenth century resulted in a dramatic change to attitudes toward female sexuality.[37] Evangelical Christianity offered women a way to rise socially by becoming exemplars of moral virtue: restraint and dispassion were signs of their civility and moral ascendancy. At the same time, there was a widening division in working roles, between men who labored away from the home and women who were increasingly confined to the domestic sphere. Carol Groneman points out that "this growing sexual division of labour was underscored by medical-scientific theories that posited the naturalness of this divide by arguing that woman's passive nature left her ill-equipped for the rough-and-tumble, competitive public world of work and politics."[38] This would seem to capture Bienville's argument precisely.

Unlike early modern writing about sexual deviance, from the Enlightenment onward there is a clear message that women must live subdued, honorable lives, cosseted in the domestic sphere, in the bosom of their families. Such medical attitudes would become far more firmly established in the nineteenth century, by such figures as the gynecologist and president of the American Medical Association Horatio Storer, the sexologist Richard Krafft-Ebing, or the British surgeon and advocate of the surgical removal of ovaries for nymphomaniacs, T. Spencer Wells. A phalanx of doctors prescribed a wide series of treatments, from diet to oophorectomy, since there was equally wide disagreement as to whether women were naturally passive or sexually insatiable. Still, the bottom line remained: women who violated social norms were deviants who inverted the natural order of things.

HERMAPHRODITES AND TRIBADES

The scandalizing and pathologizing of Marie Antoinette occurred at a time when all manner of bodily and cultural phenomena were being reworked and described with new terminology. While in previous eras differences between the sexes had been understood in metaphysical terms, in the eighteenth century they became increasingly understood in biological terms. If in the early-modern era the alleged weakness and instability of woman were understood through the figure of the biblical Eve, by the end of the eighteenth century such qualities were understood to be biologically inherent. What was once thought to be woman's natural propensity to vanity and her susceptibility to flattery became described as nervous disorder, emotional disturbance, or mental deficiency.

Part of the process of medicalizing cultural behaviors included identifying which sexual practices and what bodily characteristics were natural. Elizabeth Colwill argues that revolutionary pornographers had a hand in this process: they "did not merely reflect existing political, legal, and medical knowledge"; they also "helped to reconfigure the terrain of sexual difference, and ultimately the possibilities of sexual identity."[39] Their portrayals of the queen "flaunting a suspiciously male appendage" or engaged in homosexual acts "intervened in debates about sex and status that would circumscribe the boundaries of what came to be defined as normalcy in the modern era."[40] This seems right, and in this section I want to expand on Colwill's observations to suggest another consequence of the medicalizing of female desires and propensities. Instead of detailing how medical knowledge was used to monitor the boundary between natural and unnatural sexual practices, I concentrate on how medicine was used to police allegedly natural *political* boundaries. Defining the queen's body as pathological, her tastes as aberrant, and her sexual activities as deviant mobilized the public—more informed than ever about medical disorders—against political women.

The case of Marie Antoinette demonstrates how public women's bodies were *anatomized* in political print, in often startling detail, to reveal the physiological foundations of woman's sexual deviance. Pamphlets portrayed the queen enjoying the attentions of her companion, the "buggeress" Princess de Lamballe, but also claimed she suffered from a diseased womb, drooping breasts, and a "hideous clitoris," which as we have already seen was indicative of nymphomania.[41] This was also thought to be symptomatic of hermaphroditism and/or tribadism, or female-to-female nonpenetrative sexual contact. Hermaphrodites and tribades were distinctly "unnatural" and their pathological conditions were incurable, unlike many other conditions and diseases, which were characterized as temporarily unhealthy states. As we will see in chapter 5, for instance, a body racked by gout could be seen as an otherwise healthy body that was reacting to excess and imbalance. The accompanying pain and inflammation were signs that the body was righting itself after indulging in too much drink, rich food, and not enough exercise. But hermaphrodites and tribades were fundamentally deviant: either they were aberrations of nature (proving that in some few instances, nature could go very wrong), or they had been so corrupted by culture they were beyond repair.

In the 1790s, other public women were portrayed in various guises of sexual deviancy: some were portrayed as nymphomaniacs (the revolutionary advocate of woman's rights Théroigne de Méricourt), hermaphrodites (Jean-Paul Marat's assassin, Charlotte Corday), tribades (Princess de Lamballe), and in combinations (Marie Antoinette and her favorite, the Duchess de Polignac, were both tribades and nymphomaniacs). What made these women so dangerous—and why they were seen to deserve the death that so many of them received—was the public nature of their conditions. Scholars Mary Sheriff and Elizabeth Colwill show how these sexually deviant medical conditions intersect with the *femme publique* or the *femme-homme*.[42] Aristocratic or political women had their sexual "crimes" reiterated in pamphlets, so it appeared as if they were publicizing their own deviances and excesses. Their fame meant they could contaminate others with their immorality and unnaturalness. The public status of their private acts rendered them a serious threat to the bourgeois family, a danger to heteronormative marriage, and a peril to national stability. In other words, they endangered progressive efforts to make human relations transparent, honorable, and importantly, productive.

Tellingly, it was widely reported that when the mob attacked the Princess de Lamballe, they violently hacked her genitals from her body and then obliterated them. Whether or not such reports were true, it remains that Lamballe's sexual organs were seen to be the location of her private *and* political crimes. Like other public French women, she was represented in the press as a monster, a classification that, in eighteenth-century Europe and Britain, indicated biological aberration. So far, I have used the term *monstrosity*—a freighted term in our own and previous eras—without adequate explanation of its use in this period. It seems to me that something extraordinary happens to the meaning of this term over time. Critics and historians have documented an epistemological shift in the understanding of monstrosity in the eighteenth century. Broadly speaking, human monstrosity—conjoined twins, missing limbs, deformed facial features, skin disorders, and birthmarks—moved from the realm of superstition to the purview of science. As the understanding of generation, reproduction, and embryology developed, explanations of monstrosity relied on new scientific categories (such as the Linnaean system of classification). The process of secularizing monstrosity was accomplished, as Helen Deutsch and Felicity Nussbaum argue, "through the scientific categorization of the human," which included cataloging sexual difference.[43] Determining the etiology of disease and defect is part of the process of determining gendered categories, as well as the medical categories of pathological and normal.

On the issue of this latter topic, the philosopher of science Georges Canguilhem reminds us that such divisions are never value-free. In *The Normal and the Pathological*, a foundational text of medical theory, he refutes the widely accepted notion that historically medicine has ever *objectively* identified what is normal and healthy against what is diseased and abnormal. He argues that late eighteenth- and nineteenth-century physicians created the notion that disease was a disruption of the normal, healthy state, as if normality was not itself a malleable and contingent state. "Normal," he writes, is a "dynamic and polemical concept."[44] As the medical writing on nymphomania and the propaganda surrounding Marie Antoinette reveals, normal is constantly being created, defined, and promoted, as is abnormality and/or monstrosity. In addition, recent theoretical scholarship calls attention to the ways in which monstrosity has always been aligned with fears about difference, about corruption, and about unstable categories. Monstrous beings were by-products of a perceived breakdown of important foundational divisions, between mind and body, male and female, healthy and pathological. A central message in the scandalizing of the queen is the unacceptability of unpredictable, unknowable bodies that seemed to be "in the process of materializing as something else."[45]

There is a more than significant connection between the rage for political transparency and the ambiguity surrounding the hermaphrodite body in particular. In Britain, the famous surgeon John Hunter and the medical members of his extended family produced influential texts of comparative anatomy, in which they focused on hermaphroditism in humans and animals. Hunter's brother-in-law Everard Home and his nephew Matthew Baillie (both of whom were trained by Hunter) were keen to demystify this condition.[46] In an address on hermaphroditism, delivered to the Royal Philosophical Society, Home identified the difference between true hermaphrodites and the "kinds of monstrous production, which have been frequently mistaken for a complete mixture of male and female."[47] Home was exercised that observers, even trained physicians, often misdiagnosed bodies as hermaphroditic, and he wanted to define the condition clearly. He warned readers that hermaphroditism "has hardly ever occurred in the human subject," yet there were a number of women claiming to have this condition.[48] Individuals whose constitutions were not properly stamped with gendered attributes spent their lives deceiving others, unless they were carefully observed "so as to have their defects discovered."[49]

Home outlined two types of genital "malformations" that tended "to mislead the judgment respecting sex."[50] The first was an enlarged clitoris, which was alleged "to grow to an immoderate size in warm climates, and to resemble a penis."[51] Although Home dismissed some anecdotes about the female penis as exaggeration, he referred to eyewitness accounts that told of African women with masculine faces and voices, flat breasts, and two-inch-long clitorises that, when handled, became erect. (In chapter 5, there is more on the relation between politics, the British monarchy, and the myth surrounding the enlarged genitals of the Hottentots.) The second malformation to which Home referred was uterine prolapse. This is a condition in which, most often as a result of childbirth, the uterus becomes displaced and extends out of the vaginal opening, at times resembling a penis. Both Home and Baillie described how those who suffered from a prolapsed uterus were "mistaken for that species of monstrous formation called hermaphrodite."[52]

These two types of conditions were abnormal, but more than that Home suggested that there was something inherently deceptive about women who presented these symptoms (and as doctors pointed out, women rather than men pretended to hermaphroditism). Ideas about the ins and outs of "true" hermaphroditism could be discussed at length here, but I want to highlight the point about deception. The hermaphroditic body—whether true or simulated—was monstrous not only because it was "unnatural" and different from the "normal" body but because it was untrustworthy and inherently deceptive. To press this point further: Home refers to cases of duplicitous women who attempted to cash in on their exceptional status by deceiving the public in order to gain money, renown, or sex. In one of his examples, he describes how a young French woman with a prolapsed uterus made four hundred pounds by posing as a hermaphrodite and exhibiting herself "as a curiosity in London." But after he inspected her—himself "induced by curiosity"—he "discovered the deception" and she was forced to flee back to France.[53] Indeed, Home betrays a particular aversion to French women; he is among several physicians who recount a well-known French case about a false hermaphrodite who hoodwinked physicians. As they believed she had a penis, she was then free to wear men's clothes and to take up a trade.[54] What is remarkable is the level of discomfort with women who seem to cross gendered boundaries, both biologically and socially. What is clear is that biological uncertainty is as much a problem as the resultant obscuring of dress codes and defined social roles. What is also clear is the physician's faith that science—and women's true natures—would out them.

The "debunking" of human hermaphroditism at the end of the eighteenth century left the medical community with something of a dilemma. Physicians had accounted for the supposed female penis by identifying it as an enlarged clitoris. They now had to account for that grotesquely large clitoris, which appeared as an anomaly of nature. As Richard Sha explains, "Because the clitoris might, even to the trained eye, pass for a penis" and because it breaches the "key physiological law" that bodily form must be allied to function (and the enlarged clitoris seemingly had no biological function), physicians were left with two choices. Either they had to admit that "physiology is founded upon an error or the clitoris must be made monstrous, an example of form that has no function except to deceive."[55] Physicians chose the latter: they pathologized the clitoris by linking it with the other forms of monstrosity, including tribadism, nymphomania, and masturbation. The anxieties surrounding the perceived violation of physiological categories motivated efforts to assign characteristics to the clitoris that were also assigned to female "nature" or "character" in general. Marie Antoinette's allegedly enlarged clitoris signifies that she is at once unnatural, monstrous, and foreign (an Austrian!), yet so typical of her kind. Like her body, she is disorderly and threatening, yet with some effort, containable.

In *A Mechanical and Critical Enquiry into the Nature of Hermaphrodites* (1741), James Parsons links foreignness with anatomical monstrosity. He describes how in Asia and Africa women had large clitorises, which he deems a "useless Part" of the female anatomy, unlike the uterus. They are, he writes, "most commonly very long, and the People knowing that the Length of them produces two Evils, *viz.* the hindering the Coitus, and Womens abuse of them with each other, wisely cut or burn them off while Girls are young."[56] Writing some years later, the surgeon William Hunter uses a slightly more measured and dispassionate vocabulary in his approach to the subject. Yet, similar attitudes reveal themselves in a particularly telling lecture on sexual desire and female reproductive organs. Hunter makes clear to his audience that it was "impossible" for a woman with an enlarged clitoris to have sex with another woman because nature had shrouded it in a skin that could not withdraw like the skin around an erect penis.[57] The same biological system that seemed to make copulation between two women possible (an enlarged clitoris) also ensured that it was impossible (constraining skin). Hunter linked hermaphroditism with lesbianism yet like other doctors also insisted that a woman could never *properly* replace a man sexually. A tribade—a word that originates from the root *to rub*—was ineffectual because she could only do just that. Rubbing herself against another woman, she could never penetrate, procreate, or one presumes, satisfy.

Parsons and Hunter express a view of lesbian anatomy that was standard until at least the twentieth century. In her work on the history of sexuality, Lucy Bland sums up a tradition of classifying the lesbian as both physically and socially incommensurable with the bodies and functions of normal women: "not only was the clitoris associated with female sexual pleasure separate from reproductive potential, but lesbians were assumed to be masculinized, and the supposed enlarged clitoris was one signifier of this masculinity."[58] This marker of abnormality and confused categories make it clear why the charge of tribadism against Marie Antoinette was more than simple sexual scandal.

As a tribade, the French queen had rejected the pleasures of marriage, the satisfaction of childbearing, and the delights of bourgeois domesticity. One pamphleteer contended that she was uninterested in producing children, both as a matter of choice and as a result of biological dysfunction. Since she suffered from the "descent or collapse of the womb" (allegedly caused by her lascivious life) and since she was otherwise preoccupied with her female lovers, she scoffed at the lives of virtuous wives and mothers. She had established a "fashion" of tribadism and was the head of an "anandrine sect" that envisioned a society where "Every woman was both tribade and whore / No one had children anymore, which seemed convenient."[59]

Surprisingly, the poetic form of these lines is rather sophisticated. An easy rhyming singsong rhythm builds in this poem and comes up against the jarring last phrase "which seemed convenient." This enjambment reflects what is described here: the disruption of marital harmony and domestic bliss and the destruction of the wider social fabric. The idea of nonmaternal women free from the obligations of childbearing and motherhood threatened the family; women who desired each other, but neither husbands nor children, were that much more dangerous. Besides threatening the moral and social order, tribades were not producing the next generation of citizens for the new republic. (One thinks here of the comments Napoleon was reputed to have made some years later about how the most praiseworthy women were those who produced the most children for the nation.)⁶⁰

These representations of Marie Antoinette became so publicly accepted as factual that by 1793 they could be used as official evidence against her. They guaranteed that the progression from pamphlet to scaffold would be remarkably quick. At trial, she was accused of committing acts of incest on the body of her son. Her enemy, the shrewd editor and journalist Jacques René Hébert was a member of the Paris Commune and was appointed the second substitute of the *procureur* of the commune, which meant he had authority over the imprisoned royal family. Hébert testified that Antoine Simon, the shoemaker who supervised her imprisoned son Louis, had caught the eight year old engaging in "indecent pollutions." Hébert testified before the tribunal that the boy, "whose health was deteriorating daily, was surprised . . . in an act of self-abuse, fatal for his condition; when . . . [asked] who had taught him this criminal ruse; he replied that he owed his familiarity with the fatal habit to his mother and his aunt [Elizabeth, the king's sister]. . . . It appears the two women often made him sleep between them; that acts of the most unbridled debauchery were committed there; that there is no doubt, from what Capet's son has said, that an act of incest was committed between mother and son."⁶¹

Thus the two "mothers" transmitted to the nation's heir, not only a political hatred for liberty and for the French people, but a private debauchery that profoundly affected the dauphin's health. Driven by their own uterine furors, they had drained him physically. In fact, it was reported that one of the sickly dauphin's testicles was damaged as a result of performing the acts of self-pollution he had learned from his female carers. *Le Moniteur Universal* announced that "the shameful scenes between the mother, the aunt, and the son" had infected the dauphin with a "venom [that] now runs through [his] veins."⁶²

Hébert exploits these remarkable images of the queen as a sort of vampire figure who contaminates her innocent young victims. In his court testimony against the queen and her sister-in-law, he states, "There is reason to believe that th[eir] criminal *jouissance* was not at all dictated by pleasure, but rather by the political hope of enervating the physical health of this child, whom they continued to believe would occupy a throne, and on whom they wished, by this manoeuvre, to assure themselves the right of ruling afterward over his morals."⁶³ Hébert underscores the political motives behind the acts of incest allegedly committed by the two women. Pleasure is no motive, but feminine deceit and political ambition most certainly are. Overriding sympathy or duty or rationality, the queen and her sister-in-law had attempted to gain political influence by taking control of a young boy, by destroying his morals, and by bending his will by manipulating his body: by starving it, weakening it, and destroying it.

The republican image of Marie Antoinette and Elizabeth as ambitious political women who vampirically fed off the innocent dauphin was replicated in the British press. The language and imagery used against them proliferated in reactionary propaganda, taking on new forms in a wider campaign against political women in general. The British memoirist John Adolphus was one of many English eyewitnesses who informed British readers that the young heir had confessed that his mother had "committed indecencies with him, the very idea and name of which strike the soul with horror!"[64] The queen was "in every respect immoral" and "so dissolute and so familiar with all crimes" that she had completely cast off the "quality of mother and the limits proscribed by the law of nature."[65] According to this characterization, the queen was a biological anomaly: she lacked maternal feeling, which nature dictated every woman must have. Categorizing her as "pathological" and outside the realm of normality was a way to ensure her banishment from politics. Another English witness to the trial, Helen Maria Williams, recounts how the queen and her sister-in-law were accused of attempting both personal and political forms of infanticide by endangering the life of the dauphin and by aiming "to exterminate and annihilate liberty in its birth."[66]

Such personifications of liberty were a common rhetorical maneuver. In the British journal the *Anti-Jacobin*, France was cast as a mother figure whose abject body had produced political mayhem. "Gallia" had given "monstrous birth" to a daughter she had bloodily christened "Jacobinism"; in turn, this grotesque offspring, this "Daughter of Hell," sought to destroy "Morals" and "Domestic Virtue."[67] British propagandists portrayed French republican women in strikingly similar terms. As a result of these women's participation in the revolution—itself an overturning of the natural order—maternal feeling was no longer a natural, biological certainty. Mothers could not be counted on to act as society's moral pillars, the emblems of civility, the icons of domestic harmony, or the guardians of human decency; instead they had become unnatural creatures who produced equally unnatural offspring. The Irish loyalist William Hamilton informed his readers that in France, "base strumpets, who boast . . . of their numerous band of illegitimate children" had been seen to "sit astride on dead bodies, intoxicated with wine and blood."[68] In *First Letter on a Regicide Peace,* Edmund Burke vociferated against republican mothers who made "no scruple to rake with their bloody hands in the bowels of those who came from their own" in order "to demonstrate their attachment to their party."[69] The women of the Revolution educated their offspring to become violent, sexually depraved monsters who were incapable of feeling any human sympathy or familial loyalty. The journalist William Cobbett (at that time a staunch Tory) informed his readers that French mothers were known to tie miniature guillotines about the necks of their young children in an effort to school them early in the art of brutality.[70] Through maternal influence, "assassinations" had become "the sports of children," so that "inhumanity took place of gratitude, filial piety, and all the tender affections" that should have been naturally transmitted from mother to child.[71]

The accusations against Marie Antoinette and the gendered reading of the events of the Revolution were intimately related to then-circulating medical and philosophical discourses, both learned and popular. Several crucial interpretive paradigms gave force to the accusation of maternal monstrosity in the 1790s. One of these was the enduring belief in maternal imprinting or maternal marking. References to the frightful and unpredictable power of the mother's imagination to imprint itself on her offspring stretched back to the classical age and proliferated in early-modern print culture. The belief was that mothers' fears and desires physiologically manifested themselves on the bodies of their unborn children in the form of birthmarks, deformities, abnormal hair patterns, or other physical anomalies.[72]

Various cases that were retold through the ages included the anecdote about a noble Greek woman who was accused of adultery after giving birth to a black baby. Her honor was defended by Hippocrates, who explained that while pregnant she had gazed upon a portrait of a Moor, which then manifested itself in the baby's appearance and skin color. The same explanations were offered, centuries later, to explain monstrosity. The seventeenth-century midwife Jane Sharp informed readers that "many a woman brings forth a Child with a hare lip, being suddenly frighted when she conceived by the starting of a Hare"; likewise, if a woman "lookt on a Blackmore" she may produce a dark-skinned child.[73]

Even in the age of Enlightenment, there were reported cases of maternal marking. The English translation of the physician Nicholas Venette's *Mysteries of Conjugal Love Reveal'd* testifies to how popular fears from the past became entwined with medical knowledge about the nervous system. Although this popular treatise appeared early in the century, first published in France in 1687 and translated into English in 1707, it reveals how scientific rationality does not simply dispel the anxieties that underpin superstitions. Rather these attitudes get reformulated in *light* of new scientific knowledge. Venette writes: "The Lawyers say, after some Physicians, that the Womans fancy or imagination is so quick that there is no room to wonder at her impressing the resemblance of what she passionately desires upon what she conceives. . . . The fancy or imagination is so strong in some Women, that they send the corpuscles of extraneous objects from their brain to the Infant that is forming, so that these corporeal Images communicate themselves to the tender parts of the Infant, by a train of Nerves that come from the Mothers brain."[74] Medical reasoning becomes entangled with a metaphysical language, and Venette struggles to make the connections between them. Observable, biological matter—nerves and corpuscles—are shaped by much less material things like passion, desire, fancy, and imagination (and vice versa).

Those opaque entities give rise to an overarching sense of distrust. A woman can easily pass an illegitimate child as legitimate, for she may engender a secret lover's child with her husband's characteristics, Venette writes, "by the meer strength of her imagination." By "thinking always on her Husband, when in the Arms of her lover," he explains, "she prints the Features of the Body and Characters of the Soul of him she fixed her thoughts on, upon the tender Body of the Infant she was then conceiving."[75] For Venette, this deception has clear legal implications: a woman's illicit behavior, desires, and sexual single-mindedness contravene hereditary law and make a mockery of acts of inheritance. But more than that, he proposes that woman, with her "unruly appetite" and her determination to deceive, poses a threat to the natural moral order. Her imagination, he writes, "rather disturbs the action of Nature" than being a conduit of it.[76] By short-circuiting the processes of nature, the mother is responsible for monstrosities and the disorders attendant on that child.

As I said, Venette's is an early text. Yet, some of the anxieties he expresses survive in much later writing. What is striking is that even in the age of Enlightenment, there continued to be reported cases of maternal marking, and these made their way into legitimate, learned texts. So, for instance, in his popular treatise on the science of physiognomy—examining the features of the face to "read" character—the eighteenth-century physiognomist Johann Caspar Lavater includes an illustration and description of how a pregnant woman who had quarreled with a neighbor over a haunch of venison gave birth to a girl born with hairy patches and brown fungal growths on her skin.[77] Enlightenment physicians may have been more circumspect about this theory, but they still struggled to identify the line between superstition and science, fiction and fact, the primitive and the civilized. Their attempts to understand how the mind worked upon the body, to accurately comprehend human conception and reproduction, and to delineate the female capacity for reason and sexual desire were still colored by ancient anxieties about the imagination left over from earlier centuries. Over the course of the eighteenth century, arguments about the biological effects of maternal feeling and thinking became more refined and nuanced. But in the struggle to separate legitimate, rational reservations from illegitimate fears, doctors pushed for more access to and more authority over the mother's body and her imagination. Medical science could explain monstrosity by seeing into the body, by understanding the nervous system.

By the end of the century, new theories about nature and biology, nerves and brains, emotions and imagination served to further establish similar attitudes about sexual difference as those held by Venette. Both professionalizing male obstetricians and the female midwives they were rapidly replacing emphasized physiological difference. In *A Treatise on the Art of Midwifery* (1760), Elizabeth Nihell insists that women are naturally modest, have innate maternal instincts, and "a certain delicacy of mind" that men do not have. Nihell's conceptualization of women as more modest and delicate is intended to support her defense of female midwives, but her argument about how the "bare presence" of a male accoucheur at delivery could "excite a revolution capable of stopping the labour-pains" serves to further emphasize biological incommensurability.[78] As Lisa Forman Cody points out, for Nihell as well as for the male physicians she challenged, "the relevant distinction between male and female knowledge was not so much in their different worldly experiences, but in their fundamentally different minds." Women's supposed biological delicacy and "their innate, almost pathetic desires to please husband, child, and others made them extraordinarily vulnerable . . . and consequently best suited for the protected sanctuary of the nuclear household."[79]

Indeed, there is an overwhelming sense that, as an operation of the mind, women's ability to affect offspring is so opaque it actually escapes the gaze of medicine; it defies scientific method and rational experimentation. In *The New Theory of Generation, According to the Best and Latest Discoveries in Anatomy* (1762), John Cook evaluates the contemporary debate about the possibilities of maternal impression between fellow physicians. He concludes that although the argument is not settled as to whether women can determine the internal makeup of their children or simply influence their external appearance, skin condition, and color, there is plain evidence as to women's susceptibility and nervous instability. "I have known myself," he writes, of a case where "only mentioning" a source of disappointment, "has stung the Woman, big with two Children, into a fainting Fit, introduced with a Shriek, that killed one of the Twins directly, while the live Foetus, went its full Time some Months longer, when the other came away by Degrees, Piecemeals.... And if Imagination can thus kill a Child in Utero, why may not a weaker Impression produce weaker Effects accordingly, though we cannot mechanically account for the same?"[80] Regardless of his claims to rationality and empirical evidence, Cook's case report expresses fears about the dangerous unfamiliarity of the woman's mind and emotions. His interpretation of events also underscores for his readers the sense that women are fundamentally designed to be childbearers, even though their weak nerves endanger their offspring. As such, women must be confined to the home and kept away from the sights, stimuli, sensations, and disappointments of the public arena.

Even when, in the last decades of the eighteenth century, increasing numbers of physicians rejected maternal marking outright, the same stress on women's susceptible natures and untrustworthy passions remained. The idea of maternal impressions was "unphilosophical" and "absurd," the physician John Leake stated in 1792, and the people who believed "strange examples of marks, monsters, and mutilated forms" were fanciful and unscientific.[81] (Chief among these unenlightened people who trusted in superstition over their own rational sense were women.) Leake provided clearheaded reasons why women could not be blamed for their children's diseases and deformities, but as he did so he provided further evidence of women's limited capacities. He used simple deduction: we could assume that, since "a woman's mind, from the delicacy of her bodily frame, and the prevalence of her passions, is liable to so many excesses," then many more numbers of women should produce monstrous offspring.[82] But this was not the case; in fact, historically, monstrous births were a rarity. Additionally, anatomy provided more evidence against maternal marking: since there are no nerves in the umbilical cord, it is impossible for irrational women to transmit their imaginative excesses to the child. Regardless of her unrestrained thoughts, the mother could not contaminate the child—a distinct being—with her "sensations." Only the most basic biological material, such as nourishment and blood, circulated between the two. In other words, Leake's arguments against the superstitious fog that still clung to ideas of conception and gestation do not offer a defense of women's capabilities, nor do they disclose any of the gendered biases running through medical thought. Rather, Leake simply provides a more professional, empirically based rationale for maintaining the very attitudes that had always informed the theory of maternal impression.

This medical material gives some sense of the ways that beliefs become naturalized; it reveals how long foundational ideas about gender difference remain in currency long after they are allegedly exploded. The medical discourse surrounding the subject of maternal impression was not simply a case of folk belief or bad science. It was a way of accounting for the ambiguous etiology and bewildering effects of congenital and contagious diseases. Yet it could be argued that anxieties about the frightening, suspicious, and unpredictable nature of the maternal body, fears about woman's subtle powers of deception, and suspicions about female irrationality were stronger impetuses. The idea here, to borrow Rosi Braidotti's expression, is that woman was "morphologically dubious."[83] This biologically uncertainty in an age searching for certainty gave rise to a nostalgic turn to a natural past that never existed. Nature, in all the glory of her grand design, had endowed woman with certain biological weaknesses; therefore it made sense that authority over the woman's body should be transferred from herself and her peers to the professional male physician and her husband. Only by placing woman under the authority of legal and medical practitioners could society control her desires and delimit her detrimental influence. This nostalgic turn was sold as modernity; this was a conclusion made from informed scientific speculation.

We should not miss how similar attitudes underwrite the propaganda machine surrounding Marie Antoinette. The hardening of the ideology of incommensurability and the struggle to define, monitor, and exercise authority over woman's reproductive body provided provocative conditions for her political enemies. The motivating ideas behind the "science" of maternal marking are the same as those behind the revolutionary tribunal's contention that the queen deserved death for transmitting to her son, in equal measure, a hatred for liberty and a lust for masturbation. Fears about woman's imagination and its effect on her physiology and character (specifically, the way it stimulated her to deceive) also informed representations of republican mothers who, encouraged by the atmosphere of revolutionary excess, transmitted violence and sexual deviance to the next generation.

MASTURBATION

The issue of etiology is an important one. The apprehension around such conditions as maternal marking, as Margrit Shildrick states succinctly, "speaks to a more general anxiety about *origins*."[84] Indeed, political pornography and medical writing share an abiding concern with the causes, evolution, and the cultural implications of disease. At Marie Antoinette's trial, fears about the etiology of sexual dysfunction underpinned the charge of incest brought against her. Hébert's claim that the young dauphin had been caught "in an act of self-abuse, fatal for his condition," tapped into the social neuroses surrounding masturbation. That masturbation was a key theme in medical-moral print culture in the eighteenth century has been addressed by scholars from Michel Foucault to Thomas Laqueur to George Rousseau.

John Marten's *Onania; or, The Heinous Sin of Self-Pollution and All Its Frightful Consequence in Both Sexes*, first published in 1712 and reprinted consistently throughout the century, effectively made masturbation a disease, a sin, and a source of social degeneracy. In the much-expanded nineteenth edition of midcentury, Marten lists the dire physiological effects of solitary sex, including "Loss of Erection . . . as though . . . Castrated," the loss of bodily "Moisture," "Gonnorrhea," "nightly and excessive Seminal emissions," watery ejaculate, painful urination, penile ulcers, "phimosis" (irretractable foreskin), "paraphimosis" (retracted foreskin), and "priapisms" (constant erection).[85] Besides these effects, masturbation caused muscular, skeletal, and most significantly, mental disorder—all of which could lead to an early death.

The same was true for young girls and women: in his 1779 treatise on masturbation, the German political writer, philosopher, and doctor Johann Georg Zimmermann warned that girls would "fall headlong into every possible kind of nervous illness, fevers, consumption"; additionally, "one must fear they will become whores before they are properly sexually mature or of marriageable age."[86] As this last comment indicates, these pathological symptoms were linked to a much wider set of social, political, and moral concerns. Masturbation was an unnatural practice that defiled the individual, sapped his or her health, disrupted marriages, broke up families, and weakened the social fabric of the nation.

Very quickly, this became the consensus among most eighteenth-century physicians and moralists, and masturbation's sinister status was effectively established. Scholars have debated why, for the first time in history, masturbation (male, female, and juvenile) became the focus of a medical and moral panic. What was it about the eighteenth century? Thomas Laqueur suggests that this shift was in part economically motivated: the solitary masturbating body was not a productive one. Michael Stolberg suggests that the war on masturbation reflected an intensified concern with "uncleanness" and anxieties about maintaining a sense of self-control.[87] Stolberg's focus on discipline chimes with Peter Gay's argument that, among other things, masturbation conflicted with a growing emphasis on domestic economy and frugality.[88] In *Solitary Sex*, Laqueur helpfully summarizes what he sees as the three "core horrors of sex with oneself": it was "a secret in a world in which transparency was of a premium; it was prone to excess as no other kind of venery was, the crack cocaine of sexuality; and it had no bounds in reality because it was the creature of the imagination."[89] Clearly, the secret vice was dangerous for all kinds of reasons, yet one of the most compelling rationales for why masturbation was such a cultural threat was its association with solitude, excess, secrecy, and unchecked imagination.

These associations indicate why the charge of solitary sex was such an effective propaganda tool in political struggles. In the 1790s, onanism became a political concern as well as a medical and moral issue precisely because, like other "private" acts, it was defined as contravening increasingly important social, political, and legal values: openness, transparency, communality. In France, the terms used to condemn masturbation were also used to describe the degeneracy of the court and the old regime. Revolutionaries revealed the covert sexual and political acts that allegedly took place behind the privileged walls of Versailles, and they contended that the same sense of secrecy now shrouded the silent chamber of the young Louis. The republic would annihilate such aristocratic excess by opening the royal household to public view, closing the salons where imaginations had run riot, demystifying religion and law by replacing the secret confessional and *lettres de cachet* with open legal proceedings.[90] In Britain, reformers applauded these aims and demanded their own forms of transparency in elections, in parliamentary affairs, and in the public exercise of private virtues.

The same agitation for transparency, restraint, and order also informed medical writing on masturbation. Politics and medicine shared the same suspicion of excess, immoderation, and fluctuation in feeling and sensation. An "excess in venery" and "an extravagant or disordered imagination" led one to perform an immoral act of self-pleasure, which "debilitates the body more than any other species of debauchery," wrote Dr. A.F.M. Willich in his 1799 *Lectures on Diet and Regimen*.[91] In turn, such sexual excess led to its seeming opposite, languor and melancholy; in a further twist, this sense of listless ennui led to an even more amplified search for greater sensation. Willich described how "the unhappy victim endeavours to exhilarate himself by a repetition of these convulsive exertions of his vital spirits, and thus precipitates himself into greater misery."[92] This characterization of the onanist's life, punctuated by compulsive paroxysms, recalls Edmund Burke's description of the mood swings of the revolutionary mob. As we will see in the next chapter, fluctuations between excessive sensation and a lack of feeling became a framing paradigm in both medical and political debate. Such oscillations in feeling were severely dangerous for national stability as much as for the health of individuals.

As the connection between the public and private indicates, there is a related issue here about how individual desires are reconciled with the greater good of the community. Robert Darby suggests that in a century known for the meteoric rise of individualism, it seems counterintuitive that masturbators would be vilified for partaking of an intensely individualistic act.[93] This is an astute observation; in fact, a long line of anti-onanists, including John Marten and S. A. D. Tissot, *were* worried about individualism. In their treatises, they consistently emphasized the importance of familial and social connections: masturbation was a purely selfish act that threatened domestic stability, familial happiness, and communal harmony. As Foucault's work on the history of sexuality shows, the "socialization of procreative behaviour" was a defining phenomena of this era: the process whereby reproduction became a distinctly public matter also determined that masturbation—a nonprocreative act—posed "individual and collective dangers."[94] This double threat is unfailingly emphasized throughout John Marten's *Onania:* he insists that "when the Man, by a criminal and untimely retreat, disappoints his Wife's as well as his own Fertility," he commits "what truly may be called a Frustraneous Abuse," not just of his own body, but "of *their* Bodies."[95] Sex was meant to be shared and procreative; it was a private act, but one that positively reinforced wider social connections. In Marten's opinion, a society that tolerated masturbation was the same society that encouraged adultery and, even worse, *murder.*

In the 1790s, the growing emphasis on family, domestic affections, communality, and national cohesion was shared by political writers who likewise feared the effects of disaffection, division, and independence. In novels, poetry, and prose, the family was represented as a buttress against wild political anarchy. Plots often revolved around threats to the affective family, expressive of acute fears about the degeneration of the social fabric. In her *Letters Written in France*, Helen Maria Williams celebrated the revolutionaries for reforming the family: one of the great promises of the new experiment was to restore children to parents, wives to husbands, brothers to brothers, and sisters to sisters.[96] In her *Civic Sermons*, Anna Letitia Barbauld analogized a comparable model of familial-political interdependency in a British context. The family was a single, small waterway that, as it meandered along, naturally combined its forces with numerous other waterways, feeding into consecutively larger tributaries until joining one large reservoir, the nation. Each family contributed a small but vital role in the process of nation building. And the linchpin that connected family and state? Virtue. Family members had to be vigilant and self-regulative about their moral principles, for if a "spring be pure," Barbauld reasoned, then "what proceeds from it will be pure"; however, "if it be polluted, the broader water will be discoloured."[97] Since each family had a hand in determining the state of the nation, family members had a duty to reform themselves. These arguments should be read in part as a reaction to individualism. It is instructive to read Barbauld and Williams alongside anti-onanist pamphlets and political pornography, both of which express a similar distrust of individualism. In fact, the same targeting of selfish desires, concealed imaginations, and solitary longings that occur in Barbauld's political image of the codependent waterways also occur in the medical advice doled out to Britons in these years.

Restraint, self-management, and proper outlets for desire are prescribed to counteract excess and secrecy. This may not be surprising, but what is more novel is the emphasis on public demonstration of the exercise of restraint in response to increasing suspicions about concealment and selfishness. Not only must one *appear* to be upright and "normal," one must *openly demonstrate* such uprightness and normalcy. One must demonstrate—publicly—that one is fulfilling familial and communal obligations.

FROM BIOLOGY TO LAW

The British political press expressed a deep antipathy for Marie Antoinette and for women's political participation in general. In his 1792 *Letters on the Revolution of France*, Thomas Christie pointed to the life of the French queen as justification for his support of France's Salic law, which had prevented women from occupying the throne since the sixth century. For

Christie, this exclusion had not been enough, for in reality they were only "nominally excluded" from the throne, since behind it, they were still free to govern like "a set of prostitutes."[98] Christie approved of the National Convention's decision to retain the fundamental principles of Salic law in its modernization of the role of monarchy and endorsed the convention's decision to restrict women's role even further. According to the decree of 28 March 1791, no woman could occupy the throne and no woman but a mother (as long as she remained a widow) could have guardianship of minor male heirs. By the new constitution, then, a queen was "not known as a public character" and was limited to the "sphere of domestic life," a decision that, in Christie's view, showed that the French had "manifested superior wisdom" in knowing "where to draw the line" so as not to "endanger the welfare of society."[99] This was a line that needed to be more firmly drawn in Britain.

Like many observers before him and since, Christie refered to the female body as providing "natural" and indisputable physical evidence of woman's unfitness for political participation. In this belief, he followed a tradition set down by the seventeenth-century legal commentator Jérôme Bignon, who insisted that Salic law was not "invented" but was "born with us" and "drawn from nature itself."[100] That nature had given woman a weak body was clear physical evidence of her unfitness for political participation. The French had "rightly judged" woman's physical and intellectual weakness, Christie wrote, and were right

> in not raising them out of their *natural sphere;* in not involving them in the cares and anxieties of State affairs, to which neither their frame nor their minds are adapted; in not charging them with the weight of a sceptre, which they scarcely ever sway but in appearance—with true respect for the gentleness of their *nature,* and the delicacy of their sex, they have saved them from the horrid obligation of proclaiming war, and calling forth men to battle and bloodshed; with all the other *unnatural* and shocking circumstances that attend a reversal of the laws of *Nature,* by appointing women to rule over men.[101]

This long sentence, peppered throughout with the term *nature* and its cognates, demonstrates how conceptions of inherent gendered weakness were conceived of, and represented as, physiological fact. The royal scepter, a phallic symbol of male potency, was a reminder of women's enduring lack. That women could not physically and mentally bear the responsibilities and realities of political rule was, for Christie, demonstrated by history and, more to the point, by their bodies, which were weak on two counts: first, woman's selfish passions drove them to become adept schemers who were willing to prostitute themselves in court politics; second, they were as intellectually weak, psychologically delicate, and politically ineffectual as their frail limbs. There was only one conclusion to be drawn about women and politics. To allow them to occupy positions of authority was a crime against nature that could only have, to use Christie's term, "shocking" results. As we know from the example of maternal impression, contravening nature resulted in human monstrosity.

There is a revealing contrast between the ways political writers handled Marie Antoinette and how they represented George III's consort Queen Charlotte. Although writers accused Charlotte of some behind-the-scenes manipulation, she was mostly celebrated for her decision to stay out of politics. She became a domestic and distinctly apolitical national icon. According to Christie, the contrast between the French and English queens could not have been greater, since "to her immortal honour" Charlotte had "voluntarily chosen" a life of domestic retirement.[102] Christie took the opportunity to mock his antirevolutionary political opponent Edmund Burke while viciously satirizing the idea of women rejecting domestic bliss in favor of a public role. Mimicking Burke's famously inflated prose in his theatrical apostrophe to the French queen in *Reflections on the Revolution*, Christie expressed false sympathy for "Maria Antonietta—the daughter, sister, and wife of kings—the paragon of beauty, brilliant as the morning star," who was tragically "*doomed* for ever to be a—a good mother, and a faithful wife!"[103] Though it might make "Mr. Burke . . . very angry, that a Queen should be thought *only a woman*," that was precisely what she was, and as such her true pleasures were to be found in marriage and maternity. It was "an undeniable truth that the real happiness of a Queen, is exactly of the same kind, as that which constitutes the felicity of the humblest female of her dominions."[104] In Christie's sardonic rewriting of Burke's prose, a queen was only a woman, and women were only mothers, and mothers could only be domestic creatures. This political statement is clearly buttressed by the biology of incommensurability.

Even fulsome praise of domestic women was often underwritten with the familiar charge of deception. In *The Jockey Club*, the radical libertine Charles Pigott echoes Christie—at least on this point. He argues that "we must not rank" Charlotte with Marie Antoinette, for "the former acts within a much narrower circle than the other, nor is she capable by any means, of those scandalous excesses, which stain the life of her unfortunate sister."[105] But the designation "sister" (and the way the identities of the two women are syntactically confounded) should tell us something about the real message here. For all of Charlotte's domesticity, her irreproachable moral conduct, her numerous children, her retirement from public life, her allegedly apolitical character, she still *embodies* a potential threat to the nation. Charlotte may not be as sexually debauched nor her body as deformed as that of her "sister," but she is equally determined by her biology.

Like her French counterpart, Charlotte is still motivated by greed and by a desire for power; her tactics are invariably devious. That she is a consort and thus plays some small supporting political role, no matter how far removed from the day-to-day workings of the nation, is problematic. She may have spent years "behind the curtain" of quiet domestic retirement, Pigott claims, but this was a ruse. The unsuspecting British people "universally imagined, that her cares were solely devoted to her nursery, and her popularity with the nation, was derived from an amiable modesty and disinterestedness, never meddling in public transactions," but in truth she had been "playing the deepest game of H——p——c——sy," for it was known that the "R——y——al G——e never decided on any measure, without having first deliberated with the prudent and artful C——l——tte."[106] Her shrewdness and guile knew no bounds, for over the years she learned how to play *"her game"* with ever greater "prudence and address."[107]

Pigott was expressing a common hysteria about political women and their "natures" (an anxiety that continues to surface today). Charlotte could barely help herself from conspiring to occupy the throne when her husband the king had his first bout of porphyria-induced madness, but what else could one expect? She was simply acting according to her constitutional makeup. Her ambition was only one of the "symptoms, indicating a love of power" that, in Pigott's words, was "in some degree inherent in the female mind."[108] Such a charge betrays deep anxieties about designing women who, although excluded from overt or direct political power, still managed to exercise power through the men in their lives. Biology provided a way of accounting for women and of further constraining them. The argument, as we have seen, went like this: the desire and the ability to exercise said power originates in the very biology that prevents women from having the strength or acumen to properly exercise it.

In the eighteenth century, the female body—with all its alleged physical weaknesses, its propensities to nervous disorders, its irrational sexual drives, its unpredictability, its maternal emotions—was increasingly used to determine the metaphysical, ontological category of the female "self" and the legal, moral category of the female "person." We can draw some conclusions about how and why this occurred. For many scientists and philosophers in this period, the mechanical workings of the body seemed constant and predetermined. Bodily systems were generally seen to be homeostatic; physiology and anatomy seemed fixed, invariable, and part of an inherent, essential human "nature." As we have seen (and will see further), eighteenth-century medicine tended to support biological determinism and, arguably, one of its less positive legacies has been its promotion of the following formula, put simply: our bodies = our selves.

Influenced in part by John Locke's challenge to Cartesian mind-body dualism in his account of the self as an amalgam of soul and body, physicians in this era most often conceived of the body as determining the mind and giving rise to the "self." One of the important (and, in other circumstances, positive) legacies of Enlightenment thought is the idea that the body is not separable from the self. Character, behavior and intelligence are founded in the material body. The danger, though, is that antidualist thinking can lead to biological reductionism. The emphasis on the interconnectedness of body and mind often produced (and continues to produce) a dualism of a different kind; namely, between male and female.

2 Monstrous Mothers, Constitutional Amazons, and the Medicalization of the Breast

> Women, you say, are not always bearing children. Granted; yet that is their proper business.
> JEAN-JACQUES ROUSSEAU, *Émile* (1762)

> Physical birth symbolizes everything that makes women incapable of entering the original contract and transforming themselves into the civil individuals who uphold its terms.
> CAROLE PATEMAN, *The Sexual Contract* (1988)

Paradigms of biological transmission became tied to politics in striking ways in the late eighteenth century. As we saw in the last chapter, fears that women could impart physical deviance and intellectual deficiency to their offspring circulated in medical fields as well as in the general culture. These fears greatly influenced a medical turn to the related topic of breast-feeding, since in the view of many doctors breast milk was a medium, like blood and semen, through which physical, moral, and political qualities were communicated. Historians and literary scholars have documented the ways in which breast-feeding underwent something of a revolution in Enlightenment Europe. Though medical treatises and advice manuals of the previous century often promoted maternal nursing on grounds of health, the widespread practice of wet-nursing was de rigueur, at least among those who could afford it. Women tended to make decisions about their children's feeding, and those of a certain class tended to send them out to wet nurses. However, in the eighteenth century, increasing numbers of nursing manuals began urging all mothers to breast-feed their own children.[1] There may have always been some suspicions about wet-nursing, but the widespread and concentrated medical campaign in the eighteenth century was new for its forcefulness, the profound influence it had on women's lives, and its lasting political significance.

The first rumbles of this shift are captured in the correspondence of the diarist and bluestocking Lady Mary Wortley Montagu. One particular January 1716 letter is worth quoting at length:

You tell me that our friend Mrs —— is at length blessed with a son, and that her husband, who is a great philosopher, (if his own testimony is to be depended upon), insists on her suckling it herself.... I really think that Mr. ——'s demand is unreasonable, as his wife's constitution is tender, and her temper fretful. A true philosopher would consider these circumstances; but a pedant is always throwing his system in your face, and applies it equally to all things, times, and places.... All those fine-spun arguments that he has drawn from nature, to stop your mouths, weigh, I must own to you, but very little with me. This same *Nature* is, indeed, a specious word, nay there is a great deal in it, if it is properly understood and applied; but I cannot bear to hear people using it, to justify what common sense must disavow. Is not nature modified by art in many things? Was it not designed to be so? And is it not happy for human society that it is so? Would you like to see your husband let his beard grow, until he would be obliged to put the end of it in his pocket, because this beard is the gift of nature? The instincts of nature point out neither taylors, nor weavers, nor mantua-makers, nor sempsters, nor milliners; and yet I am very glad that we don't run naked like the Hottentots. But not to wander from the subject—I grant, that nature has furnished the mother with milk to nourish her child; but I maintain, at the same time, that if she can find better milk elsewhere, she ought to prefer it without hesitation.... I do verily think that the milk of a good comely cow, who feeds quietly in her meadow, never devours ragouts, nor drinks ratifia, nor frets at quadrille, nor sits up till three in the morning, elated with gain, or dejected with loss; I do think that the milk of such a cow, or of a nurse that came as near it as possible, would be likely to nourish the young squire much better than hers. If it be true that the child sucks in the mother's passions with her milk, this is a strong argument in favour of the cow, unless you may be afraid that the young squire may become a calf; but how many calves are there both in state and church, who have been brought up with their mother's milk?[2]

This letter reveals several things about what was at stake in the growing emphasis on women's role as breast-feeding mothers. Montagu's fascinating observations testify to several important cultural changes already underway in these years: if sophisticated physicians no longer believed in maternal marking, they still had lingering suspicions about the transmission of woman's untrustworthy passions and imaginative impulses through breast milk. In addition, Montagu's correspondence charts the transfer of authority over the maternal body from women to husbands, physicians, and philosophers. Although written early in the century, the changes associated with the professionalization of physicians and surgeons are already in evidence here. There is, in this letter, a tension between independent, social, public women and philosophizing men/husbands who insist on the moral propriety and health benefits of breast-feeding.

Further, Montagu's "pedant" philosopher-husband is a caricaturized representation of the new Enlightenment moral philosopher who forged unprecedented links between private life, politics, and medicine. In fact, this husband seems almost to anticipate Jean-Jacques Rousseau. Like Montagu's "great philosopher," Rousseau's own philosophical "system" uses nature to legitimize claims as to the proper role of women. The Rousseauvian distrust of culture and the elevation of nature as the foundation of social and political relations became a dominant viewpoint in the coming years. Indeed, Montagu's comments reveal a wider emerging conflict between nature and culture that came to characterize this century. Montagu is deeply suspicious of the uses to which reconstructed views of nature were put. She criticizes the belief that a return to nature is an antidote to a degraded culture, as if pure nature existed or as if culture was a bad thing. The trappings of culture—as supplied by milliners and mantua-makers—were signs of society's progress, not its disintegration. As Montagu suggests, nature could not be divided from culture anyway. These issues feature in this chapter. Nature became a bridging concept linking medicine, moral philosophy, and politics in the eighteenth century. Physicians, moral philosophers, and political writers made arguments about the relationship between nature and culture in ways that had tremendous effects on woman's everyday experience and their roles in political culture.

By the revolutionary 1790s, the advocacy of breast-feeding had become a distinctly political act and the mother a locus of intense moral-medical debate. By the turn of the nineteenth century, the breast had become an iconographic organ over which medicine and politics met. The historian of science Londa Schiebinger observes that in "an age that looked to nature as the guiding light for social reform," the breast and breast-feeding became a cultural sign of woman's proper alignment with nature and nurturing.[3] Along with Ruth Perry, Julie Kipp, Laura Brace, and Rebecca Kukla, Schiebinger has shown how unprecedented civic significance was attached to breast-feeding in this period.[4] Enlightened motherhood, as most effectively delineated and disseminated through countless advice manuals and medical treatises on maternal breast-feeding and wet-nursing, placed an inordinate emphasis on the female breast as the first means of inspiring familial attachment, which would eventually grow to patriotism. Moralists, philosophers, and physicians argued that breast-feeding was a natural act that fulfilled a higher cultural purpose. Breast-feeding was sold to women as their natural function, but medicomoralists also insisted that it expressed higher virtues such as good will, loyalty, and affection. Maternal breast-feeding counteracted those distinctly modern and anxiety-producing emphases on independence, individualism, and the related problem of disaffection.

ROUSSEAU, NATIONAL REGENERATION, AND THE BREAST

According to some sources, before the French Revolution, less than 5 percent of Parisian babies were breastfed by their biological mothers.[5] However, in 1793, the French National Convention ruled that mothers who did not breast-feed their children were ineligible for some types of state funding. This legislation was meant to counteract a social atmosphere, described some years earlier by Rousseau, in which there were no longer "fathers, mothers, children, brothers, or sisters" but only individuals who "are almost strangers" and each of whom "thinks of himself."[6] Rousseau's pro-family and anti-individualistic stance was part of a larger eighteenth-century anxiety about the rise of self-interest, to the detriment of community. Elizabeth Wingrove argues that characterizing breast-feeding as natural *and* as socially virtuous was a way of recruiting women to the service of a wider "dynamic of care and control that figures the body politic."[7] On the surface, then, it may appear that women had a significant part to play in the reforming of the body politic. To support such a view, one could point to the iconographic bared breast of Liberty (as seen in the images of Marianne) or to the symbol of the lactating breast in newly commissioned republican architecture. The artist Jean-Louis David designed a Fountain of Regeneration for the 1793 Festival of Unity and Indivisibility, which was erected on the site of the Bastille. The fountain represented nature in the form of the Egyptian goddess of fertility, Isis, and featured numerous spouting breasts, which symbolized the virtuous and selfless fostering of a new republic—the creation of a national family. It was expected that a similar scene would play out in the privacy of each home.

Undoubtedly, the iconographic status of the breast, and the ideology about nature and nurturing that supported it, owed much to Rousseau's midcentury writing. It was largely through his influence that the breast-feeding mother became a particularly potent symbol of national regeneration not just for French republicans in the 1790s but also for British political reformers. He fused woman with nature and motherhood with modern politics, thereby endowing the maternal body with new political and moral meanings. In his educational treatise *Émile*, he waged war against the practice of wet-nursing, declaring that mothers who sent their children out to be nursed were responsible for every instance of national depravity that "follows in the train of this first sin." From this one act of maternal refusal, "the whole moral order is disturbed" and "nature is quenched in every breast." If only mothers would "deign to nurse their own children," he declared, there "would be a reform in morals; natural feeling will revive in every heart; there will be no lack of citizens for the state."[8] Amalgamating political, medical, moral, and sentimental language, Rousseau insisted that the newborn required his *own* mother's milk in order to mature into a true patriot. Elsewhere he explained: "The newly-born infant, upon first opening his eyes, must gaze upon the fatherland, and until his dying day should behold nothing else. Your true republican is a man who imbibed the love of the fatherland, which is to say love of the laws and of liberty, with his mother's milk. That love makes up his entire existence: he has eyes only for the fatherland, lives only for the fatherland; the moment he is alone, he is a mere cipher."[9]

The mother is the conduit to nature, and her milk is the means by which her male child imbibes fraternity and acquires feelings of loyalty for family, community, and nation. Her milk is the first step to cultivating patriotic masculine republicanism, which connected the generations, with each successive patriot-father becoming the head of a small domestic circle of wife and children. On these points, if not others, Mary Wollstonecraft's vision of the political importance of hearth and home coincides with Rousseau's. In the *Vindication of the Rights of Woman* she aligns breast-feeding with political and moral reform, so that the woman who "neither suckles nor educates her children, scarcely deserves the name of a wife, and has no right to that of a citizen."[10] Nursing cemented the foundational bond between mother and child, from which grew similar attachments between husbands and wives and between citizens and their state.

Ever the advocate of nature and the adversary of artificiality, Rousseau pits maternal breast-feeding against the degradations of culture. It is important to recognize, though, that Rousseau's nature, like that of the many republicans and reformers who succeeded him on both sides of the Channel, is a civilized, principled, ordered nature. He does not advocate a relapse to, or a resurrection of, a precivilized or savage (no matter how noble) state of nature. A more complicated idea of nature informs his promotion of breast-feeding. The philosopher of reproductive ethics Rebecca Kukla helpfully describes the Rousseauvian-inflected goals of 1790s French revolutionaries, who searched for a more genuine, affectionate, and organic means of connecting citizens. For them, "the mother and child joined by milk became the symbol of the just Republic itself, which nourishes its citizens via a natural bond rather than protects them via a set of artificial conventions between separate individuals." The mother's milk was a means of achieving what might be termed a kind of "second nature": that is, lactation was a means "to *perfect* rather than just *preserve* nature."[11] In the cultured world of enlightened Europe, an authentic or original nature no longer existed, so preservation was impossible; as such, Rousseau and his followers promoted an *idea* of the natural that suited their political and moral ends.

In Britain, nature determined many questions about women's reproductive health and childrearing practices. In a raft of late eighteenth-century pamphlets, medical instruction about nursing and childrearing is buttressed by a clear moral and social agenda. William Cadogan's hugely influential *Essay upon Nursing and the Management of Children from Birth to Three Years of Age*, which was published consistently from 1748 to the end of the century, is a prime example. In the revised ninth edition of 1772, Cadogan praises the great progressive strides medicine has taken in the century, which he says owes to the new emphasis on nature. In the battle against disease and the management of health, nature ultimately determines prevention and cure. "Let us consider what Nature directs," he writes, "if we follow Nature, instead of leading or driving it, we cannot err. In the business of Nursing, as well as Physick, Art is destructive."[12] With this philosophy in mind, Cadogan asserts that breast-feeding, as the most natural of practices, is the key to establishing the health of the child and the restoration of the new mother's weakened body. The child becomes healthy and fit through proper nursing, or it becomes sick and weak through bad nursing. In a postscript to his *Essay*, Cadogan warns mothers of the serious injuries that follow from a refusal to breast-feed. He recounts how one respected lady reproached him because her child had died, even though according to her she had followed the strictures in his book. The problem, he insists, is that she had followed every one of his instructions except the most important one: she had "dry-nursed" (not suckled) her child.[13] This fatal error, warns Cadogan, led to the inevitably disastrous result.

Moreover, breast-feeding was as much a key to a mother's good health as her baby's. In fact, according to Cadogan, breast-feeding would alleviate some of those "hysterical nervous cases" that women were physiologically predisposed to, including, one would suppose, nymphomania. But those who refused to nurse endangered their own life, since forcing back milk "often lays the foundation of many incurable diseases."[14] An abundance of breast milk was a humoral redundancy that led to degeneracy in the body, which if left unchecked corrupted "the whole mass."[15] This is only one example of how moral discourse about degeneracy, corruption, contamination, and excess gave support to health warnings about disease and death. There were many others.

In *Principles of Midwifery* (1785), Dr. John Aiken insisted that neglecting to breast-feed was a "violent deviation from the line of nature [that] cannot take place with impunity."[16] Still other physicians were more specific and admonitory about the effect of diverging from nature. In his 1794 *Essay on the Management, Nursing and Diseases of Children*, the physician William Moss similarly set duty and nature in opposition to the artifice and selfishness of modern culture. Like Cadogan, he warned of the detrimental effects on woman's health if they attempted to deny their biological destinies. Women had to heed "human nature" and "suffer the dictates of reason to prevail over fashion or caprice," since any deviation from these "laws" would result in "injury."[17] Indeed, Moss placed great emphasis on biology as destiny—so much so that he insisted that women's health problems, particularly those that hindered or prevented breast-feeding, were a direct result of culture's pernicious influence. Weak constitutions, nervous complaints, a lack of milk, or inverted nipples were *not* the result of nature but of social fashions that, over time, had caused alterations in women's bodies. His principle was that "whenever constitutional *inability* occurs, it may always be deemed *acquired* and *artificial*, and not *natural*."[18] In fact, Moss was so keen to promote breast-feeding that his arguments took a rather bizarre turn. He contended that since women's characters were so naturally passive, they could not be held accountable for their refusal or seeming physical inability to nurse. Their innate timidity, he explained, meant that they would easily submit to husbands and parents who advised them to deny the "powerful impulse of nature"—an impulse to nurse.[19] Often such advisors seemed to have the woman's best interests at heart, but young mothers who followed their misguided advice were making grave errors.

Often these types of advice manuals read like a war on culture and, more specifically, on fashionable ideas about bodily beauty. The manuals target the aristocratic practice of cultivating a beautiful décolletage, which well-to-do women would display as a symbol of status and good taste in a décolleté dress. Décolletage was as important in grooming as, say, the creation of elaborate hairstyles and wearing just the right hat to show it off. Women devised various ways to stem lactation, including applying lint and ointments to the breasts, in an attempt to reduce their size and sagginess. As Cadogan observes, one of the reasons why husbands might advise their wives against breast-feeding was a desire to preserve the beauty of their wives' breasts.

Strategically, Cadogan was happy to appeal to the same sense of female vanity he criticized, in an attempt to counter and alter current fashions. If his arguments about moral responsibility and the health benefits of nursing were not convincing enough, then he would take in hand the conceits and concerns of the softer sex. Women may think that nursing destroyed "a little of the beauty of the breast," he explained, but having a quiet and contented child was a worthwhile trade-off: men would look past a sagging bosom, but they could not endure a screaming child. In an ironic twist, Cadogan urged women to appeal to their husbands' own brand of masculine vanity: "a Man of sense cannot have a prettier rattle (for rattles he must have of one kind or other)" than a child who is quietly sated from breast-feeding.[20]

Cadogan empathized with wives who felt pressure to keep their husbands from seeking out greener pastures. He acknowledged the importance of a wife's physical attractiveness and the reality of unwelcome bodily changes resulting from pregnancy. But he insisted that the general consensus about droopy breasts as a side effect of nursing was to some extent misguided. The unattractiveness of postpregnancy breasts was more often a result of a mother's propensity to gain weight and to generally let herself go. Similar arguments were put forward by other physicians and moralists, who pressured women to realign their ideas of beauty so that maternity might be seen as appealing. In his *Letters to Married Women*, Hugh Smith also opposed the seductive influence of fashion and the current ideas of taste. He urged his female readers to ignore insinuations "that your bosoms are less charming, for having a dear little cherub at your breast."[21] Like Cadogan, he argued that a wife's attractiveness was linked both to her demonstration of maternal self-sacrifice and to the demonstration of bodily self-control and moral restraint. This, he insisted in no uncertain terms, was the real way to keep a husband from wandering.

Such comments signal important transitions in the ways that women's roles were defined. For one thing, there is a shift in emphasis, from the view that a husband's love and admiration were inspired by woman as social being, to the view that husbandly affection should be tied to woman as domestic being. This transition, and the arguments made in support of it, advocated a new form of female subservience. Woman's role was still to please, but not as hostess, accomplished beauty, or clever and witty *salonnière*; rather, women were now expected to perform purely as domestic creatures whose primary roles were to give birth, to feed babies, and to provide a blissfully tranquil retreat for husbands otherwise engaged with the business of public life. A corpus of treatises and manuals were also part of the well-documented shift of authority over women's bodies, from women themselves to professional male doctors. A strong appeal to nature went far to legitimize this transfer of authority: vague but powerful, *nature* became a paradigmatic term, used not only to determine healthful and wholesome practices but also to legitimize normative social roles, to manage bodies, and to transfer decision making from women to their husbands via their physicians.

Breast-feeding took center stage in this transfer of authority, as evidenced in Cadogan's recommendation that every father should be sure "to have his Child nursed under his own eye, to make use of his own reason and sense in superintending and directing the management of it; nor suffer it to be made one of the mysteries of the *Bona Dea*, from which the Men are to be excluded."[22] Women's bodies should be under the purview of men of reason, since biology determined that women were much less capable of exercising their "own" reason. Again, the emphasis is on transparency; everything must be open, visible and managed. In her reading of Cadogan's statements, Rebecca Kukla rightly notes that "enlisting fathers in the surveillance of the maternal body" gives some indication of how the mother's body was moved "into a domain of social concern," where it then became an object "of surveillance and accountability" in the public sphere.[23] Once women were safely ensconced in the domestic realm, they became the objects of managing doctors, legislators, and moralists—*within* the very public space they had so recently vacated. Cadogan's highly influential arguments demonstrate how, as Ruth Perry argues, the concentration on the breast in the eighteenth century effectively colonized women's bodies to serve patriarchal ends.[24] For instance, men achieved greater control over the lineage of inheritance: confined wives were faithful wives. Meanwhile, their husbands were free to hold political office, to receive recognition for their accomplishments, and to move at liberty in salons, clubs, pubs, coffeehouses, theaters, and parliament.

In light of all of this, it would seem very difficult indeed to interpret maternal breast-feeding as part of a dynamic of woman's empowerment. Yet some scholars have done just that. In particular, Rebecca Kukla identifies something positive about the new status accorded the maternal body as an object of social concern. In her interpretation, the "publicizing" of woman's maternal role and the political, cultural, and medical attention bestowed upon the breast-feeding body is a sign of how mothers obtained some social influence and recognition. She reads an affirmative angle to Rousseau's writing on motherhood and the part he plays in "the project of forming human nature into a civic project appropriately monitored by public institutions, rather than just a private process governed by the logic of maternal excesses and restraint."[25] That pregnancy and breast-feeding practices became governed by reason and public monitoring is, for Kukla, a beneficial step, and indeed, I agree that the Enlightenment emphasis on rationality, scientific evidence, and empirical research did much to dispel superstition and poor health care. However, from the medical treatises of the first half of the century to the philosophy of the latter half, she detects an "elevation" of the maternal body, so that by the 1790s the lactating breast is elevated "into a social symbol." The breast, she argues, thereby takes on a "power . . . to heal and create proper social bonds."[26] I would not use the same language of empowerment to describe the use of the breast as social symbol or to characterize the refashioning of the breast-feeding body.

The intersection of moral philosophy and medical science on the issue of maternity and breast-feeding marks a particularly problematic turning point in the history of the body and gender. Historian Elizabeth Colwill is right to observe that in this era doctors produced "ever more precise physiological bases" to buttress the notion that "woman's strength came to reside in maternal love."[27] Just what kind of "strength" that was—if indeed we can use that word, or the word "power"—has always been open to debate. There is a troubling continuity between medical manuals advising women of their biologically defined roles and Rousseauvian moral philosophy, which insists that nature dictates woman's suitability for motherhood and domesticity. As insightful as Kukla's study otherwise is, I would argue against her suggestion that the breast became a source of woman's political power. The monitoring and governing of the maternal body, by patriarchs, physicians, and the masculinized republican state, are not a sign of empowerment or influence. Instead, the husband becomes a wife's conduit to the outside world, while she remains tied to the home through breast-feeding and the duties of childcare. The role of familial and national regeneration supposedly ascribed to mothers is not a political or public one (even if on rare occasions it was packaged as such). Women could have a hand in moral and social reform only by maintaining or reestablishing their supposedly close biological proximity to Mother Nature. The "elevation" of the breast-feeding mother is only indicative of her further eviction from public spaces and from political debate, quite simply because that elevation is purely emblematic. The lactating mother is a *symbol* of regeneration, not an active participant in the work of nation building, parliamentary reform, or institutional restructuring.

This is not to say that physicians were incorrect in asserting the health benefits of nursing. Indeed there were more than nutritional benefits to breast milk: women who sent their children to wet nurses suppressed their flow of milk; we now know that this suppression diminishes the positive contraceptive effects of lactation. As a result, those who sent their children to wet nurses could find themselves constantly pregnant, while ironically, wet nurses gained the contraceptive benefit and had lower birth rates. Under the old system, well-to-do women were often "tied to perpetual pregnancy and poor mothers to perpetual suckling."[28] Still, my concern here is with the negative effects attendant on the medicalization of the breast and the "elevation" of the breast-feeding mother. The resulting types of social and cultural pressures to conform to models of motherhood are much more difficult to measure, but I would argue that women's breasts became signifiers of biological destiny as they never had before—and this had detrimental effects. In this era, women's breasts, both maternal and nonmaternal, were represented as signs of women's biological *limitations*.

The case of Georgiana, the Duchess of Devonshire, effectively illustrates my arguments. Her political and personal lives have been well documented by Amanda Foreman and others, but I want to briefly address two 1784 caricatures in which her breasts are a focal point. In contrast to the majority of caricatures that portray Georgiana on the campaign trail for the Whigs, in public streets, and in alehouses, in these pictures she is in the home. Figure 2.1 presents the seated duchess offering a bared breast to a fox (Whig leader Charles James Fox) who is dressed very much like her own neglected infant. To the left, a cat, dog, and kitten mimic the scene, indicating how much this is a world turned upside down. Significantly, Georgiana's expression and Fox's pose, with his paw across her lap, recalls the medical argument that breast-feeding is an acceptable source of sensual pleasure for mothers. But rather than a baby, it is a notoriously hard-living, philandering liberal politician who provides the pleasure. Georgiana's torn sympathies and divided loyalties are indi-

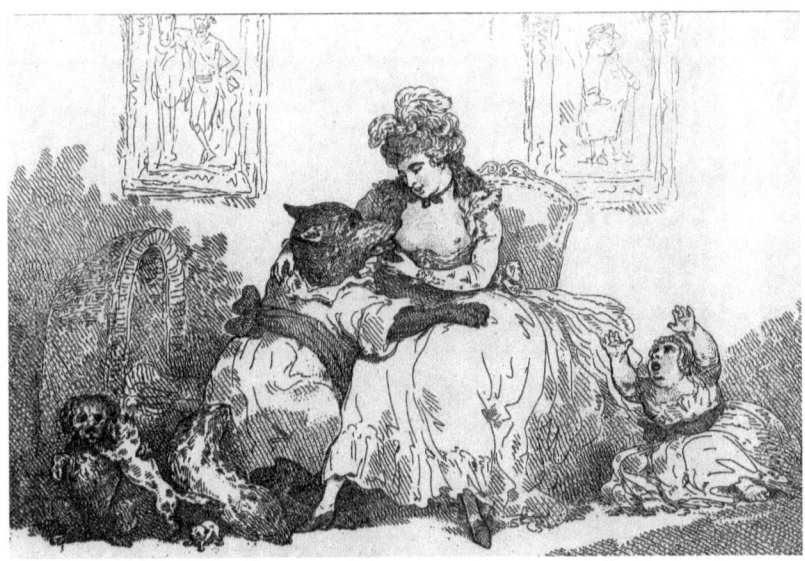

Figure 2.1   Thomas Rowlandson, *Political Affection* (1784 © Trustees of the British Museum, London)

cated by the competing portraits above her head, one of her husband and one of Fox.

Figure 2.2 is an image that appeared in the *Rambler's Magazine,* and it presents a very different, reformed Georgiana. In the *Duchess of D—— in the Character of a Mother* (1784), politics are banished; with her smiling husband by her side, the duchess contentedly suckles her child. At the duke's feet is the *Treatise on Getting and Nursing of Children,* which, according to the cover, he has authored himself. The duke is recruited in support of the professionalization movement, which saw physicians displacing midwives and male-authored advice manuals replacing traditional forms of oral knowledge. The duke has regained control over his wife's body, as advised in the very type of treatise that appears here. There are the same kinds of domestic objects in this image as in figure 2.1: the empty cradle, the pictures on the wall, the seated duchess with bared breasts. But here the duke has stepped down from the portrait to appropriate control over the domestic space. This is a world turned the right side up: the mother has returned home; the child has replaced the politician.

These images appeared on the heels of a press flurry about the duchess's decision to breast-feed her daughter. In the previous year, the

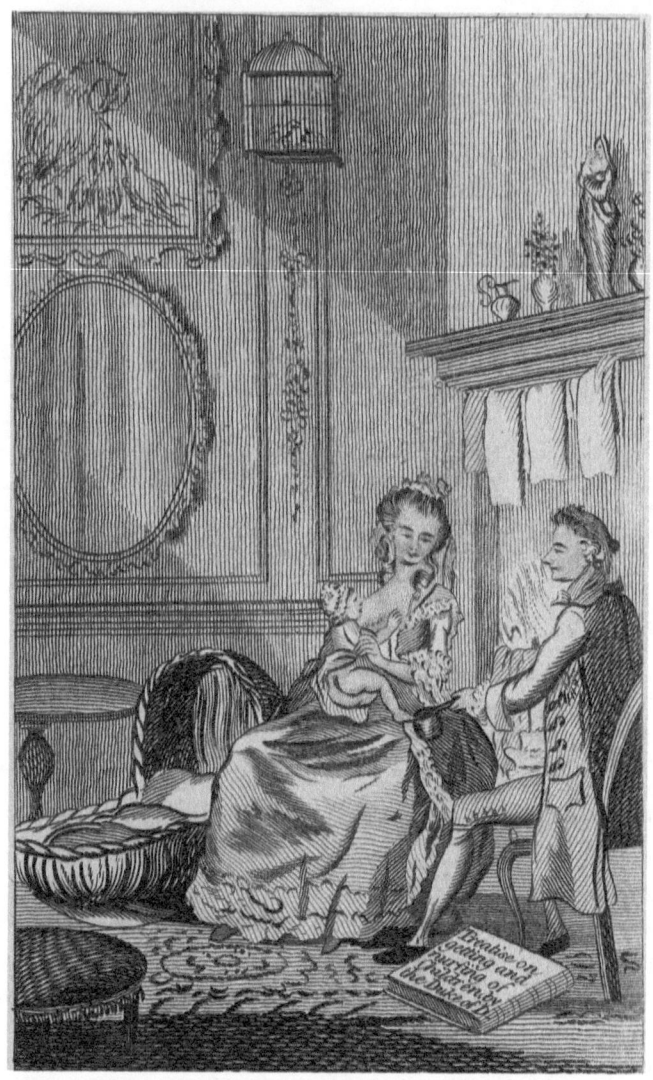

Figure 2.2 Anon., *Duchess of D—— in the Character of a Mother*, from the *Rambler's Magazine* (1784 © Trustees of the British Museum, London)

Rambler's Magazine congratulated the duchess on her choice but used the opportunity to send an unambiguous message to readers about woman's proper duties: "Her grace deserves commendation for this, but it is rather a reflection on the sex, that females in high life, should generally be such strangers to the duty of a mother, as to render one instance to the contrary so singular a phenomenon."²⁹ This commentary was seconded by Charles Pigott, who was happy to inform readers of his *Female Jockey Club* that the duchess, having had "her sensibility" awakened by Rousseau, went against fashion to nurse her own children.³⁰

As this language and the images reveal, breasts and breast-feeding had become potent markers of woman's biological incapacity for politics, signs of her unsuitability for public life and signifiers of her potential to contaminate the echelons of political decision making. The images of the duchess also demonstrate the growing sense that women were properly the objects of professional and domestic management. The caricatures and advice manuals made women the focus of the all-seeing eye of public opinion. As we will see further, the growing consensus was that according to the nature of women's bodies they had no place in politics.

REPRESENTING THE POLITICIZED BREAST

In political texts of the 1790s, there was congruence between the medical idea of maternal marking and the propagandistic use of the breast as a motif for the transfer of dangerous political ideas. Time and again, British reactionaries used the image of the French breast that produced blood instead of pure milk as emblematic of the dark side of republicanism. Like the bloody breast, the revolutionary interpretation of the ideals of equality and liberty deviated profoundly from natural law and order. The Scottish conservative Thomas Hardy (not to be confused with the radical shoemaker of the same name) and William Cobbett (before he became a supporter of Thomas Paine) both employed the image of the monstrous mother infecting the next generation through breast-feeding. In the same way that "the republic was suckled with blood," Hardy declared, so had French babies "sucked in blood with their mother's milk."³¹ By contrast, Cobbett employed the emblem of the English breast to represent communicable patriotic feeling. While the French obviously hated their own nation, he and his loyal compatriots were politically motivated by "that love of his country which every true-born Englishman sucks in with his mother's milk."³²

In another antirevolutionary pamphlet, this one authored by a "Member of Parliament, and of His Majesty's Privy Council," Tom Paine's efforts to reform the British constitution are characterized in similar terms. His attack on Britain's unwritten charter—the people's national birthright—was an attempt "to poison a mother's milk."³³ William Godwin and his *Enquiry Concerning Political Justice* are painted with the same brush as Paine and his *Rights of Man*. According to the conservative W.C. Proby, if Godwin's "abstract principle of universal good" and his emphasis on "public utility" were "sucked in by the infant with the mother's milk," Britons could be sure that the milk would produce a prejudiced, unenlightened, and disaffected individual. Children who were "inculcated" with Godwinian principles would form a new generation of unrecognizable Britons who resembled the robotic, unfeeling Spartans of the ancient world.[34]

The politicized breast as a monstrous medium of anarchy, violence, disloyalty, and disaffection proliferated in visual culture. Whether overt or subtle, intentional or unintentional, these images visually marked out woman's biological difference and portrayed her as a political liability. In previous decades, breasts had been portrayed in graphic satire in a fairly uniform representational style, but they became much more particularized in 1790s caricatures. A whole set of bodily characteristics were aligned with political qualities, so that the breast became the bearer of signs about woman's limitations in the public sphere.

In the double image in figure 2.3, two opposing types of women's breasts are heavily endowed with political value. On the left, the withered, milkless breasts of the aristocratic woman signal the decline of the ancient regime. They are desexualized and unproductive; their sag is due to lack of use rather than breast-feeding. The aristocratic breasts represent the type of woman censured by Rousseau: her elevated position takes her from the home, into salons and society, and away from domestic duties. In the same way that the old regime starved her citizens, this woman withholds nourishment and refuses motherhood. Her monstrosity is her sociability—her "publicness"—and this monstrosity registers in her masculinized body, with its angular facial features and firmly set jaw. The partner image is just as damning. The female democrat is also masculinized, but this is indicated by a distinct lack of cleavage. Her flat chest is a linked to her participation, like that of her fellow female republicans, in the male sphere of politics. The female democrat is a political Amazon, for she has voluntarily traded motherhood for politics, sacrificing her maternal "nature" for the hurly-burly of public life. Though political opposites, both women are equal in one crucial respect: they have no proper role in the future of the new republic.

Perhaps the most iconic and skillfully executed image of the politically inscribed body is James Gillray's *Un Petit Soupèr, à la Parisiènne: or, A Family of Sans-Culotts Refreshing, after the Fatigues of the Day* (figure 2.4). Printed on 20 September 1792, while newspapers were relating

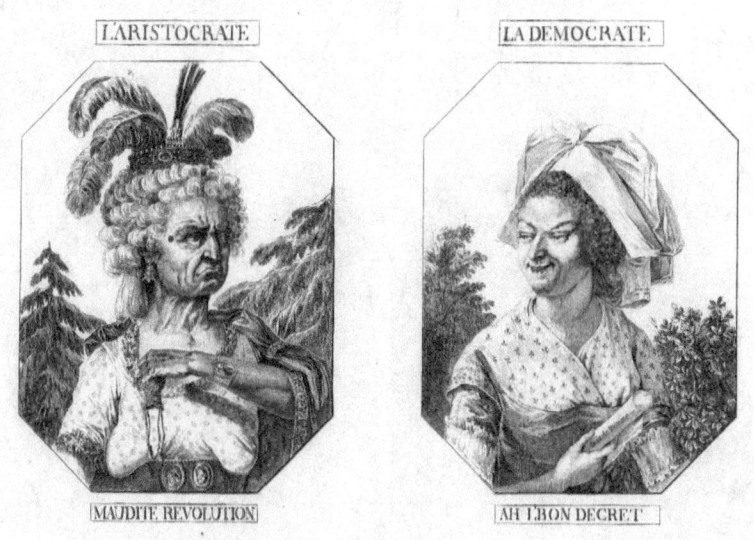

Figure 2.3   Anon., *L'aristocrate; la democrate* (1790 © Trustees of the British Museum, London)

the shocking news of the violence committed by Parisian women in the Paris massacres, Gillray's image portrays a simple peasant family at a cannibal's feast. Diana Donald, Richard Godfrey, Ronald Paulson, and Timothy Morton have all addressed how in this image Gillray transforms the communal table—the symbol of domestic felicity and the emblem of the most routine of activities—into a monstrous communion of shared depravity. But I want to revisit this image to focus on how women's bodies not only record the perils of republicanism but also testify to the problems of political women in general. In a twisted version of maternal protectiveness, Gillray's mother figure delicately "bathes" the sacrificial child, an action that under different circumstances might attest to her dedication. Instead, she facilitates depravity. Maternal care is still evident in this act of domestic labor, but it has become horribly deformed by revolutionary principles. As in Cobbett's description of republican mothers who suckle their children on blood instead of breast milk, the mother figure oversees her fattened little monsters gorging on a bloody meal of entrails. With her less-than-human feet, her masculinized features, and her shapeless body, we are meant to be repulsed.

Women's breasts also figure in this domestic world turned upside

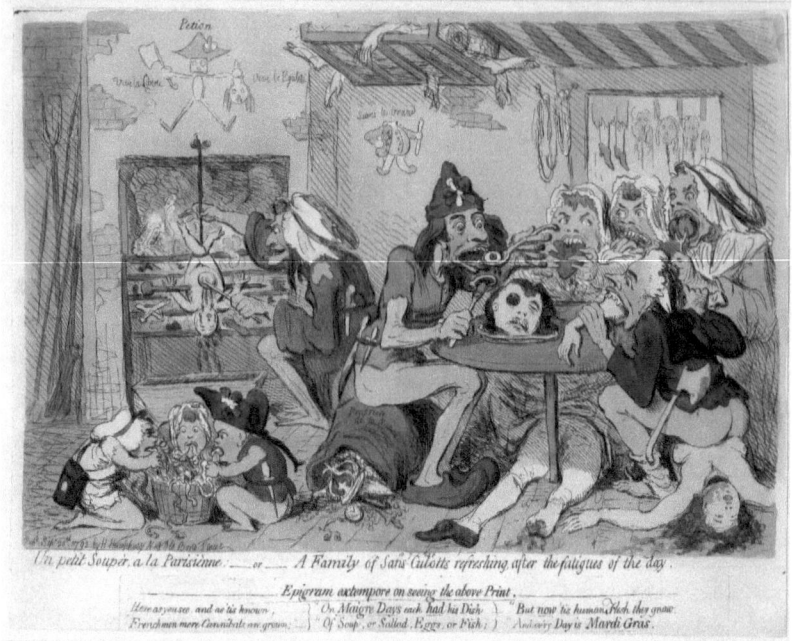

Figure 2.4 James Gillray, *Un petit Soupèr à la Parisiènne: or, A Family of Sans-Culotts Refreshing, after the Fatigues of the Day* (1792 © Trustees of the British Museum, London)

down. The opposite of Rousseau's image of motherhood, Gillray's women make a monstrous mockery of a long history of maternity portraiture, including representations of *Maria lactans* or the *Madonna del latte*, stretching at least as far back as the medieval period. Historically, the full breasts of *Maria lactans* signaled domestic purity, bountiful nourishment, comfort, and regeneration. The full breasts of the youthful dead woman in the lower right corner have become a seat for a cannibalistic sansculotte. As such, these otherwise sexualized breasts signify an inversion of desire and duty, for they are neither a source of sexual allure (the male figure is content only to use her as a seat) nor a means of nourishing the next generation. In the republic, violently asexual men and hungry children have a taste for something rather more ghastly.

In political propaganda in this period, even the fecund, maternal breast becomes threatening when attached to a political woman. The voluminous, fleshy, sagging breasts of clamorous fishwives and slovenly laboring women appear everywhere in the graphic art of Gillray and others. George Cruikshank's *Belle-Alliance, or the Female Reformers of*

Medicalization of the Breast / 67

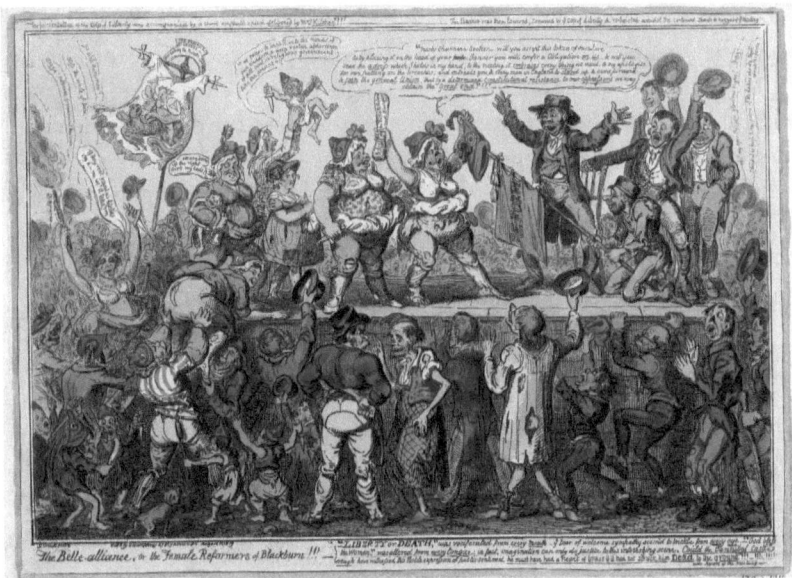

Figure 2.5 George Cruikshank, *The Belle-Alliance, or the Female Reformers of Blackburn!!!—* (1819 © Trustees of the British Museum, London)

Blackburn!!!— (1819) (figure 2.5), a satire on British female reformers, is one such example. The politicized fishwives have breasts that may testify to their (rightly) having suckled their own children and perhaps those of others, but the point is that these biologically productive women are, like animals, determined by the most basic of impulses. They are breeders foremost. As such, they are *naturally* preoccupied with their physical appetites, with having crude, grunting sex (one imagines) and with churning out litters. Their lives are mapped out according to the constant cycle of pregnancy and childbirth, which makes them incapable of the type of careful, reasoned, intellectual deliberation that political participation requires.

The Belle-Alliance was published in 1819, but it makes important references to the French Revolution; in particular, to the idea of the masculinized female democrat. The women wear the *bonnet rouge*, or cap of liberty, and to the left of the stage, slightly above the crowd, a woman resembles the frenzied maenad of the Revolution. With dagger in hand, she proclaims in a vulgar and foreign-sounding accent, "If they von't grant us Libeties vhy d——me ve'll take 'em." On the stage, a little to the right, a bony woman brandishes a child, who, suckled on lawlessness and rebellion, also wields daggers. The bony woman articulates the pledge of her laboring compatriots: "We swear to instill into the minds of our children, a deep rooted abhorrence of all civil or religious government like the present!!" The language plainly expresses the dangers embodied by the politicized working-class woman. She transmits irrationality, disorder, and hostility to an impressionable and captive next generation. A very fat woman follows, with child roughly tucked under her arm, thus freeing her hand for a bottle of liquor. Her speech testifies to her mannish and vulgar ways: "We are some of the right sort my lads!"

Representations of what might be called "overly" maternal breasts, which are obviously fecund or large and slack from nursing, indicate where woman's legitimate role lies. This is brought home most clearly in a reputed encounter between Napoleon and the writer and *salonnière* Germaine de Staël. The memoirist Madame Campan records how, at one particular reception, Napoleon overheard Madame de Staël taking an active part in a discussion of "de haute politique." He allegedly strode up to her and stared straight at her décolleté and inquired loudly "whether she had suckled her own children"—intimating by his tone that it was obvious that she had.[35] By doing so, he publicly announced a disinterest in the estimable political pedigree of a woman who had attended meetings of the Estates-General and the National Assembly, had been an ambassadress, had held salons attended by important diplomats (among them Talleyrand and Narbonne), and had shared ideas with the philosopher Benjamin Constant. This may be anecdotal evidence, but the fact that it was consistently reported substantiates a certain attitude about women's bodies and abilities. The maternal bosom was a biological marker that signaled woman's incapacity for politics. Like other women, Staël was publicly humiliated as an interloper in a male sphere.

In her study of the biological and ideological roles of French women in the Revolution, Lynn Salkin Sbiroli argues that scholars have neglected "the importance of the concept of regeneration, particularly in its relationship to biology and medicine, in defining women's roles." Regeneration, she points out, "came to signify a promised social reform" based on an adherence to biological and moral laws. The central icon of regeneration was the "good mother" who would nurture the reformed nation.[36] Sbiroli refers to France, but British moral reformers advocated a similar vision of regeneration. They rolled maternity, morality, loyalty, and domesticity into an iconic image of the good mother. This mother was both a buttress against revolution and the inaugurator of a program of national moral renewal, which begins in the home. In the same way that French and

British propagandists produced Marie Antoinette as the symbol of the degenerate body of the political woman, they also produced her opposite. Conservative biographers turned loyal French wives and mothers who had lived through the Revolution into emblems of regeneration and propriety for English-speaking readers. These women, or at least the print version of these women, were used to align British women's bodies with the virtues of hearth and home. Memoirs, eyewitness accounts, and biographical texts memorialized women who had demonstrated markedly feminine, domestic qualities in the face of revolutionary excess, namely by heroically refusing to participate in politics and choosing instead to act as antidotes to the madness and violence of the Terror. They were celebrated for retrenching themselves in the home and providing maternal protection for their children and emotional support for their beleaguered husbands.

A key text in this moral regeneration campaign was the English translation of Louis Du Broca's popular *Interesting Anecdotes of the Heroic Conduct of Women previous to, and during the French Revolution* (1804). A clear theme runs through this much reprinted little book: although there were very few examples of politically informed, knowledgeable, or influential women in revolutionary France, those women were both an anomaly and a problem. Since women's involvement threatened peace, productivity, and general happiness in the home, it also seriously disrupted the smooth functioning of the body politic. But those who refused the call of politics were Broca's moral exemplars, such as the wife of the minister Clavierie. She may have been publicly known for her "talents" (which remain unnamed), but she was celebrated most "for that sweet and modest character which had always kept her aloof from public affairs."[37] Only when her husband was imprisoned and facing death did she involve herself publicly, and that was only to beg for his release.

Broca's interpretation of the life of the politically astute salon hostess and influential member of the Girondist faction, Madame Roland, is even more edifying. From an early age, Roland was shaped by Rousseau's educational writing on proper feminine virtues as well as his philosophical writing on equality and democracy. But Broca ignores the latter set of ideas and highlights the former. According to Broca, when Roland was imprisoned as part of Robespierre's elimination of the Girondists, she may have spoken from her jail cell "with the extent and greatness of mind of a man of the first order of talent," but when she thought of the sufferings of her husband and child, naturally "the susceptibility of her sex gained the ascendance."[38] Roland receives a similar treatment by the anonymous author of the 1797 *Biographical Anecdotes of the Founders of the French Republic*. She is a woman whose great fortitude in the face of death only faltered at the moment her husband and daughter "came across her mind."[39]

For both authors, the very fact that Roland was such an anomaly provided evidence that by nature women were not intended for politics. As is typical, Roland's public role is explained in terms of morality: it is not that she is herself politically astute but that her quietly exemplary life provides a gentle example to political men, reminding them of their moral failings. In an attempt to emphasize her uprightness and to urge male politicians to bolster their civic virtues, the author of the *Biographical Anecdotes* praises Roland's humble resilience but suggests that more was expected from male politicians. "While the only woman" among the Girondist faction "was more than man, the men, generally speaking, were less than women!"[40] The exclamation mark ending this statement is a telling punctum: as admirable as Roland had been, she was most remarkable simply for her uniqueness, her exceptional status. This simple comment reveals another powerful current of political propaganda. The charge that men "were less than women" intimates that female ability was inherently "less than"; thus, less was expected of them. As such, their presence in the political sphere necessarily disrupted the manly performance of public duty.

AMAZONS AND SODOMITES

In the atmosphere of rapid social and political change that characterized the 1790s, the fear that women would become like men and men like women engendered the trope of the Amazon. In political writing in this decade, actively political women were portrayed as following in the tradition of that ancient all-female society of infanticidal warriors who reputedly cut or burned off one breast to enhance their archery skills. If the useless breasts of aristocrats, the flat breasts of republicans, and the pendulous breasts of fishwives were emblems of political incompetence, then the single breast of the republican Amazon signaled a particularly acute political danger. The hermaphrodite and the nymphomaniac were troubling enough in a world that increasingly looked to nature as the foundation upon which to build an ordered, transparent society; the female Amazon was all the more disquieting. In an era in which medicine and its male practitioners were obtaining ever greater sway over the female body, the Amazon rebelled dangerously against such management. She reversed this transfer of authority. If nature was the touchstone for the medicomoral enterprise of this period, then the Amazon refused to be determined by nature. This was a woman who ferociously defied nature by chopping off the part of her body that most characterized femininity and signaled her biological destiny. She refused to be subservient to male authority and freely (and violently) altered her own body. The Amazon turned biological incommensurability on its head: if her female organs marked her as politically inadequate, then she would remove that organ.

Reactionary propagandists employed the figure of the single-breasted mythical Amazon to capture how unnatural, violent, and perverse politicized women were. In the new world of revolutionary France, women shed what were otherwise thought to be inherent female qualities to take on masculine characteristics. In Henry James Pye's anti-Jacobin novel *The Democrat* (1795), republican women were savage, physically hideous beings who had no interest in having men as husbands, fathers, and brothers but rather saw them as fellow soldiers. One of Pye's characters, a "classic amazon," followed in the footsteps of the mythical Artemis, who joined men in battle and "behaved with proper spirit" as she sunk the ships of her enemies.[41] An even more acerbic characterization appeared as an "eyewitness" account of a French all-female club in a 1792 issue of the British magazine *Bon Ton*. In "The Amazons, a Parisian Society," a British journalist described the goings-on of a monstrous, sexually aggressive, and weapon-carrying club of republican Amazons. These brazen women, who were more than willing to "give up their persons to the indiscriminate enjoyment of every man who wishes for the possession of them, did not desire to cleave to a husband, to find domestic security and to nurture children."[42]

Crucially, journalists tarred specific female political figures with this characterization. Isaac D'Israeli's 1805 satirical novel *Flim Flams!* is an attack on the political radicalism and unconventional personal relationship of William Godwin and Mary Wollstonecraft. D'Israeli's Wollstonecraft is a female philosopher who revolted against her womanly softness and gave free reign to her irrational impulses. She had banished natural female qualities, including "sympathy and daylight," from "the dark room of the Amazon!"[43] The fictional Wollstonecraft compromises her moral and philosophical principles when she falls head over heels for a smooth-talking and distinctly unsuitable young artist who wants to paint her nude. Through this representation of Wollstonecraft, D'Israeli challenges Godwin's arguments about reason and passion. In his *Political Justice* (1793), Godwin contends that the body's unruly passions and unreasonable desires could become contained and overruled by a rational mind, if humans were properly free to exercise their rational minds. The Amazonian Wollstonecraft is a reminder that the exercise of reason is the purview of enlightened men, not women.

Politicized women emasculated men, as illustrated by Wollstonecraft's shamelessly embarrassing flirtation, carried on right under Godwin's nose and in his own house. The sexual excessiveness of Amazonian women and the acuteness of their violent urges were matched by the weakness and inefficacy of feminized male republicans. Woman had the ability to render man "more womanish than she," Rousseau warned; particularly a woman with political ambitions. But why would women want to emasculate men? The answer, according to Rousseau, is that when women discovered their bodily and mental incapacities, they were sorely disappointed. When they realized they were "unable to make themselves into men," they turned their resentment into making men "into women."[44] This theme underpins the satirical hyperbole and bloody detail of the *Bon Ton* article referred to above. In "The Amazons, a Parisian Society," the anonymous author describes how the Amazonian club of "maids, wives, widows, wantons, and vestals" solemnly promised "to exterminate by every possible means, all men that favour royalty, aristocracy, and inequality." As part of their inauguration ceremony, new society members performed what is described as a horrifying "act of emasculation" involving the removal of the sexual organs of their male enemies. The women's intention, it is explained, was to "separate and destroy" those "parts of the human body" necessary for "the perpetuity of the species."[45] This was certainly *one* way that scheming women might render men scepterless.

These satirical anecdotes betray a deep anxiety about political and cultural change, which seemed as much a violation of nature as the Amazon herself. Feminist Marilyn Yalom considers why the Amazonian body became such a hideous signifier of a reversion of order: Her "missing breast creates a terrifying asymmetry," Yalom writes. "One breast is retained to nurture female offspring, the other is removed so as to facilitate violence against men."[46] In a world in which time-honored structures and institutions were being torn down, this was one more violation of established boundaries. British commentators insisted that by taking on masculine roles, Amazonian political women forced men to take up female roles. In fact, woman's newfound aggressiveness inversely rendered men the sexually subservient partners of other men. In French pamphlets, Louis XVI was portrayed as unmanned by a sexually aggressive wife; he had trouble producing heirs; he was politically impotent; and he desired men. In *The Royal Dildo* he is unable to satisfy a wife who is "so often starved" of sexual attention (and children) because he prefers to ejaculate "into secret places that make Nature blush."[47] French republican satirists linked acts of sodomy with a lack of productivity and with sexual and political impotence. In the old regime, the bodies, morals, and politics of men were corrupted, in part because they had been rendered effeminate by women who had asserted themselves in public life. The message was that men who sought to reform a damaged nation and to defend the new republic had to ensure that Amazonian women were excluded from political participation.

The male counterpart to the Amazon was the sodomite. Like other appropriable icons in this period—the breast-feeding mother, the emblematic Marianne, the cannibal, the Amazon—the sodomite was also adopted and adapted by almost every political faction. One particularly notorious tract, *Les enfans de Sodome à l'Assemblée Nationale* (1790), targeted members of the transitional government body (June–July 1789) that existed between the fall of the old Estates-General and the establishment of the National Constituent Assembly. This tract satirizes the perceived ineffectualness of a political group that was not fully of the new regime; these men were more interested in negotiating with the king than with fully instituting democracy in a manly way. Their willingness to compromise was equated with feminine subservience and homosexuality. The tract lists the clerical and aristocratic deputies of the National Assembly who allegedly participated in homosexual acts and presents visually graphic scenes of sodomy between deputies. Beneath one tableaux, for instance, the caption reads, "This masculine trio, with its ingenious tastes, recalls for you the readers the games of true buggers." The "wrongs" done to each other mirrored "the wrongs done . . . to France." These "defective and effeminate" men formed a stark contrast against the "healthy" republican, who could boast a "male and vigorous constitution."[48]

This hybrid medicopolitical vocabulary creates links and oppositions: a healthy physical body is linked to conventional, productive heterosexuality *and* to the dedicated republicanism of the bourgeois male. In contrast, a weak and pathological body is associated both with nonprocreative sex (now demarcated as abnormal) and with the collaborative spirit of old regime peers. Sodomites violate what art historian Ewa Lajer-Burcharth describes as "the body as the Republic wanted it . . . a signifier of social unity and coherence: men as brothers united by fraternal embrace; women as noble mothers caring for their children." I would count the sodomite, along with bloody mothers and sadistic Amazons, among the bodies the republic not only feared but had to excise, at least in part because it was, to use Lajer-Burcharth's phrase, "a metaphor of social, political and psychic fragmentation."[49] The sodomite was a constant reminder of how easily orderliness could tip into disorder and seemingly stable arrangements collapse into disarray.

Similar fears underwrite British eyewitness accounts of the disturbing incidents of gender-role reversals in the upside-down world of the French republic. The eponymous memoirist of the *Narrative of the Incarceration of Count O'Neil, and the Massacre of His Family in France* (1814) informed his readers that "a strange metamorphosis" had taken place in France, so that "men have become furious as tygers, and women as wolves."[50] Indeed, the French revolutionaries had so "entirely changed the national physiognomy" that France and its people were no longer recognizable.[51] Not only were women acting as ferociously as men, but French men were violently emasculated at the hands of other men. Count O'Neil recalls how, when he was imprisoned at Pontivy, he watched his cellmate, a merchant shipman, "stripped naked" by French guards allegedly looking for concealed coins. The brutality of the guards knew no bounds and they "were even guilty of indecencies toward him, which, out of a regard to the beauteous part of the creation," O'Neil must "decline to name."[52] Avoiding the patina of sexual perversion with his silent-but-not-silent description, O'Neil explains how all over France men had descended so far into debauchery that they had adopted the practice of raping men as if they were women. He recalls overhearing an old man who, upon witnessing the destruction of his village, remarked that "God knows the times are changed; Frenchmen are not Frenchmen—but we are French women."[53] This is a fear-inducing sentence. Sodomy acts as both sexual act and as a metaphor that captures a whole other category of fears: about the rapidity with which profound social and political change can happen and about the British Isles being invaded and penetrated by the French. In addition, the sodomite is a sign of the shakiness of categories more generally. He threatens, for instance, national and European identities that have built up around the culture of chivalry and masculine civic virtue (of the martial Roman type, not of the Spartan or Athenic, which were infused with same-sex eros).

Such propaganda played on existing homophobic fears. The British government exploited these fears and, according to historian Anna Clark, were responsible for increasing the number of public executions for sodomy in order "to distract the people from radical unrest."[54] These deeply threatening cultural images must be read, not only in light of legal clampdowns, but with reference to medical strictures against sodomy. According to Clark, the 1790s heralded a more focused political and legal repression of sodomy than in earlier decades (although there were trials against sodomites and "molly" subculture throughout the eighteenth century).[55] In the medical world, a similar campaign had been underway for some time, which linked men who rejected conventional codes of masculine behavior and sexuality with the spread of disease. The surgeon Jonathan Wathen's 1763 translation of Herman Boerhaave's *Lectures on the Lues Venerea* classed buggery as one of the most "shameful diseases" that destroyed the body and demeaned the human character: when "indulged to a more than brutal excess" (as it was in places like Africa), it led to a particularly virulent form of pox [syphilis]."[56] The disruption of one boundary led to the destruction of other boundaries. To violate gendered sexual roles was to violate moral boundaries, national boundaries (disease spread across borders from Africa to the British Isles), and the boundary between health and disease.

In his 1772 *Treatise on the Venereal Disease*, the surgeon Nikolai Detlef Falck likewise railed against sodomy, which introduced contagion to the nation, destroyed bodies, ruined lives, shattered families, and indicated social regression. In an era in which civic virtue was a prerequisite of citizenship, and virtuous public life became coextensive with political legitimacy, sodomy was a sign of a nation heading toward irretrievable political ruin. Falck categorized sodomy, onanism, and the use of prophylactics—a "disgustful and unnatural practice"—as part of a group of activities that were about secrecy, selfishness, and concealment.[57] Practicing birth control is here ranked with other sexual offences because, like them, it is a cultural practice that contravenes nature's grand plan. Unnatural acts had no place in a society deeply occupied with reforming itself. Secrecy had to be expunged from a nation on its way to establishing political and legal transparency. Furtive and perverse acts also had no place in a healthy society eager to distinguish the normal from the pathological. The ongoing battle against disease, deformity, and dysfunction required openness and vigilance.

Throughout the revolutionary and Napoleonic wars, loyalists continued to use the images of Amazonian Frenchwomen and sodomitical Frenchmen to incite a deep distrust of the republican cause and its relation to gendered bodies and their concomitant roles. The fear was that the overturning of gendered sexual boundaries would penetrate to the very center of Britishness and, in particular, would compromise a British identity closely connected to domestic ideals. One 1803 broadsheet portrays invading French soldiers attacking a family of English cottagers on home soil. Pointedly, the foreign soldiers declare that "they have called us Sodomites, and they shall not call us so for nothing; as their handsome Footmen, and Farmers, and their lusty young labourers will find."[58] This is a monstrous vision of Britain's future. Could any Briton possibly adopt any of the so-called principles of these republican sodomites? To borrow the words of William Cobbett, "Can any man with the common feelings of humanity about his heart, contemplate such scenes of horror, without execrating the revolution that gave rise to them?"[59]

The variety of texts addressed here—Rousseau's educational writing on breast-feeding, medical treatises on female reproductive issues, the caricatures of Georgiana the Duchess of Devonshire, the visual representations of aristocratic and republican female bodies, satires on Amazonian revolutionary women, memoirs about encounters with sodomitical Frenchmen—is obviously quite wide. But what these diverse texts share is their emphasis on gendered biological difference and their promotion of distinct roles based upon such alleged bodily difference. These emphases were promoted by an increasingly professionalized, male-dominated medical establishment as much as by a growing body of alarmed moralists and reactionary political philosophers. As we have seen, the intensified attention on women's breasts was part of a redefining of women's roles as maternal and domestic, in the same way that the uterus was seen as the source of women's irrationality and tendency to hysteria. Biological difference, whether real or perceived, historically has been used to define women as unsuited to politics and philosophy.

One of the political ends—both intentionally and unintentionally—of the biology of incommensurability is the exclusion of women from politics. In eighteenth-century France and Britain, medical arguments about woman's so-called maternal "nature" and her inherently unstable sexual "nature" were used to make ideological arguments about her inability to withstand the demands of public life. We have seen how medical treatises articulated biological difference; how political pornography revealed woman's sexual deviance in both visual and verbal terms; how Rousseau's philosophy assigned women a role in the body politic as the nation's breast-feeders; how caricatures became visual indicators of women's political unsuitability. In addition, we will see in the following chapters how beliefs about biological incommensurability were used to herald a new model of masculinity, which had significant political repercussions. For men to be legitimate political actors, they needed to demonstrate a code of civic virtue that was grounded in a morally upright private life. Men in this era were pressured to demonstrate, perhaps more than any other quality, restraint. The same political and medical pamphleteers who targeted women also urged men to demonstrate a manly openness about their habits and activities, appropriate to a new age of transparency. In opposition to the effeminate French male "other," the English man did not look to impress women in society so much as to carefully protect and superintend his family while fulfilling his public duties.[60]

As a final note, it is worth observing how the crossover between medicine and politics—and the resulting culture of incommensurability—has continued to affect women politically. Pierre Saint-Amand has drawn startling connections between the negative representations of Marie Antoinette and the hate-filled discourse used against Hillary Clinton two hundred years later, during the 1992 American presidential election. Saint-Amand argues convincingly that Clinton was a victim of what he calls "Marie Antoinette Syndrome," that is, the press appropriated her body and invested it with political meaning. Like the French queen, Clinton's body was transformed from an object of adoration (the press reported what she wore, who did her hair, and what lipstick shade she wore) to one of abhorrence. She became a figure of sexualized female aggression; a woman who disrupted the homosocial political status quo by unduly influencing her husband in state affairs.

Since the 1992 election, Clinton's body has become even more of a focus in print, television, and on the Web. In 2006 the sculptor Daniel Edwards produced what he terms a "presidential bust of Hillary Clinton" (figure 2.6). In an interview with the newspaper *USA Today*, he explains that he chose to present her "in a low cut gown" with "her cleavage . . . on display" as a way of "prominently portraying sexual power which some people still consider too threatening."[61] So, in an image that he characterizes as subversive and empowering, the political woman *still* becomes defined through her body, her sexuality, and specifically her breasts. In this image and in other images, Clinton's body is anatomized; her breasts, like other parts of her body, signal her unsuitability for politics. The Web is full of images in which her body appears in masculine guises: in one doctored photograph, which can be found on a number of political blog sites, she is captured urinating standing up, in front of a White House urinal. There are a plethora of captions to accompany such images, such as "Hillary Clinton is the man for the job."

These types of representations illustrate how political women—past and present—are subject to long-standing fears about their biology

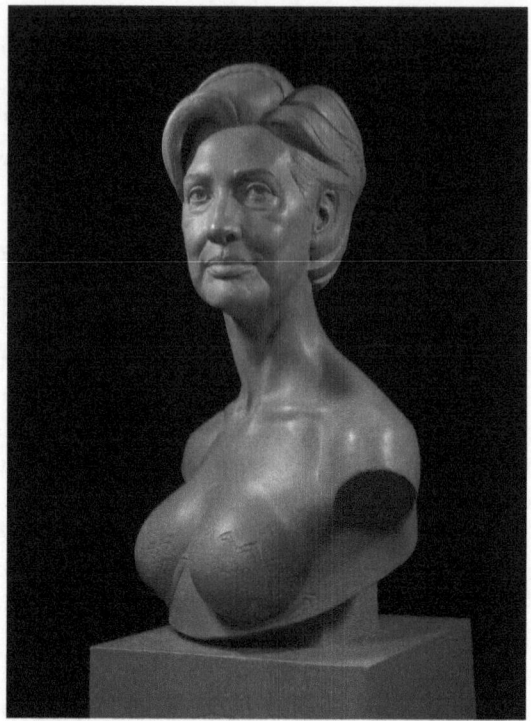

Figure 2.6 Daniel Edwards, *Presidential Bust of Hillary Rodham Clinton* (2006, by kind permission of the artist and Cory Allen Contemporary Art, New York)

and their bodies. Of course, we must protect free debate, yet there is something deeply disturbing about the way the political woman's body becomes a spectacle, "a voyeuristic enterprise for a whole nation."[62] This long trajectory of training the punitive public gaze on political women reveals "how profoundly immoveable mentalities are, how stagnant representations can remain."[63] We still lack awareness about the ways in which these types of images and exchanges are part of a disciplinary process, whereby biology is used to define sexual boundaries, to identify undesirable bodies, and to entrench gender-specific cultural roles. The pathologizing of public women's bodies has enforced our obedience to prevailing cultural norms while legitimizing the exclusion of those women from politics.

PART II

Radical Pathologies

3 Murder to Dissect

*Godwin, Wollstonecraft,
and the Pathology of Indifference*

> He might dissect, anatomize, and give names.
> MARY SHELLEY, *Frankenstein*, 3rd ed. (1831)

Two very similar caricatures circulated in the mid-1790s. One targeted the leader of the opposition, the Whig Charles James Fox, and the other took aim at the Tory prime minister William Pitt. In *A Right Hon. Democrat Dissected* (1793), Fox is displayed as a cadaver, with his body, personal life, and politics open to view (figure 3.1). His body is bisected in more ways than one; in fact, his body reveals something of a split personality. As the labels affixed to his internal organs indicate, British qualities are matched by French ones; his loyalty to the establishment is matched by an advocacy of republican principles; his conservative sentiments are matched by libertarian ideas. His self-interested brain ensures that he is more than willing to trample on morals, duties and good order, while his legs—pillars of "hypocrisy" and "fornication"—reveal a readiness to adopt a whole array of personas and "principles" in order to get what he wants. His stomach is filled with "intemperance" and his guts or intestines with "French principles" (a term synonymous with moral anarchy). Taking center stage, Fox's groin is the rather ironic seat of his "private virtues," indicating that he is motivated by his sexual appetites rather than by firm political principles. Ruled by his genitals and not his heart, Fox presents what was a conventional portrait of the Whigs in the 1790s: a party of drinkers, gamblers, and libertines whose unrestrained licentiousness paralleled their political irresponsibility, disloyalty, and inconsistency.

The second image, *A Dissection* (1797), reveals a flayed William Pitt (figure 3.2). At first glance, the prime minister appears to share some of Fox's characteristics: his heart is motivated by money and his ribs are made of "influence." The characterization of Pitt as a favor-seeking flatterer and an excessive drinker appeared often in 1790s print culture. One

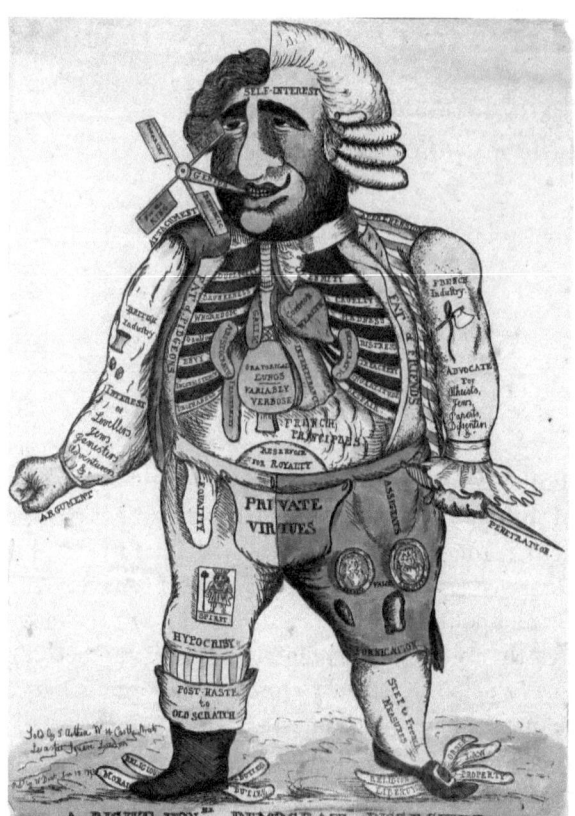

Figure 3.1 William Dent, *A Right Hon. Democrat Dissected* (1793) © Trustees of the British Museum, London)

particularly scurrilous 1795 piece appeared in the *Telegraph* and as a pamphlet titled *Admirable Satire on the Death, Dissection, Funeral Procession, and Epitaph, of Mr. Pitt*. The prime minister's bogus death is caused by a "civil war" in his stomach, between French claret and queen's cake. As he nears death, one minister suggests that his restorative treatment should follow the principle "Perish the stomach; let the constitution live!" After all, "the body politic, when afflicted with revolutionary motions, can be cured . . . only by *starvation*."[1]

But, there are also significant differences in the characterizations of Fox and Pitt. Whereas Fox is flexible, Pitt is a distinctly immoveable character: his knees may have some flexibility but his feet are firm, his

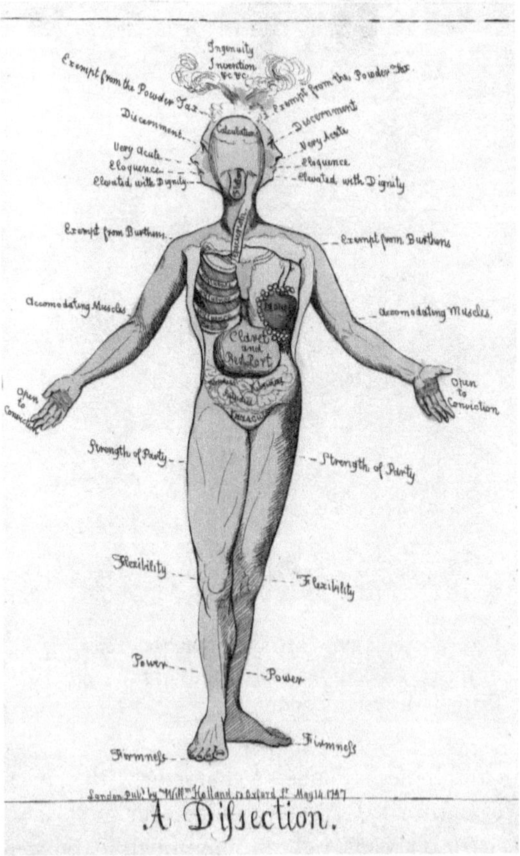

Figure 3.2 Anon., *A Dissection* (1797 © Trustees of the British Museum, London)

thighs strong, and his physiognomy shrewd. The real contrast with Fox, however, lies with the genitals. While Fox's are lustful and well used, Pitt's are labeled "IMMACULATE," in reference to his nickname "Immaculate Boy" (a tag much-loved by the Whig newspapers). His alleged sexual frigidity, his emotional detachment, and his political heartlessness were a constant reference point for papers like the *Morning Post,* which once used the descriptor "as *cold* as Mr. *Pitt*" to capture the severe drop in London's temperature.[2] Whig propagandists linked his political ruthlessness to his bachelor status and to his reputation as a sexually inexperienced loner whose spotless private life was something of a void. In James Gillray's caricature *A Sphere, Projecting against a Plane* (1792), Pitt is cast as the

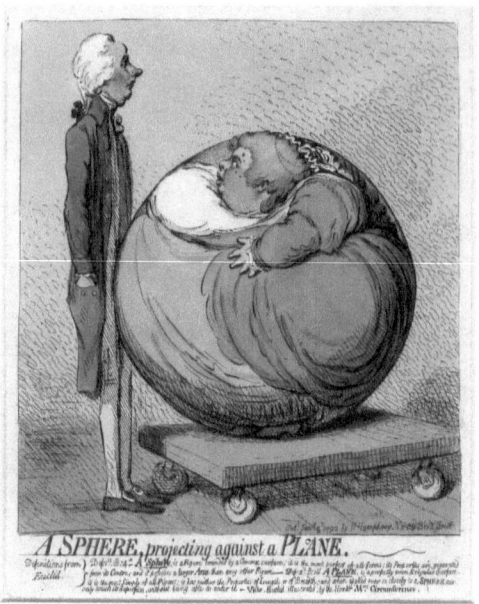

Figure 3.3 James Gillray, *A Sphere, Projecting against a Plane* (1792 © Trustees of the British Museum, London)

extremely thin and lifeless "Plane"—a character with "a perfectly even & regular Surface" (figure 3.3). "When applied ever so closely to a SPHERE," the text of the cartoon reads, he "can only touch its Superfices, without being able to enter it," a fact supported by his distinctly unsatisfied facial expression.

Pitt's inability to express or to consummate sexual desire was also the focus of another especially vulgar satire that appeared in newspapers and as a broadside in 1795. The anonymous satirist asks Pitt why, at thirty-six years of age, he remained "an enemy to the delights of Love," particularly when the possession of a woman's charms had the added bonus of "humaniz[ing] the soul."[3] In similar fashion, a 1794 edition of the *Courier* announced in a mock theater advertisement that "Signor Pittachio" would make "JOHN BULL A JACK ASS," by performing "A SOLO ON THE VIOL D'AMOUR."[4] It went on to describe how Pitt would play with himself for the amusement of the public in a one-man show. He was, after all, only capable of feeling for himself (quite literally). In light of the depth and breadth of late eighteenth-century anxieties over masturbation, this was a particularly damning representation. In another mock playbill, Pitt's

"Prettygirlibus indifferentissimus" and the fact that he had not "engaged any female performers" were incontrovertibly linked to his political cudgeling of the British public.[5] The same asexual character appeared in the *Admirable Satire on the Death, Dissection, Funeral Procession, and Epitaph, of Mr. Pitt.* "Suffice it to say, that the marks of *sexual* distinction," the satirist reported, "were not easily to be discerned" when the body was examined.[6] In defense of their man and in reaction to these types of charges, a discomfited Tory press consistently announced Pitt's impending marriage to Eleanor Eden, the daughter of Lord Auckland—but this was an event that never happened.[7]

According to the opposition press, Pitt's lack of passion was intimately connected to his willingness to sacrifice British citizens on foreign battlefields and, as the 1795 Two Acts had shown, to use the long arm of the law to quell free speech. The spurious account of his "dissection" linked his pathological body parts to his lack of sympathy for fellow Britons. The satirist described how "the appearance of the *heart* was so remarkable" that the anatomists paid special notice to this medical curiosity: "The *pericardium*, or membrane, in which the heart is inclosed, was much distended; but what is most singular is, that the liquid which it contained was frozen into a solid lump. No application of heat could dissolve it; but by pouring a large quantity of wine upon it, and after wards touching it with gold.... The heart was very cold to the touch, and very hard."[8]

As this passage indicates, Pitt's image was represented as part and parcel of his political ideology (as was the case with Fox). Pitt's personal life chimed with the increasingly popular view of the Tories as a rigid, calculating, and cold-hearted party.[9] These two political personas—the immoral hedonist and the frigid bachelor—emerged roughly along political party lines in the first half of the 1790s and were confirmed in the wake of the 1794 Treason Trials. For all their differences, both men illustrated how individualism threatened cooperative ties, familial bonds, and wider communal relations. A contingent of reformist and conservative pamphleteers railed against the "vanity of aspirers to profligate distinction" like Fox, as well as against the selfishness of unfeeling bachelors like Pitt.[10]

The radical utilitarian philosopher William Godwin would seem to have very little in common with either Fox or Pitt. Ironically, however, he was characterized in the press as a sort of amalgam of both. He was at the same time sexually immoral *and* frigid. On the one hand, he advocated a form of free love and rejected marriage, family, and monogamy; on the other, he was a coldly unfeeling and allegedly virginal figure who was only interested in his clinically rational philosophy. The point is that the characterization of these three public figures—as similar or different as they are—places them firmly outside the bounds of then-contemporary definitions of British manliness. The revival of chivalric codes of duty and obligation were an increasingly significant aspect of masculinity in this period. In addition, as Tim Fulford points out, chivalry "became recognisable as a manipulable code which the middle and labouring classes could deploy and redefine for their own ends."[11] Among other things, chivalry was redefined as the open demonstration of private virtue, patriotism, paternalism, and an affectionate marriage that recalled medievalist notions of manorial feudalism and courtly love.

Pitt and Fox were anatomized in the press for their failure to fulfill this emerging model of masculinity, but the case of Godwin was quite different. He was accused of being something of an anatomist himself. His political opponents, alarmed by his single-minded devotion to a philosophy that subscribed to a mechanical law of cause and effect and that posited rationalism and impartiality as the basis of all human action, described him as a scientist. Godwin's materialist values were in direct opposition, they suggested, to masculine, chivalric ideals. More specifically, they alleged that Godwin's political philosophy—which refused rule-bound practices such as contracts, property ownership, and marriage—had induced him to perform a singularly undignified, immoral, and unchivalrous act. He had performed a type of public autopsy of his own wife.

It is well known that when Godwin published his *Memoirs of the Author of "A Vindication of the Rights of Woman"* in January 1798, a mere four months after Mary Wollstonecraft's death as a result of complications in childbirth, he became one of the most reviled figures in the loyalist press. Almost without exception, reviewers of the *Memoirs*, whatever their political persuasion, were shocked at his candid detailing of his wife's pursuit of the married artist Henry Fuseli, her pregnancy (resulting from her affair with the American adventurer Gilbert Imlay), her attempted suicide, and finally, their own sexual relationship and resulting second pregnancy. It is equally well known that the *Memoirs* devastated Wollstonecraft's posthumous reputation as a thinker and writer and seriously damaged the first stirrings of a feminist movement in Britain. True to form, the *Anti-Jacobin Review* led the onslaught against the radical couple. In one of its more venomous responses, a reviewer accused Godwin of holding back biographical truth, for surely the "concubine" Wollstonecraft had even more "amours" than he recorded. Although

"Mary's theory" of female equality seemed a new philosophy, the writer argued that her key precept—"the right of women to indulge their inclinations with every man they like"—was "as old as prostitution." Rather ruthlessly, the magazine then listed "Wollstonecraft" under the heading "Prostitution" in its index for 1799.[12] In the years following the publication of the *Memoirs*, the *Anti-Jacobin* continued its offensive, proclaiming that "no modest woman could reputably associate" herself with a woman who was "A LIBERTINE SYSTEMATICALLY AND ON PRINCIPLE."[13]

Since 1798, scores of readers have blamed Godwin for instigating this attack on his dead wife. They have puzzled over Godwin's frankness—a word he used often in his canon—and have castigated him for his detrimental authorial choices. Rehearsing that debate is not my aim. Instead, I want to focus on an overlooked but important aspect of the public reaction to the *Memoirs*. One of the most effective accusations leveled against Godwin was that he had transgressed the inviolability of human life by performing a public dissection of a loved one for a *scientific cause*. Godwin's decision to share the medical details of the complications around Wollstonecraft's delivery and her subsequent death from puerperal, or childbed, fever provided conservatives with a whole set of biographical-medical facts. These facts where then promptly employed in a successful campaign to brand the couple's politics as imperiling to marriage, hostile to British identity, and threatening to political stability. That this campaign was so successful tells us something significant about the changing relationship between medicine and political culture and about public anxieties surrounding materialism, empiricism, and the value of the human.

PERFORMING AUTOPSIES IN PRINT

Of course, Godwin had come under fire for his philosophy in the years before publication of the *Memoirs*. In the mid-1790s, he had been satirized in the press as a "new philosopher" who in his own work famously described marriage as a fraudulent institution and "the worst of monopolies."[14] Like *Jacobinism* the term *new philosophy* was largely undefined and indefinable; this nebulous label encompassed individualism, antistatism, sexual freedom, and "any transgression against the institutions or manners of the *status* quo."[15] Anti-Godwinian literature took aim at what was perceived to be the fundamentally nihilistic nature of new philosophy, which as Matthew Grenby describes it, "expresses itself simply as the absence of all constraint."[16] One of the most frightening aspects of this abnegation of order was a rejection of marriage—the social cement of society—and along with it, cohabitation and monogamy. In *Political Justice*, Godwin notoriously describes marriage as an institution sanctioned by church, state, and family that, "by despotic and artificial means," legitimized the possession of one human being by another. It was a relationship founded on "the most odious selfishness," which had the effect of multiplying "our vices." Personal judgment, said Godwin, not legal and religious obligation, should dictate when someone begins and exits a relationship. Personal candor about desire would prevent the type of clandestine and deceitful behavior that marital obligation and moral strictures gave rise to.[17]

Alongside the image of Godwin as an amoral nihilist who advocated free love, there emerged a somewhat contradictory picture of him as a politically, philosophically, and personally frigid individual—somewhat reminiscent of Pitt's persona. This particular aspect of Godwin's public self became entrenched after January 1796, when he published *Considerations on Lord Grenville's and Mr. Pitt's Bills* in response to the notorious "Two Acts" of 1795, which included the Seditious Meetings Act and the Treason Act.[18] In this pamphlet, Godwin characterized the meetings of the London Corresponding Society and the political lectures of fellow reformer John Thelwall as "well adapted to ripen men for purposes, more or less similar to those of the Jacobin Society of Paris."[19] In retaliation, Thelwall attacked Godwin in the preface to the second collected volume of his lectures, *The Tribune*.[20] Ironically, Thelwall attacked Godwin using the same grounds on which Pitt had been attacked. Despite Godwin's full social calendar and a renowned love of company and conversation, Thelwall represented the unmarried forty-year-old philosopher as a disaffected loner. According to Thelwall, marriage would have enabled Godwin to formulate more judicious political views. Godwin's pamphlet was "proof," Thelwall argued, of "how great and how dangerous . . . the life of domestic solitude" could be. For Thelwall, conjugal affection inspired fraternity, solidarity, friendship, and kinship; marriage enabled an individual to recognize, to appreciate, and to "inspire that generous sympathy—that *social ardor*, without which a nation is but a populous wilderness."[21] The unmarried life led to selfishness, vanity, and philosophic and political insularity. Thelwall's arguments tapped into cultural suspicion of an emerging individualism that seemed to jeopardize family ties. Bachelorhood was perceived as a manifestation of narcissistic tendencies. Footloose and fancy-free, bachelors were at liberty to pursue individual pleasures, without obligation. By rejecting traditional and permanent relationships, they undermined the resulting network of dependencies and duties that produced a sense of social cohesiveness (a particularly important quality in this politically tumultuous era).

This argument and its vocabulary indicates how closely Godwin's private life was becoming wound around his philosophy; only two years later, this link would be put to use in the service of a moralizing campaign. Thelwall characterized Godwin as an abstract, theoretical thinker, whose habit of taking long, deeply contemplative walks through London was a sign of his disconnection from the hurly-burly of everyday life. This image also occurred in the press in the mid-1790s; for instance, in the spring of 1795, the *Morning Chronicle* reported that the introspective Godwin had been struck down by a man on horseback on Oxford Street and as a result had "received a violent contusion in his face, which was also much cut."[22] Picking up on this lampoon, Thelwall invoked the image of Godwin as a sightless perambulator, a *"philosopher"* whose remoteness rendered him "only a *walking* index of obsolete laws and dead-lettered institutes."[23] Godwin, in this view, is a "singular man" whose "scrupulous avoidance" of popular debate shows how prolonged solitude tends to "deaden the best sympathies of nature, and encourage a selfish and personal vanity, which the recluse philosopher . . . mistakes for principle."[24] Thelwall portrays Godwin as politically ineffective and personally untrustworthy, but even more to the point Godwin's cold Enlightenment rationality and his lofty philosophizing separate him from regular citizens who valiantly struggle along in the fight for equality and individual rights. Thelwall accuses Godwin of attempting to appease the establishment by separating himself—the philosopher—from honest, working radicals. From this point on, the characterization of Godwin as a cold intellectual would beleaguer his political endeavors in ways that he could not have anticipated. The nadir of his reputation came, however, with the 1798 publication of the *Memoirs* of Mary Wollstonecraft. Of course, many things about this confessional work were construed as morally and politically dangerous, but I am most interested in certain alarmed reactions to particular passages in which Godwin gives a seemingly dispassionate account of the medical details surrounding Wollstonecraft's death from childbed fever. It makes sense to begin with a brief synopsis of the pertinent sections here.

Godwin recounts how on Wednesday, 30 August 1798, Wollstonecraft went into labor and a female midwife was called to attend her. All seemed well, so he went off to study in his apartments (he kept a separate residence for that purpose). Things did not proceed as planned, however:

> It was not till after two o'clock on Thursday morning, that I received the alarming intelligence, that the placenta was not yet removed, and that the midwife dared not proceed any further, and gave her opinion for calling in a male practitioner. I accordingly went for Dr. Poignand, physician and man-midwife to the same hospital, who arrived between three and four hours after the birth of the child. He immediately proceeded to the extraction of the placenta, which he brought away in pieces, till he was satisfied that the whole was removed. In that point however it afterwards appeared that he was mistaken.[25]

From here, Godwin recalls how Wollstonecraft suffered fainting fits, lost a fair deal of blood, and experienced great pain. The next morning, she asked for another doctor, George Fordyce, to attend her; after his examination on Thursday afternoon, Dr. Fordyce pronounced (incorrectly) that the patient was in recovery. He was overheard telling "a mixed company" that Wollstonecraft's case supported his belief that pregnant women should employ females as midwives.[26] Since "appearances were more favourable" on Friday morning, Godwin left to attend business in "different parts of the town."[27] On Sunday, 3 September, Godwin made several calls, only to return in the evening to find Wollstonecraft in an alarmingly deteriorated state. He expresses regret at leaving her and vows to stay with the patient who, it is now clear, is in serious trouble. She suffers a second shivering fit:

> Every muscle of the body trembled, the teeth chattered, and the bed shook under her. This continued probably for five minutes. She told me, after it was over, that she had been a struggle between life and death, and that she had been more than once, in the course of it, at the point of expiring. I now apprehend these to have been the symptoms of a decided mortification, occasioned by the part of the placenta that remained in the womb. At the time however I was far from considering it in that light. When I went for Dr. Poignand, between two and three o'clock on the morning of Thursday, despair was in my heart. The fact of the adhesion of the placenta was stated to me; and, ignorant as I was of obstetrical science,—I felt as if the death of Mary was in a manner decided.[28]

Godwin then gives specific details about the doctors involved and their various treatments. Readers are told how, by the following Monday, there was fear that her disease would spread, and so "Dr. Fordyce forbad the child's having the breast, and we therefore procured puppies to draw off the milk."[29] The obstetrician Dr. Clark also attended her, along with the surgeon Mr. Carlisle, who recommended the wine diet. Finally, Wollstonecraft died on the morning of 10 September.

The initial reaction to and subsequent legacy of this relatively brief section of the *Memoirs* is revealing. To scores of observers, nothing illustrated Godwin's inhumanity, unnatural character, and political unsuitability more than his systematic and public dissection of the medical circumstances surrounding Wollstonecraft's death. Contemporary reviewers were appalled at the cold precision with which he relayed such graphic detail, as if he were a man of science rather than a loving husband. The *European Magazine* expressed its horror that Godwin gave the public entry into "the last fatal scene of her life" and provided his audience with "a very minute, and in some particulars a disgusting, narrative" of her labor, illness, and death.[30] He had authored his own wife's disgrace and indecently violated her privacy, but even more than that he had willingly performed a public autopsy of her body in order to make a political and philosophical statement. In doing so, Godwin inadvertently demonstrated that his socially maladaptive behavior was directly related to his political philosophy.

Godwin's opponents consistently characterized his brand of utilitarianism as more of a *scientific* cause than a political one. In his 1801 anti-Jacobin novel, *The Infernal Quixote*, Charles Lucas pronounced the *Memoirs* a perversely "scientific work," while the *British Critic* labeled it "a medical statement."[31] These descriptions indicate how and why Godwin's biographical ventures were seen as so problematic: his candor, impartial tone, and scrutinizing methods were not a departure for him; but now his philosophical impartiality merged with medical impartiality. Indeed, his 1790s body of work demonstrates a penchant for anatomizing the naturalized beliefs of his fellow Britons and for dismantling the ideological foundations of established cultural institutions. He plumbs the deepest psychological recesses of his characters in his 1794 novel *Caleb Williams*, as befits his own writing practice. Godwin describes how his imagination worked most effectively when he was analyzing "the private and internal operations of the mind" and when he applied his "metaphysical dissecting knife in tracing and laying bare the involutions of motive, and recording the gradually accumulating impulses."[32] A number of scholars observe how this same methodological predilection underwrites the *Memoirs*. Tilottama Rajan, for instance, notes how Godwin's decision to publish Wollstonecraft's correspondence together with her biography established "a contiguity between corpus and corpse."[33] Mitzi Myers sees the *Memoirs* as an extension of Godwin's interest in "psychological dissection," a manifestation of his desire "to get inside his subject's skin, to understand how and why she developed as she did."[34]

Even more germane is Angela Monsam's characterization of the *Memoirs* as an "autopsical biography," a hybrid genre that prefigures Victorian "scientific autobiography."[35] This is in many ways an apt and useful description; moreover, her claim that "Godwin's clinical approach . . . is intentional" is evidently right, as is her conjecture that Godwin's interest in science would lead him to "a more in-depth understanding of anatomy as time progressed."[36] Yet at least part of Monsam's reading is overly speculative and too focused on pinpointing intentionality. Many of her observations rest on a theory that the *Memoirs* was *intentionally* "modelled after contemporary medical writings, particularly dissection reports," even though she admits to a lack of material evidence.[37] Moreover, determining whether Godwin was well read in the medical treatises of the time or whether he intentionally replicated the methodologies of contemporary anatomists is a peripheral issue here. The more significant point is that his political opponents interpreted his method as if he *had* copied the anatomists; moreover, the way that denunciations of Godwin mirror contemporary public criticisms of surgeons and anatomists is much more remarkable. How the public perceived Godwin's project is significant to our understanding of the development of political culture and its relationship to medicine. Anxieties over issues surrounding dissection and scientific materialism, combined with the reigning atmosphere of political urgency in the late 1790s, make sense of *why* Godwin's views seemed so dangerous; it helps us understand *how* Wollstonecraft's posthumous reputation could become so damaged by his revelations about her illness and death.

THE SCHOOL OF FLESH AND BLOOD

This section recontextualizes the *Memoirs* by placing the work within the wider context of eighteenth- and nineteenth-century developments and debates in the rapidly changing field of anatomy. At least two points about visual representation are worth considering here. The first concerns transparency in this era: anatomists, physiologists, and surgeons made the body newly visible through a range of materials. Dissections in anatomical theaters, wax models, engravings, and huge collections like that amassed by the Hunter brothers were accessible not only to professionals but increasingly to laypeople. Scholars have shown how the

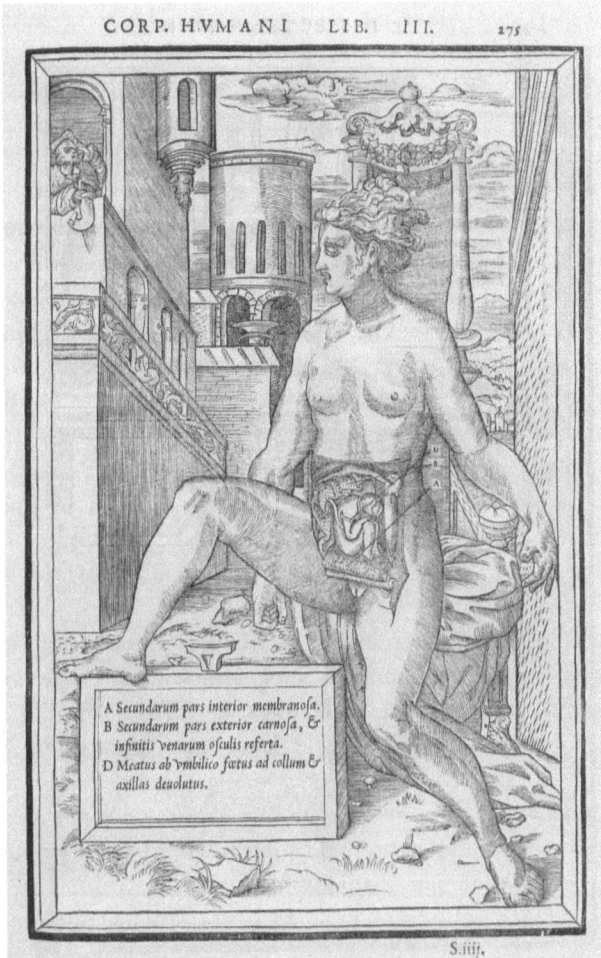

Figure 3.4 Pregnant woman with fetus showing, from Charles Estienne, *De dissectione partium corporis humani libri tres* (1545, by kind permission of the Wellcome Library, London)

growing importance of the science of anatomy, as well as increased public access to anatomical specimens, rendered "the body's previously invisible depths now seemingly transparent to a general public."[38] The second and related point concerns a shift in the art and science of anatomical representations of the female body in this era.

In Renaissance anatomical texts, such as Charles Estienne's 1545 *De dissectione partium corporis humani libri tres* (figure 3.4), reproductive imagery is part of a whole pictorial narrative. The pregnant female is not portrayed in the manner we have since become used to: her body is neither objectively nor disinterestedly presented. The emphasis on clinical distance that will come to characterize Enlightenment and post-Enlightenment medicine is absent. In this image, the biblical David spies on his lover Bathsheba, who not only is very much alive despite being flayed but rather seductively displays her sexual organs and developing fetus to the spying David. Groomed, posed, and surrounded by the stuff of life—urban buildings and the profusion of nature—she is both an aesthetic object and part of an organic environment. It should be said that this type of representation was partly determined by Renaissance printing technology. Woodcuts were reused in often completely unrelated publications. In this case, Estienne reworked a woodcut originally used in a semipornographic book of sexed-up biblical love lives. He simply opened up Bathsheba's midsection. Notwithstanding the ins and outs of early-modern print technology, this image indicates a mode of physiological representation that is symptomatic of an organic, holistic view of the body.

There are unexpected similarities between Estienne's image and some of the highly stylized anatomical images produced in the eighteenth century, such as Jacques Fabien Gautier d'Agoty's 1773 *Anatomie des parties de la generation de l'homme et de la femme* (figure 3.5). Although more than two hundred years separates these aesthetically dissimilar images—one a woodcut engraving and the other a colored mezzotint—they both present a stylized female subject. As in the previous image, d'Agoty's pregnant woman is anatomized, but she also has an identity. Her composed face is differentiated; she gazes serenely out at us, as any other portrait sitter. Her body may be flayed at the abdomen, but she is otherwise intact, groomed, and beautifully posed. She is part of a visual narrative that merges the aesthetic with the scientific, imagination with reality, openness with opacity, and life with death. As for the work itself, it is "painterly," calling attention to its own status as art.

Yet the differences could not be more pronounced between this 1773 image and the engravings by the Dutch medical illustrator Jan van Rymsdyk, which appear in William Hunter's 1774 *The Anatomy of the Human Gravid Uterus Exhibited in Figures*. Figures 3.6 and 3.7 depict an altogether different form of anatomical image. In the trajectory of anatomical representations, this was part of a new way of looking and representing, which transformed the body into an almost purely scientific object. Art historian Martin Kemp labels Hunter as the most

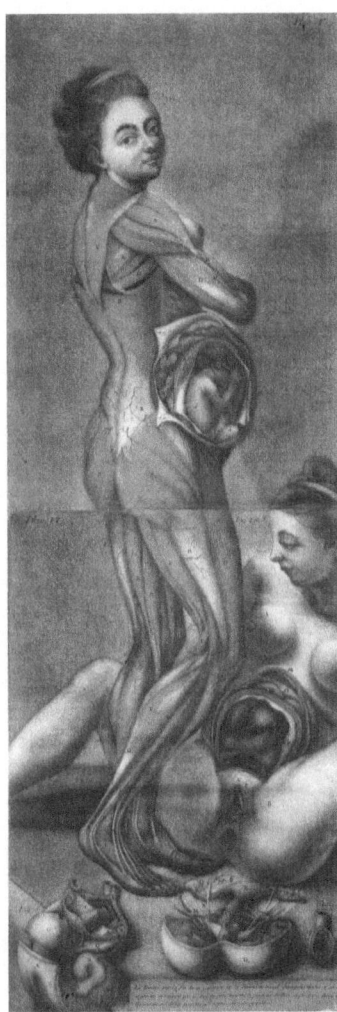

Figure 3.5 Standing and seated pregnant women, from Jacques Fabien Gautier d'Agoty, *Anatomie des parties de la generation de l'homme et de la femme* (1773, by kind permission of the Wellcome Library, London)

prominent among the "extreme advocates of the 'flesh-and-blood' school of illustration" but also points out that Hunter's desire for objectivity and Rymsdyk's unflinching style were part of a larger movement.[39] The anatomical images of the gravid, or pregnant, uterus were symptomatic of a late eighteenth-century "belief in the need for illustrations to portray a direct, uncompromising and (as far as possible) unmediated image of a form as it actually could be seen in all its reality."[40] This particular form of anatomical realism was part of a still wider shift toward aesthetic realism, which as Kemp explains, "signaled the intellectual commitment of

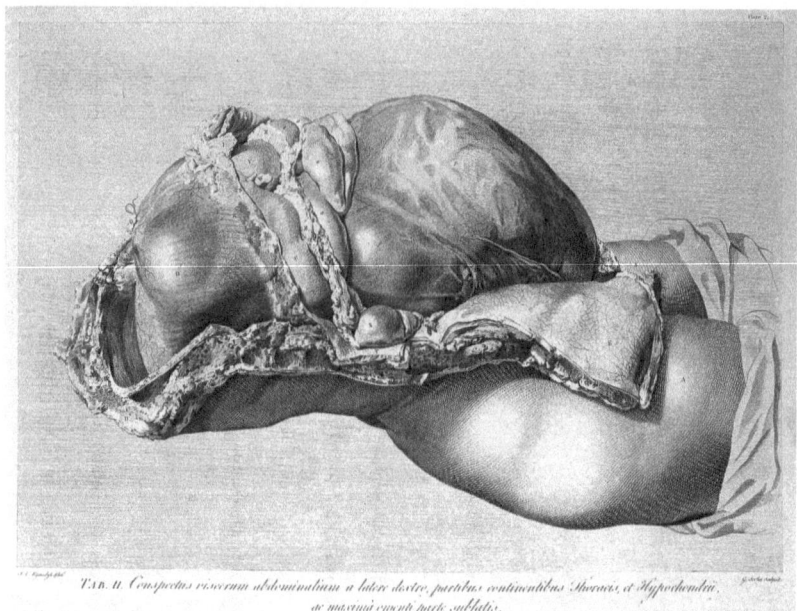

Figure 3.6   Abdominal viscera, from William Hunter, *The Anatomy of the Human Gravid Uterus Exhibited in Figures* (1774, by kind permission of the Wellcome Library, London)

the anatomist to an uncompromising empiricism which shows everything 'exactly as it is.'"[41] Indeed, these images, which express an Enlightenment faith in the eyes as the most accurate sense organ, exhibit an unwavering commitment to reality and truth over the fanciful or merely imaginative. In this canonical treatise on obstetrics, women's bodies are depicted objectively, impersonally, and accurately; in fact, it is hard to exaggerate how carefully each anatomical feature is captured in its raw reality.

Jan van Rymsdyk recorded everything as he observed it, as precisely and as realistically as the engraver's art would allow. (In one of his images, the window in the dissecting room where the artist worked is reflected in the chorion, or outermost membrane, that covers the fetus.)[42] Tellingly, Rymsdyk describes the methodological differences between his illustrations and that of painters. While they work at a "medium distance" from their subject and use "art" to represent the "effects" of nature, he works much closer, bringing the subject "so near the Eye" so as to reveal "every minute Part" of real nature.[43] This statement has unexpected connections to Edmund Burke's warning, sounded only the year before, about the

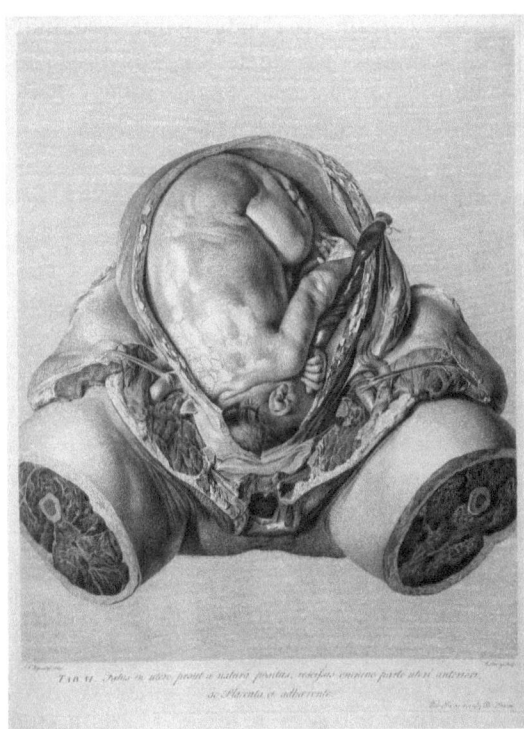

Figure 3.7 "The child in the womb, in its natural situation," from William Hunter, *The Anatomy of the Human Gravid Uterus Exhibited in Figures* (1774, by kind permission of the Wellcome Library, London)

effects of tearing away the "drapery of life" (a phrase I will return to on a few more occasions). On the one hand, in both medicine and politics there was a move to strip away ornament and artifice in order to expose reality, to see things as they really were. On the other hand, there were those who, like Burke, were deeply anxious about losing the adorning manners, customs, and tastes that beautified and gentrified human existence.

The organization of Hunter's anatomical atlas is also important. Turning each page of this enormous volume, the viewer follows the steps of dissection: each successive plate portrays another layer of skin and flesh excised from an increasingly depersonalized body. As skin and tissue fall away, the human subject loses its identity and becomes less recognizable *as* human. Extraneous parts—skin, legs, hair—are literally hacked off to get to the body's center. Our eyes are made to ignore the external body and to focus on the interior instead. Hunter and Rymsdyk isolate their anatomical subject from "the stuff of life" that are part of d'Agoty's Renaissance image and they tear away the painterly drapery that beautifies that earlier anatomical illustration. They isolate the womb from the rest of the body, thereby erasing the body's expressive, individualized exteriority, which is so much a part of d'Agoty's picture. This invites the viewer to penetrate progressively deeper into human flesh, closer and closer to the fetus, the site of geniture that had previously been unviewable.

Paul Youngquist has noted that "the processes of reproduction become clearer and clearer" in Hunter's volume; until, in the penultimate image, it is as if "the female body dies to science and motherless fetuses float in empty space."[44] In his less affirmative reading of Hunter's project, Youngquist characterizes these images as a map of the transformation of a pregnant woman into a mound of abject flesh "without history."[45] Youngquist records the sense of disquiet, past and present, surrounding the opening of the physical body and the public dissection of a "life." To some twenty-first-century observers, as well as their eighteenth-century counterparts, Hunter's empirical method appears dangerously uncompromising and disrespectful of human life. As we will see, the same was said about Godwin's utilitarian approach.

To Hunter and his contemporaries, the most prized anatomical subject was the pregnant female body—the body traditionally protected by codes of respectability, modesty, and decency. Hunter's images obviously have important medical purposes, but they also seem to signal a certain kind of trespass into the body—specifically, a body that, according to gender (female) and social role (motherhood), had been thought of as a body closed to the public gaze. To a lay audience, it is as if anatomists and engravers have reduced woman to a bodily husk, within which is hidden the empirical evidence needed to understand biological function. The anatomist's historical fascination with "the heremeneutic slipperiness of the maternal body, balancing precariously between life and death" is, according to critic Courtney Wennerstrom, an indecent one.[46]

In fact, the type of single-minded eagerness Wennerstrom identifies in many eighteenth- and nineteenth-century surgeons is clearly evidenced in Hunter's account of obtaining a pregnant cadaver. Hunter recalls how that particular body provided him with "the first favourable opportunity of examining, in the human species, what before he had been studying in brutes." He goes on to explain how "a woman died suddenly, when very near the end of her pregnancy; the body was procured before any sensible putrefaction had begun; . . . a very able painter . . . was found; every part was examined in the most public manner, and the truth was thereby well authenticated."[47] In Hunter's passage, the pregnant woman is not a unique person, or someone's beloved, or someone with a history; rather, she is

Murder to Dissect / 99

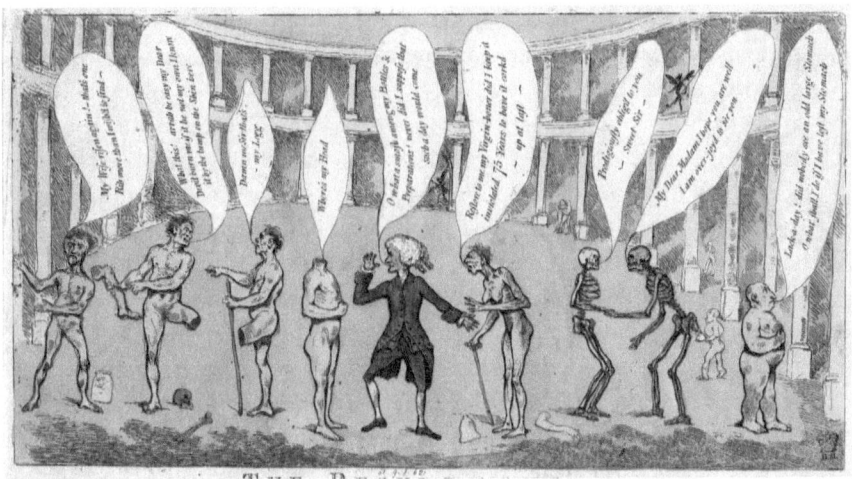

Figure 3.8 Thomas Rowlandson, *The Resurrection* (1782 © Trustees of the British Museum, London)

"the body." Hunter's concerns are purely material: she is only decomposing matter. There is none of that Burkean cultural drapery to protect her from being cut, probed, flayed, and displayed, or to use Hunter's words, "examined in the most public manner."

Without doubt, women appear in anatomical images not just as subjects of scientific study but also as objects of the sexual gaze of male physicians and readers. There is a discomfort with looking at the body in this way. It may seem a prurient activity; the viewer experiences a scopophiliac pleasure from visually penetrating the vulnerable, lifeless body of the woman under examination. Thomas Rowlandson's 1782 cartoon *The Resurrection* (figure 3.8) suggests precisely this. In this image, Hunter's scientific explorations invade, degrade, fracture and violate. Rowlandson depicts Hunter in his famous anatomy school on Great Windmill Street, Soho, London on the day of resurrection (a play on the term given to body snatchers, or "resurrectionists," who trafficked illegally in bodies retrieved from graveyards). The poor souls who, in the name of scientific progress, had been prevented from being buried intact search for their missing parts. Notably, the lone female figure plaintively mourns her irretrievable spotless virtue, which, she says, was kept "inviolated 75 years," only "to have it corked up at last." Her demand that Hunter "restore to me my Virgin-honor" aligns dissection with sexual perversion.

In the public imagination, anatomists were often thought of as predatory and a little too enthusiastic about their scientific pursuits. As in Rowlandson's satirical print, contemporary writers and artists linked resurrection and dissection with sexual immorality, female vulnerability, and the demeaning of the human. Anxieties about dissection, and medicine's wider aims, continued to build in the years following publication of Godwin's *Memoirs* of Mary Wollstonecraft. These fears would come to a head with the 1827–28 William Burke and William Hare murders (the two Edinburgh men sold the corpses of seventeen murder victims to surgeons for dissection). Although occurring some years after publication of the *Memoirs*, the literary output inspired by the Burke and Hare crimes reveals the tangled relationship between literature, medicine, public opinion, and scandal. Gothic narratives about the dark side of medicine proliferated in journals, such as Charles Lever's "Post-Mortem Recollections of a Medical Lecturer" (*Dublin University Magazine*, June 1836), the anonymously authored "The Victim" (*New Monthly Magazine*, December 1831), and the enormously popular *Passages from the Diary of a Late Physician* (serialized in *Blackwood's*, 1830–37). In "The Victim," for instance, a medical student encounters his colleague's recently "burked" fiancé on the dissecting table. He lusts after her beautiful naked corpse and, before he cuts her, kisses her and falls asleep on her body. In a testament to her beauty, he sketches her image for posterity, so he can keep her close to him always.[48] This is just one example of the sexualized portrayals of anatomists that appeared in popular gothic writing in these years.

To many observers, the coldly rational approach of anatomizing surgeons was matched by their passionate, obsessive attachment to science. And the collateral object of this obsession was most often female—a circumstance observed by disconcerted contemporaries such as Ann Millard, the widow of a resurrectionist who, in the first decades of the nineteenth century, protested against a culture of dissection that approached the bodies of women with both a clinical detachment and a voyeuristic desire. Even seemingly heartless "practitioners of medicine" must "shudder" at the idea, she wrote, "that the remains of all which was dear to him, of a beloved parent, wife, sister, or daughter, may be exposed to the rude gaze and perhaps to the INDECENT JESTS of unfeeling men, and afterwards be mutilated and dismembered in the presence of hundreds of spectators."[49]

Millard's appeal to the sympathetic side of doctors expressed prevailing fears about the facelessness of medicine. The concern was that medicine removed the female subject from her constellation of human relations and roles. The highest of woman's alleged virtues—honor, dignity, modesty—were stripped from her in the same way that her flesh was stripped from her bones. Millard expressed an anxiety that—under the anatomist's knife and subject to his anonymous, scrutinizing gaze— dissected women became reduced, to borrow Paul Youngquist's phrase, to "existentially anonymous, interchangeable husks of flesh."[50] This clinical detachment of the scientist is the very thing that, as Courtney Wennerstrom observes in her reading of Millard's passage, "enables the pornographic conflation of utility and arousal" that is "implicit" in the dissection of female cadavers.[51] Whether or not these critical appraisals of the aims and effects of surgeons such as Hunter are well founded, whether dissection was in some way a sexually titillating and degrading enterprise, is another issue, for another project. The point here is that many contemporary opponents of dissection held these views, as do some twenty-first-century critics.

Yet, the language of Millard's appeal is also problematic. We have already seen how other seemingly ethical appeals to nature had the effect of narrowing and normalizing social roles. Millard suggests that the woman on the dissecting table is only worth protecting from anatomists and the public gaze *because* she is someone's "parent, wife, sister, or daughter." Like other critics of dissection, Millard implies that woman's "value" is diminished *because* she is no longer prized for her maternal and feminine qualities. My point is that the anatomist's most fervent critics made the same claim for an inherent, biologically based "nature" as the very same anatomists and surgeons these critics challenged. As we will see, developments in anatomy and physiology, as well as the anxieties about those medical developments, were employed from both sides of the debate against political figures like Wollstonecraft. The same conservative-minded individuals who criticized medical research were also willing to use new medical knowledge to strip women of their political identities and to obscure the value of their work.

OVERSTIMULATION, APATHY, AND ENNUI (OR THE PROBLEM OF TOO MUCH INFORMATION)

This discussion may seem some way off from Godwin and the *Memoirs*. Yet, the cultural anxieties attendant on medicine's progressive infiltration of the female body provide an absolutely integral context to the reception of Godwin's texts and the afterlife of his ideas. If physiological and anatomical knowledge, and beliefs about pathology and normalcy, migrated from medical treatises to the realm of moral reform and political debate, then the *Memoirs* sits squarely in the middle of these overlapping concerns. There are significant connections between the way the public conceived of the aims, procedures and outcomes of anatomical dissection and the way they interpreted less physical but equally insidious forms of trespass into the body—and one of these was Godwin's textual intrusion.

Godwin's opponents were most disturbed by the affinity they perceived among three things: the principles of utility he had outlined in *Political Justice*, the disastrous effects of living by those principles (as demonstrated by Wollstonecraft's private life), and the rise of medical materialism. Anti-Godwinians (who were alarmed by the philosopher's emphasis on rationality and utility) aligned themselves with scientific vitalists (who were alarmed by how medical materialism aimed to locate thought and feeling in physical processes). As scholars point out, the division between vitalists and materialists has never been cut-and-dried; many thinkers were somewhere in the middle on this issue. Generally, however, those who believed that human vitality was God-given, separate from and superadded to the body, felt threatened by materialists who identified the source of life in the body's biochemical processes. Materialists challenged the vitalists' belief in a transcendent mind or an immaterial soul separate from the brain and nervous system.[52] According to vitalists, materialism submitted the wonder of divinely created human life to the microscope's lens; anti-Godwinians viewed the philosopher's emphasis on utility and rationality in similar terms. Godwin's philosophy rendered the ascendant human equally susceptible to the degradation of dissection and empirical measurement. The loosely connected group of vitalists, antirationalists and anti-utilitarians accused materialists and rationalists of erroneously and/or immorally attempting to reduce the human to something merely material and mechanical.

At the turn of the nineteenth century, *material* and *mechanical* were key terms, with an important pedigree and a considerable future. Throughout the 1790s, Edmund Burke used these words to great effect in his fight against French republicans and British radicals. In his *Reflections on the Revolution*, he describes republicanism as a "barbarous philosophy, which is the offspring of cold hearts" and as a *"mechanic philosophy"* that relies on "that sort of reason which banishes" the patriotic sentiment and national pride "that create in us love, veneration, admiration, or attachment."[53] The species of reason promoted by modern philosophers eliminated human affection and dependency, which bound individuals into compacts, communities, and nations. Philosophies founded on rationality were "barbarous" because they substituted cold calculation for affection, emotion, and loyalty.⁵⁴ Burke specifically targets republicanism as his detested strain of mechanic philosophy, but it would be fair to say that the social and political manifestations of republicanism and Godwinian utilitarianism would be, for Burke, basically the same.

Some decades later, *mechanical* became a keyword for conservative thinker Thomas Carlyle, who in his essay "Signs of the Times" blamed Benthamite utilitarianism, the rise of political economy, and the increasing popularity of medical materialism for turning society into a conglomerate of disconnected, disaffected, and apathetic individuals. He took aim at French ideologues who attempted to locate thought in the brain's mechanical functions: the materialist physiologist Pierre Jean George Cabanis sought to "open our moral structure with his dissecting-knives and real metal probes" and then to submit "it to the inspection of mankind, by Leuwenhoek microscopes, and inflation with the anatomical blow-pipe."⁵⁵ In *Sartor Resartus*, Carlyle equated the mechanical activity of eating with the grinding indifference with which human relations were conducted in a utilitarian society. If the political economists and rationalist philosophers had their way, he warned, the transcendent soul would be reduced to "a kind of *Stomach*"—that most lowly and insensible organ.⁵⁶ Carlyle's bodily language reflects the dethroning of the sacred and the soulful in favor of the material. Again, Carlyle's spleen was not aimed directly at Godwin, with whom he had little contact, but rather at later utilitarians like Jeremy Bentham and, to a lesser extent, James Mill and John Stuart Mill. Still, Carlyle targeted a tradition of thought to which Godwin belongs. In his correspondence, Carlyle describes Godwin as a "rational, instructed, but cold" writer of history and he pronounces the *Memoirs*, which he read in 1839, "a tragedy, a deep tragedy which I cannot get out of my thoughts."⁵⁷ I include these comments because their rhetoric echoes that of Carlyle's own ideological predecessors, who attacked Godwin in the 1790s and after. That Britain would become a mechanized society composed of alienated individuals who felt no union with or empathy for one another is a symptom of a modernity steeped in scientific method, reason, and utility.

Godwin's contemporaries were deeply troubled that his clinical approach in the *Memoirs* grew out of his clarion call to "general utility." His decision to publicize the details of Wollstonecraft's life accorded with his belief that utility should be the basis of all human action. In a very pragmatic way, Godwin intended her life to provide salutary examples for the improvement of society. But reactionaries appropriated and deflated his aims, scoffing at what they saw as a gross miscalculation of human nature and morality. They effectively avoided addressing Godwin's challenges to various forms of corruption and to social and political coercion. They sidestepped his charge, for example, that *"government by its very nature counteracts the improvement of original mind."*[58] Anti-Godwinians used bombast and satire rather than accurate or rigorous argumentation to undermine a philosophy they found contemptible (a tactic that Carlyle has also been accused of). Anti-Godwinians had the added bonus of being able to use biographical detail—which Godwin had himself provided—to deflate his and his wife's political aims. "The *utility*" of Wollstonecraft's life, the *Anti-Jacobin* declared, was that it showed the public what it was "wise to avoid," namely sexual independence and a lax attitude to marriage, modesty, and morality.[59] Similarly, the reviewer for *The Scientific Magazine and Free-Mason's Repository* contended that one could only conceive of the *Memoirs* as "useful" in the sense that the book clearly demonstrated the degree to which the repulsive *"moral sentiments* of Godwin" and the shocking *"moral conduct* of Wollstonecraft" were directly related to "their principles and theories."[60] A philosophy of utility demanded of its practitioners the same profound emotional detachment as that required of surgeons. As the poet Robert Southey observed, the moral majority accused Godwin of "having a want of all feeling in stripping his dead wife naked."[61] Godwin could gaze with equanimity on the most horrifying aspects of life, but a civilized mind embraced beauty, goodness, and decorum; it recoiled from the ugly reality of bodily decay, disease, and death.

Godwin's writing was particularly dangerous because the language he used had contagious effects. The *Monthly Mirror* offered a detailed explanation of how the apathetic language of the *Memoirs* gave rise to a similar sense of apathy and indifference among readers. In Godwin's description of his wife's death, "there is little to interest the feelings," because

> her labour, and the circumstances attending her death, are too minutely described.... There is a frequent repetition of the same occurrences: this gives that sort of *ennui*, which, to the generality of readers, must render its perusal very desultory and insipid. It is easy for many minds to comprehend the nature of a dangerous and trying labour; and when once we are led into all the minutiæ of this state, our pity for the afflicted object is mingled with astonishment at the cool precision of the person who describes it. This observation holds particularily in the present instance—for as Mr. G. was her husband, he might, with as much credit to himself, have left all the minutiæ of the case for the memorandums to the medical men who attended her. Surely it is not necessary in a plain simple biographical composition

to alarm one's readers with a recital of circumstances not immediately understood by every head, and not sufficiently dignified to heighten the awful catastrophe of the scene.[62]

Quite simply, then, knowing more meant feeling less. Rather than predisposing an audience to feel sympathetically toward Wollstonecraft, details about her body, the birth, and the ensuing disease gave rise to emotional indifference. Readers not only found it impossible to *feel,* they also distanced themselves from the shock of such coldly medical but also vividly repellent information. It was art rather than hard fact that inspired feeling. Disease and death needed to be presented as tragedy through a carefully crafted narrative that focused on the *emotional* effect of loss rather than on the corporeal particulars. The pathological human body needed to be cloaked—not laid bare in all its monstrosity. Individuals had a duty of care to ensure that the memory of their loved ones was pleasing and that their bodies were kept undefiled by curious strangers and unfeeling surgeons. A mourning husband who sought to memorialize his wife had a responsibility to ensure that the reading public had a similarly affective reaction. (The fact that Godwin was too distraught even to attend Wollstonecraft's funeral was one detail consistently overlooked by critics).

The *Monthly Mirror*'s claim that readers would experience "ennui" and thus respond apathetically to the *Memoirs* is a serious indictment. Borrowed from the French and refashioned to suit the psychosomatic conditions of eighteenth-century British culture, "the malady of ennui" came to describe a nervous disorder that plagued well-read, world-weary, and well-to-do moderns.[63] A precursor to modern-day depression, ennui—or its sister nervous disorder, melancholy—was something of a cultural obsession throughout this period. The influential Scottish school of medicine had much to do with the pathologizing of ennui; particularly notable in this respect was the work of John Brown, whose 1795 *Elements of Medicine* caused duels in Edinburgh and riots on the Continent. Brown proposed a formula of health and illness that was rather ingenious in its simplicity: The body had to be in balance, he argued. Too much or too little stimulus produced either a deficiency or a surplus of "excitability." These imbalances would then result in diseases of excess (in the case of the former) or debility (in the case of the latter). Following from this formula, then, a restoration of health required a "diminution of excitement *in the case of* diseases of excessive stimulus, and encrease *of the same excitement* for the removal of diseases of debility."[64] Brown's diagnoses and prescriptions emphasized consistency and balance; he defined a healthy body as one that strayed as little as possible from an emotional median.

It could be said that something like a Brunonian system of medicine underwrites the *Monthly Mirror* review cited above. The journalist's argument is that Godwin's "cool precision" and the "minuteness" of the gory details he provided of the "awful catastrophe" of his wife's death had the effect of producing "astonishment" in his audience. In turn, this astonishment overstimulated the reader, thereby producing ennui. As in Brown's account of excitability and debility, the overly stimulated readers reacted passively and became incapable of feeling sympathy. In other words, Godwin had essentially contaminated his readers with the pathology of indifference. An encounter with the *Memoirs* made readers as detached as Godwin himself, even when confronted with the vision of a dying wife and mother—and detachment was very dangerous, personally and politically. Although of different genres, Brown's medical treatise and the *Monthly Mirror* review demonstrate an escalating suspicion of excess and a simultaneously growing confidence in moderation and balance (about which we will see more in chapters 5 and 6).

Cultural suspicions about apathy, ennui, and excessive sensation took on a political twist in the 1790s. In fact, there are important links between John Brown's medical treatment of ennui, the reader response to the *Memoirs*, and Edmund Burke's linking of apathy and hysteria in his *Reflections on the Revolution in France*. Burke argues that an ennui-ridden nation is one that had left off its most important defining qualities: chivalry, loyalty, affection, dignity, and honor. In her reading of this text, Anne Mallory uses a suitably scientific terminology to make the case that boredom occupies an essential position in "Burke's taxonomy of political affect" and in his "anatomy of revolution."[65] Burke contends that apathetic individuals search for sources of external stimulation in order to feel sensation; as a result, their ennui tips into its opposite. Suddenly overstimulated, their boredom and lethargy give way to the type of histrionics that produce revolutionary fervor. That the French populace became overstimulated is clearly indicated by the events of the Terror, in which merciless compatriots willingly sacrificed each other to the guillotine. But there is an end to the violent fervor, for the initial drama of revolution—which excites torpid individuals to violence and hysteria—*must* eventually give rise to an aftermath of disaffection and estrangement. Burke describes a frighteningly reactive chain of extreme emotional swings in the body politic. A productive and stable nation needed to avoid either an excess or a deficiency of excitation. This balance could only be achieved through cooperation between people who were bound by a social contract and who felt something for one another, even if that feeling was based solely upon shared national identity. A civilized state could only be achieved, and more to the point maintained, when that shared emotion stayed steady. Governments could not suffer from extreme "nervous" swings as had the government in France, where the mood fluctuated wildly from acute apathy to excessive excitability. Change should only be carried out gradually.

The ideas about excess and moderation that circulated through medical and political discourse are closely tied to issues surrounding national identity. In the revolutionary years, political ennui was closely bound up with issues about national and familial cohesion. Accusations about inducing ennui tapped into established ideas about the English physiology. Although conceptions of national identities constantly evolve, certain characterizations of Englishness have prevailed. In the popular satire *The History of John Bull* (1712), the Scottish doctor and political satirist John Arbuthnot categorized the English as having a tendency toward the "Choleric."[66] According to neohumoral theory, that meant they were abundant in yellow bile, which indicated an energetic temperament that, if stirred, would descend into much stronger emotions. The image of Britain as a nation of industrious and honest people who, though usually reticent, did not suffer fools gladly has been a lasting one. This characterization was exploited fully at the end of the eighteenth century by radical pamphleteers who wanted to rouse national sentiment.

In his *Thoughts on the Probable Influence of the French Revolution on Great-Britain* (1790), the reformer Samuel Romilly praised his compatriots for their support of the storming of the Bastille. The English might be characterized by a certain "indifference," but they were also a loyal and sympathetic people who had a very low tolerance for injustice and misery, wherever it was found. Thus, when they viewed the beginnings of revolution in France, they could not help but be moved: "Who, indeed, that deserves the name of an Englishman, can have preserved a cold and deadly indifference, when he found a nation, which had been for ages enslaved, rousing on a sudden from their ignominious lethargy, breaking asunder their bonds?"[67] The English may be much less passionate than southern Europeans, but injustice inspired "bilious" indignation. As a reformer, Romilly put the charge of ennui to different political uses than Burke: he classified lethargy, or inertia, as the most reprehensible aspect of the French character under the old regime. *Ennui* was a romanticized term that licensed corrupt aristocrats to neglect their duties and encouraged tyrants to exercise arbitrary authority. The great body of the people had a vital energy, however, which would drive them to rid the nation of the apathetic upper classes.

Yet for conservatives, Godwin's candid confessions not only inspired ennui; they were also distinctly un-English in character. His cold rationality (which prevented him from feeling real sympathy), his seeming nonchalance about matters of the heart, his lack of chivalric sentiments (loyalty, protectiveness, devotion, fidelity), and his surgical detachment in the face of tragedy all made him appear unnatural and unfamiliar. After 1793, Godwin's character, his opponents suggested, was more foreign than the most inhuman French Jacobin. He would be more at home in the company of the Parisian *tricoteuses*, those notorious women who sat knitting, day after day, at the foot of the guillotine during the Terror. Their reaction to the daily round of gory performances alternated between vociferous rage and morbid nonchalance.

RATIONALITY, IMPARTIALITY, AND THE CRIMES OF SADISTS

After publication of the *Memoirs* in 1798, writers returned to and reviewed some of the more contentious statements Godwin had made five years earlier in his once-celebrated *Political Justice*. In effect, his arguments were reconsidered through the lens of his personal confessions. In their reassessment of this influential work of political philosophy, reactionaries targeted the empirical, rational language of his formulation of the "good" as the pursuit of pleasure and happiness while avoiding pain and "misery." Godwin's was a deeply misguided attempt, they argued, to reduce human ethics to a formula and to rationalize what could not—and to many observers should not—be rationalized.

That Godwin had taken rationality too far was clearly illustrated by the ethical dilemma he proposed in his chapter "Of Justice." This dilemma, which has since become known as the "famous fire cause," asks, if an individual had to choose between saving either the philosopher François Fénelon or his or her own mother from a burning building, who should be saved?[68] In later editions of *Political Justice*, Godwin substituted a valet for the mother, but the answer remained the same: the morally correct action would be to save Fénelon, since he invariably contributed more to the general good of society than either a family member or a servant. As Godwin suggested, a servant or family member may as easily be a fool or prostitute, so to be obliged to save them was to exercise false judgment.

"Suppose the valet had been my brother, my father or my benefactor," Godwin reasoned, even "this would not alter the truth of the proposition." It stands that "the life of Fénelon would still be more valuable than that of the valet; and justice, pure, unadulterated justice, would still have preferred that which was most valuable. Justice would have taught me to save the life of Fénelon at the expense of the other. What magic is there in the pronoun 'my,' that should justify us in overturning the decisions of impartial truth?"[69]

This dilemma expressed in precise terms a critical point of contention for anti-Godwinians—and much of the debate hinged upon the term *my*. For Godwin, *my* signified an irrational partiality based on proximity rather than rational choice. To choose Fénelon was to emancipate the individual from inhibitive, arbitrary, and thoughtless obligations. However, for reactionaries, this partiality was the glue of society: *my* was less about possession and ownership (as Godwin posited) and more about belonging and kinship. For conservatives, *my* signified human connection and indicated that humanity had evolved from its dark, selfish, and isolated origins. In contrast, Godwin's emphasis on impartiality and autonomy appeared to them a product of abstract reasoning as well as appallingly heartless.

Reactionaries considered Godwin's *Memoirs* of Wollstonecraft illustrative of the sentiments underpinning his famous fire cause; they reinterpreted his emphasis on justice as impartiality as a form of rational logic gone mad. In a 1798 anti-Godwinian pamphlet titled *Modern Philosophy and Barbarism*, W. C. Proby re-presents the same fire scenario but makes it personal to Godwin. Influenced no doubt by his reading of the *Memoirs*, Proby offers a version of the fire cause in which a husband must choose either to save his wife ("the dear object of his heart") or to rescue "a citizen of splendid talents and exquisite mental attainments, whose exertions are of infinite service to the state."[70] There are several conclusions to draw about Proby's "citizen of splendid talents": First, the more overt suggestion is that Godwin is the husband in the dilemma and Wollstonecraft the wife he chooses to let burn. There is also an implicit secondary inference that the citizen who is saved by Godwin *is* Godwin himself. The inflated and rather sarcastic adjectives—"splendid," "exquisite," infinite"—that describe the worthy citizen satirize the ideals of the Godwinian philosopher. In this reading, the ideal "citizen" is a sort of *estranged* Godwinian double, a product of utilitarian philosophy who, like Godwin himself, only feels passionately about his philosophy. There is yet a third alternative: the accomplished citizen could also be a perfect stranger. That Godwin would suggest that we should save a person for whom we feel either indifference or loathing, rather than a wife or family member, demonstrates a wish to erase affection and gratitude from the national character.

Whichever interpretation one subscribes to, the fact remains that the *Memoirs* illustrates the famous fire cause in action. According to Proby, this little book demonstrates how, by decimating "the ties of private affection" and "substituting in their stead the chains of public good," Godwin's barbarous system "would destroy civilization."[71] Like other alarmed reactionaries, Proby recasts Godwin's anecdotes and reinterprets his emphasis on justice as impartiality as ridiculous but still deeply threatening. More to the point, Proby makes personal Godwin's distinctly impersonal ethical dilemmas.

What are we to make of this contradictory image of Godwin? Of the unusual pairing of rationality and passion that he embodies? Certainly, even after his marriage in 1797 and the publication of the *Memoirs* in 1799, Godwin continued to be represented as sexually disinterested—as cold as Mr. Pitt, it might be said. But while he did not feel normal sexual desires, philosophy thrilled him. He was single-mindedly devoted to rationality—a dangerous thing to be in postrevolutionary Europe. Godwin's brand of "enthusiasm," Charles Lucas pointedly declared in his 1801 anti-Jacobin novel, *The Infernal Quixote*, was "deaf to the calls of nature."[72] The pamphleteer Thomas Green represented the Godwinian philosopher as a "heated" individual who felt "unbroken constancy" and "infuriate ardour" for his project, while harboring "hatred . . . intensely inflamed by the blast of zeal" for the things that typically inspired strong emotion: "friendship, patriotism, parental affection, filial piety, confidence, fidelity," and "conjugal union."[73] The *Memoirs* was philosophical enthusiasm put into practice, but it was an enthusiasm for cold detachment and personal solitude. Godwin uncompromisingly insisted on an absolute frankness that, contrary to English values, overrode marital or affective obligation. He willingly promoted his philosophical cause by sacrificing his wife's memory (just as Proby's Godwinian husband would forfeit his wife to the fire).

This double-sided representation of Godwin's character is highlighted in Isaac D'Israeli's *Flim Flams! Or the Life and Errors of My Uncle and the Amours of My Aunt* (1805). In this satire Godwin is characterized as the coldly frigid "Uncle" who obsessively retreats into "philosophical solitude" to conduct experiments, while "Aunt" Wollstonecraft is left to pursue her own pet projects.[74] Although D'Israeli's Godwin might be nonchalant about his wife's sexual history and her intellectual pursuits, he is extremely jealous of his own pursuit of reason. His "violent passions," we are told, are only "expressed by angular positions," or logical activities. When an artist named "Countour"—an overblown sentimental character whose lasciviousness is disguised as connoisseurship—admires the figure of "Aunt" Wollstonecraft, it seems Godwin may finally be susceptible to jealousy of a more personal nature. Yet when he demands an end to his wife's artistic liaisons, he reads her ensuing tears *not* as a sign of disappointment and despondency but as a chemical and biological process. "Tears are nothing more than secretions by the lachrymal glands, mucilage and common salt!" he exclaims.[75]

Although Contour wants to capture her unenhanced splendor, Godwin can only gaze on her naked form "like an *anatomist*" or a man of science who believes that "the true beauty" of woman "lies on the *inside*, and not the *out!*"[76] (This recalls the Hunter-Rymsdyk anatomical drawings, where the external body, and along with it individual identity, is literally peeled away to reveal internal organs and other biological matter.) Godwin is an anatomist and a chemist rather than an affectionate husband; he interprets his wife's symptoms as signs of disease and not as heartbreak—a politically strategic representation on D'Israeli's part. Godwin sets out to cure his wife of her *"sentimental* vertu" with what she, in protest, describes as his "inhumanity" but that is ultimately demonstrative of the "triumph of the severer sciences."[77] The rationalist Godwin prescribes a purgative and a course of bleeding for a condition others would diagnose as unrequited love and unsatisfied desire. Medicine, in Godwin's mind, would purge his wife's/patient's body of her "criminal wishes"; it would eradicate her of "peccant humour"; it would "purify" her "loose thoughts" and "cool the unnatural heat of [her] body."[78] Sexual interest, desire, pleasure, and human emotion are medicalized and reinterpreted through Godwinian philosophy as purely material ailments.

This representation casts Godwin in the same league as figures with whom he would otherwise have little in common. For instance, although personally and philosophically the Marquis de Sade may seem worlds away, his reputation bears a striking resemblance to Godwin's. In fact, what was known and understood about Sade's work, life, and reputation helps us understand something about how and why critics represented Godwin as they did. Namely, Sade's writing demonstrated the dangers of "scientific" enthusiasm. In his novels, he links rationality and scientific thought with sexual compulsion. A panoply of characters defer to rationality on questions about human motive, desire, and character, and the consistent privileging of reason over sympathy gives rise to extreme violence and sexual deviance. In *La nouvelle Justine* (1797), for example, the monk Clement believes that "perfecting ... the science of anatomy" is the key to understanding "the relationship between man's constitution and the tastes which have affected him."[79]

How far the man of reason will go is indicated most, however, by the ruthlessly ambitious surgeon Rodin of Sade's *Justine* (1791). He repeatedly rapes his adolescent daughter Rosalie in an attempt to prime her for the anatomical experiments he will conduct on her body. "Anatomy," Rodin proclaims, "will never reach its ultimate state of perfection until an examination has been performed upon the vaginal canal of a fourteen- or fifteen-year-old child who has expired from a cruel death."[80] Rodin's partner and student, Rombeau, marvels at his mentor's dedication to medicine and suggests Rodin's own daughter as object of their sadistic studies. Unperturbed by social niceties or familial connection, Rodin agrees: sacrificing his daughter is nothing, since he finds "it odious" that such "futile considerations" could "check the progress of science."[81] The body holds the secrets to human nature, and the way to access those secrets is through dissection (or vivisection); in the name of progress and the common good, as Rodin repeatedly states, the individual may need to be sacrificed.

We can never know how many English readers Sade had, nor what their responses were. Likely there were few in the early nineteenth century. Yet Sade's narratives and the types of statements made by characters like Rodin and Rombeau give context to the reception of Godwin's writing; they also clarify why apprehensive observers might draw connections between anatomy, materialism, utilitarianism, and sexual sadism. In the public imagination, the projects of William Hunter, William Godwin, and the Marquis de Sade appeared frightfully allied.

Readers past and present have read Sade's fiction as confessional. Of course, we want to be cautious about reading novels through the lens of biography and, certainly, we should be suspicious of pat statements about authorial intention. Yet the fact that statements made by Sade's fictional characters have become so entwined with his life is itself revealing. Readers have interpreted the monk Clement's statements as explanations of Sade's alleged attempt to vivisect the beggar Rose Keller (who became known as the "femme vivante disséqué"). This incident is recorded by Réstif de la Bretonne, who claims, ironically, to dissect Paris night life in the same way as a surgeon applies his knife to the "anatomy of a corpse" in his *Nights in Paris*.[82] He reports how Sade took Keller to a room in his house where he performed anatomical experiments, with the intention of dissecting her before an audience. Preparing to open her body to view, Sade purportedly demanded, "Who wants this unfortunate being in the world? She can do nothing and will serve to reveal to us the mysteries of the human structure."[83] This language expresses an obsessive desire to flay and to infiltrate the depths of the body, in order to understand human nature while at the same time satisfying the curiosity, aspirations, and desires of the anatomist. According to other reports, Sade also had a penchant for strapping women down, flagellating them, cutting them, and pouring wax into their wounds. His mother-in-law wrote to Horace Walpole that once caught for these crimes, he had "claimed to have done a fine thing and to have rendered the public an important service, viz., the invention of an ointment which heals wounds quickly."[84] Medical progress demands sacrifices: inflicting pain brings about the discovery of cures. In the eyes of an anxious public, medical science was uncomfortably linked with covert sexual urges and a taste for violence. Sadistic impulses turn *utilitarian*, at least according to the erroneous understanding of that term.

The accuracy of these anecdotes is not the point; the fact that they circulated among the public is. They convey insights about fears surrounding science, experimentation, and the limits of human sympathy. That an individual's desire to understand the mysteries of the human structure could override sympathetic feelings was deeply appalling to the public imagination. Suspicion circulated around medical objectivity and empiricism: these Enlightenment inheritances could turn diabolical. In the twentieth century, Simone de Beauvoir's comments on Sade indicate how long-standing these suspicions have been. For Beauvoir, Sade was so "enveloped" in his "own experience" that the existence of "the inner presence of other people" was completely "foreign" to his understanding.[85] Fraternity is, for Sade, a completely illogical and unreasonable construct, since there are no essential or obligatory bonds between individuals. For the self to be so removed from others on a personal, emotive level is to threaten the very idea of community and civil society.

Beauvoir's reading of Sade echoes public reactions to Godwin at the turn of the nineteenth century. Like Sade, Godwin's private life was viewed as selfishly solitary and his writing as promoting an end to affective connective ties between individuals. Unlike Sade, Godwin may have emphasized duty in his philosophy, but he also insisted that political or moral obligation cannot be grounded in any social contract. The only criterion for moral or political obligation is general utility. Clearly, these two figures—one an egoistic, sadomasochistic pornographer and one a supposedly frigid but loose-moraled utilitarian rationalist—are in many ways oppositional. Yet their contemporaries interpreted their lives as similarly frightening manifestations of Enlightenment reason and, more specifically, as representing the blind immorality of scientific pursuit. We can see how—in the imagination of their contemporaries—the crimes of sadists, the practices of anatomists, and the cold textual autopsies performed by biographers could seem much more interrelated than we, as twenty-first-century observers, might at first think.

WOLLSTONECRAFT AND THE QUESTION OF FEMALE EMBODIMENT

Negative public attention did not stay focused on Godwin. The same moralists who were so outraged by his autopsical biography of Wollstonecraft reopened her life for further dissection. In fact, her body, illness, and death became points of particularly heated debate about the nature of woman and her political capacities or incapacities. Conservatives argued that one of the salutary lessons gleaned from Wollstonecraft's miserable life was that biological differences between men and women could neither be denied nor inverted. Just as Godwin's canon was reconsidered in light of the revelations of the *Memoirs*, so too was Wollstonecraft's. One of the points of contention in her writing, as much now as at the turn of the nineteenth century, centered around the oppositions of nature/culture and reason/emotion.

In her 1792 *Vindication of the Rights of Woman*, Wollstonecraft suggests that what was thought to be biologically inherent in woman's "nature" was often a product of culture. Suggestively, she proposes that if women "were allowed to acquire more understanding," they would not "always remember that they are women."[86] Women *become* "enfeebled"; their "weakness" is "artificial"—not natural. In fact, she argues, "Nature is counteracted" in a society that sees women as "born only to rot procreate and rot."[87] If females were not socialized to act, indeed to *be* a certain thing, if their bodies were not always referred to as evidence of their incapacity for rationality, and if they were not always pressured to conform to norms of gendered behavior, then they would exercise their reason and their bodies as freely as men. Wollstonecraft then extends this list of factors that contribute to the ideology of biological difference. The culture of sensibility, the cult of domesticity, the gendered emphasis on fashion and beauty, the pressures of the marriage market, and Rousseauvian ideas about restricting women's education have made women physically, mentally, economically, and socially dependent. In turn, their dependence has ensured their exclusion from the public sphere.

At the same time, Wollstonecraft also insists that women have domestic responsibilities. She famously chastises them for leaving off their roles as good wives and mothers, and she often identifies gender-specific qualities and behaviors. *Vindication* is peppered with references to female appetites and desires—and the struggle between denying them and satisfying them. She cautions against homoerotic contact between girls and insists upon habits of modesty, which include solitary bathing and other issues of hygiene. In her fiction and travel memoirs, she describes the particular pleasures and pains of living in a female body. These pains are highlighted in her unfinished novel *Maria; or, The Wrongs of Woman*, which was posthumously published by Godwin in 1798. An outline of one of Wollstonecraft's proposed endings to the novel provides a tragic synopsis of her eponymous heroine's end and a snapshot of what a woman's life might entail: "Divorced by her husband—Her lover unfaithful—Pregnancy—Miscarriage—Suicide."[88]

Wollstonecraft's seemingly contradictory statements about sexual biological difference have been a perennial point of debate among her critics. Her dual emphasis on reason and desire, intellect and the body, has led modern-day feminist scholars to identify a marked ambivalence in her writing. According to Mary Poovey, Wollstonecraft "vacillat[es] between denying her female feelings altogether and falling hostage once more to the very categories she was trying to escape."[89] Often, this ambivalence is interpreted as evidence of the problems women writers face as they attempt to write female-embodied experience *and* to express themselves in a "masculinist" prose that appeals to reason (allegedly the purview of male writers) over emotion (aligned with female writing). In recent years, "back-to-the-body" feminism has sought to reclaim the female body and to promote female-embodied writing—and Wollstonecraft has been made into a standard bearer for this reclamation movement.

Ashley Tauchert and Mary Poovey argue that Wollstonecraft fluctuates between a desire to claim "male" rationality for women and a desire to give voice to a maternal or female-embodied subjectivity.[90] This latter aim, Tauchert explains, is an attempt to redress historical inequalities that privilege supposedly male-specific characteristics grounded in bodily difference. She suggests that Wollstonecraft's work responds to what Moira Gatens describes as a "public sphere [that] has historically been an almost exclusively male sphere" because it has developed on the assumption "that its occupants have a male body."[91] Since the male body is "the norm or standard of the liberal individual," women can only be considered legitimate citizens if they "elide their own corporeal specificity" to fit into this male world.[92] According to Tauchert, Wollstonecraft adopts this strategy of bodily denial: in her early, "pre-maternal" and "manly" writing (including her two *Vindications*—*Vindications of the Rights of Men* and *Vindications of the Rights of Woman*— and her *Historical and Moral View of the French Revolution* of 1794), Wollstonecraft presents a rational masculinist identity to the world. Only as a result of pregnancy and becoming a "mother of a daughter," Tauchert argues, does Wollstonecraft adopt a positively female-embodied form of writing. [93]

However, I want to take issue with these readings and with the attempt to turn Wollstonecraft into an advertisement for female-embodied writing. She is, after all, a vociferous proponent of reason and rationality. Poovey's comment, in particular, draws a clear opposition between female and male feelings and assumes that rationality is a male category, and thus one that women somehow need to escape. This assumes the view that female embodiment is in tension with "masculinist" writing and with the assumptions, categories, and demands associated with the male sphere. The great dilemma in Wollstonecraft's writing is *not* that it lacks "female feelings" but that she was and is expected to have something called "female feelings"—that are oppositional to male reason. In more general terms, this suggests that all women share the same group of feelings: What of specificity and diversity here? What about the great range of human emotion and opinion? Wollstonecraft's writing challenges the idea of inherent gendered characteristics and contests naturalized views about the gendered dimensions of emotion, character, desire, and intelligence.

For Gatens, Tauchert, and Poovey, the female body may be a starting point of resistance or protest, but I would argue that the critical emphasis on female embodiment replicates the very same conservative attitudes surrounding women's bodies and abilities that have been detailed in this and the previous two chapters. This strain of feminism shares with eighteenth-century medicine a desire to identify certain biological traits as inherent or natural rather than cultural. Feminism that disregards social-constructivist views of gender, and instead grounds gendered emotion and bodily desire in biology, plays right back into the tradition of biological incommensurability identified here. The concept of female embodiment and writing through the female body falls into the trap of essentialism.

In fact, the biologically based assumptions about the female body put forward by some feminist critics are strikingly similar to those mobilized against Wollstonecraft in a conservative, reactionary campaign that largely silenced her arguments after 1798. The Cornish author and clergyman Richard Polwhele's satirical long poem *The Unsex'd Females* (1798) represents female authors as hysterical, immoral, irreligious, insubordinate, masculine, violent, grasping, shrill, and dangerous to good order. As harbingers of radical Enlightenment philosophies and French political ideas, they endanger political peace and social stability. Polwhele's deeply personal tarring of specific female writers and artists—Anna Laetitia Barbauld, Mary Robinson, Charlotte Smith, Helen Maria Williams, Ann Yearsley, Mary Hays, and Angelica Kauffmann—indicates something of the many cultural barriers they faced. More to the point here, Polwhele insists that Godwin's description of Wollstonecraft's final days reminds readers that she "died a death that strongly marked the distinction of the sexes, by pointing out the destiny of women, and the diseases to which they are liable."[94] Women's bodies were prey to a completely different set of afflictions than men; it follows that they were bound for a different set of roles. As their physiology indicated, they were destined for motherhood rather than public life. It was, as E. P. Thompson wryly observed, rather "convenient that this most rational of women, who proclaimed the equality of sexes and who attempted to live her principles in free marriage . . . should have died in childbirth."[95] To conservatives and their readers, her death appeared as writing on the wall: philosopher-women could no longer play the part of men. Her body had made that clear. We should be aware of how similar attitudes can underpin twenty-first-century attempts to locate female feelings, characteristics, and desires in the gendered body. The view of women as maternal beings whose principle role is childbearing and childrearing remains a biologically deterministic one. Such sexual branding reduces women to a sum of their reproductive parts.

Polwhele's statements about the division of the sexes might not have been particularly new, but his rhetorical strategy—of using the intimate details of Wollstonecraft's private life and her medical history to buttress his arguments—was more novel. Rather than address her philosophy, he used gender-specific illness to discount her intellectual capabilities and political aspirations. Other conservative writers had turned their attention to Wollstonecraft's work in the 1790s, but after Godwin's revelations her corpus of writing was resurrected only to be dissected in light of new biographical facts. Reviewers targeted her writing on issues surrounding the human body and morality, especially passages that seemed to offer an overly rational or scientific approach to those subjects. One of these was her 1789 translation of German educator Christian Salzmann's *Elements of Morality for the Use of Children*. In the "Advertisement" to the volume, Wollstonecraft described this "very useful production" as "a rational book" that offered readers "a well-digested system" of pedagogically useful narratives.⁹⁶ These seemingly innocuous descriptors—"rational," "useful," and a "well-digested system"—gesture toward precisely what reviewers would find so disturbing ten years later, following publication of the *Memoirs*.

The following passage on the issue of children's "chastity and impurity," from Salzmann's *Elements*, raised reactionary hackles: "Impurity is now spread so far that even children are infected, and by it the germe of every virtue, as well as the germe of their posterity, which the Creator has implanted in them, is destroyed. . . . The most efficacious method to root out this dreadful evil, which poisons the source of human happiness, would be to speak to children of the organs of generation as freely as we speak of the other parts of the body, and explain to them the noble use which they were designed for, and how they may be injured."⁹⁷ The argument that parents should speak candidly with their children about sexuality and should caution them against masturbation was, in the opinion of some of Wollstonecraft's detractors, as destructive as the practice itself.

Crucially, critics assumed or pretended that the author of this passage was Wollstonecraft and *not* Salzmann. Three pages following the passage above, Salzmann addresses female readers directly, writing "*your* sex has undeniably more tenderness than *ours*."⁹⁸ The gendered pronouns clearly indicate male authorship, yet after 1798 reviewers continued to accuse Wollstonecraft of penning salacious tracts. The reviewer of Godwin's *Memoirs* for the *British Critic* wrote, "In the account of her last sufferings, which seem to have been indeed uncommonly severe, her husband does not scruple to specify the exact circumstances of the case, which, though more suited to a medical statement than a book of memoirs, intended for general perusal, *is exactly conformable* to the *Elements of Morality written by Mrs. G herself; in the introduction to which she urges the propriety of making young persons, particularly girls, intimately acquainted with certain parts of anatomy,* generally thought to be unfit for their contemplation."⁹⁹

Besides the direct reference to Salzmann's text, there is also a more oblique reference to the *Vindication of the Rights of Woman* and in particular to Wollstonecraft's assertion that she had "conversed, as man with man, with medical men, on anatomical subjects; and compared the proportions of the human body with artists."[100] The *British Critic* reviewer accuses her of being as much a rationalist empiricist as Godwin. That she would cast herself as anatomist led her detractors to place her among those rationalists who, in the words of Polwhele, plucked "each precept cold from sceptic Reason's vase."[101] As someone who dealt in inappropriate subjects like anatomy and who approached such matters as children's sexuality with bare-faced candor, she deserved the clinical treatment she received at the hands of her rationalist husband. In this respect, Wollstonecraft and Godwin ended up being accused of committing very similar crimes. Anatomy was as much an inappropriate subject for young girls as it was for woman-philosophers or husbands who viewed their wives as bodies rather than as objects of affection. Both Wollstonecraft and Godwin were attacked for improperly using the yardstick of utility to measure institutions like marriage and to quantify inestimable phenomena like human emotion.

In *The Unsex'd Females*, Polwhele also invokes Salzmann's infamous passage when he decries "Mary Wollstonecraft's instructions in Priapism."[102] Polwhele's remark makes strategic reference to eighteenth-century hysteria about masturbation and degeneracy. The condition of priapism, or having abnormally persistent penile erection, as an effect of solitary sex. As a distinctly pathological activity that fell well outside the normal course of human relations in the eighteenth century, masturbation was a pathology with profound cultural/ideological implications. In an era in which medicine "became the voice of morality," onanism was a key target of physicians, educators, and philosophers who sought to create "a new ethics grounded in nature and reason."[103] Polwhele interprets Wollstonecraft's educational and political writing as purposely and insidiously undermining the medical and moral "pedagogization" that, as Foucault notes, took center stage in "the war against onanism" in this era.[104] Ironically, the same Salzmann who Wollstonecraft translated also wrote in depth on this subject, warning readers that onanism was a disease that, like a parasite or a thorn, worked its way into the body but never stayed confined to one part. Worse, onanism spread out from the host, to poison the entire social fabric. According to Polwhele, Wollstonecraft's ideas about female equality and her advocacy of liberty contaminated her followers and students in a similar way.

Polwhele's reference to masturbation is connected to his satirical portrayal of Wollstonecraft as the icon of overweening sensibility. He describes her as a "love-sick maid," thereby linking to the idea that masturbation and sensibility shared the same origin. As G. J. Barker-Benfield observes, physicians and moralists viewed masturbation as a pathology that developed from overcultivated sentiments, an excess of emotion, a susceptibility to impression, and an ardor for affective stimulation.[105] The culture of sensibility and onanism were understood as products of physical, emotional, and intellectual stimulation and imaginative excess in a world in which luxuries and gratification were increasingly accessible. Sensibility and onanism were both born out of an increasingly individualistic society that privileged personal expression and particularized human sensation.

In addition, Polwhele's description of Wollstonecraft's body as a diseased "pale form" mirrors representations of the waning masturbator or the languid, overly nervous or sensitive artist/intellectual/philosopher. In a study of the physiological analogies used in sentimental discourse, Ann Jessie Van Sant points out that excessive sensibility, believed to originate in an "organic sensitivity" of the heart, brain, or nerves, rendered the individual vulnerable to emotions.[106] In turn, this vulnerability—to which women succumb much more than men—led to disease, decline, and death. Vulnerability is a key concern for Polwhele, who envisions the spread of Wollstonecraftian influence—sexual libertinism and political radicalism, to be precise—among unsuspecting and impressionable young women. In *Vindication*, Wollstonecraft expressed reservations about women studying botany, yet Polwhele accuses her of tutoring her impressionable students in "a little plant adultery," instructing them in "the prostitution of a plant" and rather ironically, he describes a scene of Wollstonecraftian females attempting to "dissect" a plant's "organ of unhallow'd lust."[107]

These accusations tapped into an ongoing debate about the appropriateness of botany for women.[108] Polite publications like Jean-Jacques Rousseau's *Letters on the Elements of Botany Addressed to a Lady* (trans. 1787) and Priscilla Wakefield's *Introduction to Botany in a Series of Familiar Letters* (1796) yoked botany with appropriately moral lessons. But in his popular *Botanic Garden* (1791), Erasmus Darwin linked the overt sexuality of Linnaean botany to radical political and scientific arguments.[109] He made clear his support for the French Revolution, as well as for Enlightenment materialism. He suggested that human emotion and character were products of physiology—an argument that his detractors interpreted as atheistic. In "Loves of the Plants," one of the two poems that comprise this work, he used an overtly sexual discourse to anthropomorphize the fertilization of plants, partly with the aim of representing human sexuality as a natural process. It would be fair to say that aligning a public woman with botany after Darwin was likely to have detrimental effects on her reputation.

Notably, Polwhele has Wollstonecraft "dissecting" plants, in a sexualized context. Once again then, dissection is linked with illicit sex and also captures the anxiety about scrutiny, probing, and the penetrating inquisitiveness of scientists, skeptics, and female botanists. Polwhele's characterization is another expression of the anxiety motivating William Wordsworth's famous maxim that moderns would "murder to dissect" in their craze for knowledge. Polwhele's comments also reveal the struggle between a Godwinian transparency, frankness, and rationality on the one side and a traditional emphasis on modesty and decorum on the other. That Wollstonecraft would express her willingness to take on the role of the anatomist in the same breath as she declared her intention to dispense with "the absurd rules which make modesty a pharaisaical cloak of weakness" reverberates uneasily, as did Godwin's utilitarianism, with Burke's influential warning that if given the chance, unchivalrous republicans, reformers, calculators, and sophists would tear away the "drapery of life" to reveal the ugly reality of the material world beneath.[110] The ugliness of material reality—corporeality, human sexuality, decay, death, and all the things medical men dealt with—was much closer to things like anarchy, nihilism, violence, and rampant immorality than might first appear. In the eyes of reactionaries like Burke, what Wollstonecraft termed "absurd rules" were absolutely integral to a civilized society and the sole means of preventing Britain from commencing on the same downward slide into national degeneration as had France.

NERVOUS DISORDERS, THE CULTURE OF SENSIBILITY, AND RADICAL WOMEN

Godwin represented Wollstonecraft as a woman of sensibility. In the *Memoirs*, he insists that she was "endowed with the most exquisite and delicious sensibility" and he surmises that her mind might have been "of too fine a texture to encounter the vicissitudes of human affairs."[111] Quite simply, her weakness was that she felt too much. To a creature of such sensitivity, "pleasure is transport and disappointment is agony indescribable."[112] Unfortunately, Godwin's language also resonated with less positive views of the cult of sensibility, in damaging ways. Godwin's characterization of Wollstonecraft as a woman whose "sensibility of . . . heart would not suffer her to rest in solitary gratifications" chimes with characterizations of the Rousseauvian radicalized woman of loose morals, who appeared in antirevolutionary novels in the 1790s.[113] Godwin's emphasis on acute emotions echoes the medical language of treatises on nervous disorders, particularly relating to sexual hysteria, "hypochondriacal affection," or "hysteric passion." Physicians who warned readers of the dangers of physiological predispositions to sexual excess described patients who were alternatively transported by exquisite pleasures and plunged into despairs of the blackest kind.

Hysterical susceptibility was the dark side of the eighteenth century's emphasis on the expression of delicacy and sentiment. In his discussion of the gendered dimension of the eighteenth-century culture of sensibility, G. J. Barker-Benfield couples the positive qualities associated with female sensibility, such as "intellect, imagination, [and] the pursuit of pleasure," with negative ones, such as "physical and mental inferiority, sickness, and inevitable victimization."[114] These latter qualities, he points out, cast "severe doubt on the effectiveness of the female will."[115] I would add another negative quality to this list: female sensibility became aligned with an incapacity for political and philosophical pursuits. Moreover, sensibility became associated with nervous ailments. Whereas in previous centuries mysterious attacks and disorders had spiritual or metaphysical explanations, eighteenth-century doctors of reason located their source firmly in the body's physiology.

Early in the century, having exquisitely receptive nerves—like demonstrating one's sensibility—was seen as a sign of taste and status. In *The English Malady* (1733), George Cheyne argues that "Fools, weak or stupid Persons, heavy and dull Souls, are seldom troubled with Vapours or Lowness of Spirits" in the same way that thoughtful and sensitive individuals were.[116] But by midcentury, the definition of *nervous* and its cognates changed from connoting strength (as in *nervy*) to denoting, according to Samuel Johnson's Dictionary, "weak and diseased nerves." Later in the century, in the tradition of Cheyne, Dr. William Cullen pinpoints the nervous system as the origin of what he termed "neuroses" (diseases that manifested themselves physically and psychologically but had no obvious physiological origin). These newly identified but vague disorders—melancholia, hypochondria, splenetic moods, imaginative excess, mania, and other nervous ailments—resulted from a fault between brain and body. Indeed, Cullen blames the ebb and flow of nervous stimuli to the brain as the cause of extreme swings in mood and perception.[117] Thomas Beddoes, the physician and friend of Samuel Taylor Coleridge, outlines the way that passions, fears, and thoughts gave rise to physical pathologies that were difficult to classify. In his *Hygeia* (1803), he summarizes postmortem findings of autopsies performed on melancholics. Among other things, their skulls were overly thick or thin in certain parts, and the membranes of the melancholic brain were often inflamed and contained watery liquid.[118] At times mental affliction was seen as a product of culture, but as this type of material reveals, there was a move to find biological bases for mental and nervous disorders.

This emphasis on nervous system pathology had profound repercussions for women in particular: their vaporish tendencies, mental derangements, and splenetic moods were another sign of the incommensurability of male and female bodies. Indeed, medical manuals insisted that while women's bodies rendered them more sympathetic and sensitive than men, this went hand in hand with physical delicacy. In turn, women were prey to emotional instability and nervous affliction, ranging from lovesickness to hysteria. Cullen explains hysteria as a "turgescence of blood" accumulated in the female sexual organs.[119] As is well known, the uterus as the biological site of hysteria has a long history since at least the classical age; Cullen's comments reveal the persistence of such beliefs.

Like Cullen, other medical writers also underscored the sexualized and gendered nature of nervous disorders and their connection to excesses of emotion or unbridled imagination. In a chapter with the revealing title "Of the Sexual Intercourse; its physical consequences with respect to the Constitution of the Individual; under what circumstances it may be either conducive or hurtful to Health," Dr. A. F. M. Willich urged restraint for both men and women. Yet he emphasized that sexual excess had different constitutional consequences for each. Semen should not be "wantonly and improvidently wasted," he cautioned, for "the ablest physiologists" had discovered that when the male body retains "this refined fluid ... it imparts to the body peculiar sprightliness, vivacity, and vigour."[120] Committing "excess with impunity" would result in diseases of the eye or consumption of the back.[121] Men's physical vigor was lessened and their nervous balance upset by too much contact with women. In other words, women sapped the vitality of men.

As for women who indulged in excessive sex, they could expect to be afflicted with loss of vision, ailments of the stomach, disordered lungs, loss of bone strength, sluggishness, as well as *"fluor albus,* violent fluxes of the menses, bearing down of the vagina, and innumerable other maladies of a disagreeable nature."[122] More serious still were the mental symptoms. Woman's whole nervous system would become "reduced to a state of extreme debility," and she would experience "hypochondriasis" (irrational anxiety about imaginary illnesses), loss of memory and judgment, and severe "imbecility," so that she would not be able to be attentive "to one object, for a quarter of an hour together," or she would see "imaginary figures" floating before her eyes.[123] Passionate women could become physically incapacitated, sexually inadequate, mentally unhinged, and delusional. Their weaker nervous systems could never recover from sexual excess.

Medical writing on women's nervous disorders was part of wider cultural attitudes that conceived of women as naturally unsuited to life in the public sphere. The portrayal of women as capable of sapping men of their masculine vitality, yet as fragile beings with enervated constitutions, was common in print culture. The moral alarm and the hyperbolic language present in the writing on women's nervous disorders also appeared in satirical and fictional writing. The polemicist and physician Bernard Mandeville provides an early example in his satirical portrayal of women's psychosomatic performances. In his fictional *Treatise of the Hypochondriack and Hysterick Diseases* (1730), the male character, Misomedon, and his wife, Polytheca, are both hypochondriacs, yet while the husband retains a rational distance from his affliction, the wife is consumed by hers. "I never dare speak of Vapours," she states, for "the very Name is become a Joke; and the general notion that Men have of them is that they are nothing but a malicious Mood, and contriv'd Sulleness of willful, extravagant, and imperious Women, when they are denied, or thwarted in their unreasonable Desires; nay, even Physicians because they cannot cure them, are forced to ridicule them in their own Defence, and a Woman, that is really troubled with Vapours is pitied by none, but her unhappy Fellow-sufferers."[124] Mandeville's characterization testifies to the belief that the nervous systems of men and women are inherently different. There are countless such examples, but this one gives a sense of why, much later in the century, Godwin's revelations about Wollstonecraft and her nerves would become such effective fodder for her enemies.

As doctors constituted the gendered human body, so they constituted the gendered self. If, as George Rousseau posits, "the nervous system became the battlefield on which civilization and its discontents would be played out," then nerves were a political minefield on which women were forced to step ever more carefully to avoid political discussions that might upset their delicate systems.[125] These conceptions informed the accounts of women's lives and their politics, whether given by reactionaries or reformers. Gender-specific physiological explanations accounted not only for Wollstonecraft's death in childbirth but also for her sensitivity and receptiveness, her chasing after sensation, her desire for public acclaim, her sexual excesses, her melancholy, her suicidal tendencies, her revolutionary philosophies, and her feminism. That there were biological explanations, founded in irrefutable nature, to account for the Wollstonecraft phenomenon must have provided alarmed observers with some assurance in the face of the challenges she presented. Wollstonecraft's female, sexually active, and pregnant body was susceptible to a realm of pathological conditions, resulting in such things as loss of judgment and a fixation on an "imaginary figure" (her unrequited passion for Gilbert Imlay). Her female nerves rendered her irrational and hysterical and drove her to attempt suicide (once by laudanum and once by jumping into the Thames). Interestingly, Wollstonecraft described her drowning attempt as a distinctly rational choice: it was not, she wrote, "a frantic attempt" but rather "one of the calmest acts of reason."[126] This, of course, is not how her life and political philosophy have been interpreted.

The medical emphases on the relationship between, on the one hand, excess and sensation and, on the other, the resulting melancholy, ennui, and despair had dire effects on Wollstonecraft's image. To suffer from such extremes of emotion—to plunge from sensation to apathy—was part of the negative image of 1790s radical protofeminists. In the *Vindication*, Wollstonecraft acknowledges how powerfully women are shaped by the culture of sensibility and admits that it is challenging for women to extricate themselves (and herself) from its seductive influence. Reactionaries and moralists portrayed not only Wollstonecraft but the writers Helen Maria Williams, Mary Robinson, and especially the early feminist Mary Hays as women victimized by the types of emotional oscillations associated with sensibility. As such, they were unable to manage the same rights and privileges for which they had publicly agitated. Much has been made of the resemblance between Hays and the characters of her biographical-fictional novel, *Memoirs of Emma Courtney* (1796). The philosophical correspondence between Emma Courtney and Mr. Francis reflects Godwin's ideas and his communications with Hays. In addition, Emma's obsession with the character Harley is also widely interpreted as a biographical portrayal of Hays's own unrequited sexual obsession with the Unitarian radical William Frend.[127] There are also connections between the unhealthy emotional state of the novel's yielding heroine and the representations of Wollstonecraft's desperately untenable passions. Like Emma Courtney, Wollstonecraft is said to have experienced excessive sensibility and overly sensitive nerves that produced acute symptoms. In the novel, the combination of sensibility, ardent emotions, and rationality led to suicide, adultery, and infanticide. These same combinations and "crimes" appear in Wollstonecraft's work and, in the case of adultery and suicide, in her own life.

Ironically, then, Wollstonecraft was accused of falling prey to the *opposite* condition as Godwin: whereas he felt nothing, she felt too much. Neither of these conditions made for good politicians. These physiological explanations for what physicians identified as diseases of culture, and what Freud will later describe as the by-products of civilization, had great impact on the representation and reception of Wollstonecraft and her work. She was a hysterical woman who belonged to a hysterical age—a self-indulgent age that would be replaced by a generation that sought to counter the excesses of their predecessors. The Victorians, if we can risk making a gross generalization, would self-identify as more disciplined, controlled, and less "nervous" than their Romantic forebears.

SOCIAL SHAME AND PUBLIC DISCIPLINE

So far we have seen how medical knowledge was used in service of a campaign against Godwin and Wollstonecraft, in the cause of morality and social order. This campaign also recruited the public to act as a disciplinary body, since there was a growing feeling that the public, and not the legal courts, was the most efficient means of winning the ongoing battle against moral deviance and political radicalism. This move is captured by the full title of one pamphlet in particular: *Thoughts on Marriage and Criminal Conversation, with some hints of appropriate means to check the progress of the latter; comprising remarks on the life, opinions, and example of the late Mrs. Wollstonecraft Godwin* (1799). This tract was addressed to Lord Kenyon, the Lord Chief Justice who notoriously demonstrated an inordinate amount of enthusiasm for criminal conversation trials, in which husbands brought suit against the lovers of their adulterous wives for the loss of property rights (since wives were legally considered their husbands' chattel). The author of this pamphlet, identified as "A Friend to the Social Order," urged readers to take up their critical role in the "civil war of lust" raging in Britain. In this war, the people could wield a valuable weapon—"SOCIAL SHAME"—that was more effective and faster acting than any legal court.[128] It was up to the public to ensure that moral, civil, or social laws regarding human relations, even if they appeared arbitrary or defective, remained safe from Godwin's rationality and Wollstonecraft's sexualized sensibility.

One of the ways that commentators recruited the public was to make heroic exemplars of those public figures who had snubbed Wollstonecraft. Reviewers interpreted Godwin's belief, stated in the *Memoirs*, that their "marriage would place her upon a sure footing *in the calendar of polished society*," as bare-faced impudence.[129] Such a comment demonstrates, they insisted, Godwin's lack of a sufficient understanding of human nature and his total disconnection from social reality. His philosophy would remove the social controls necessary to prevent men from becoming sexually voracious beasts and women their defenseless victims. Thankfully, certain well-known public figures had been exemplary in ejecting the dangerously philosophizing couple from the calendar of polished society. Journalists congratulated the actresses Sarah Siddons and Elizabeth Inchbald for refusing to receive their old friend Wollstonecraft after her 1797 marriage to Godwin. Her union with Godwin made it obvious that either she had never married her previous lover Gilbert Imlay, a man by whom she had had a child, or alternatively, that she had now become a polygamist. An *Anti-Jacobin* writer wrote that although "the morals of the great" were not as "correct as they ought to be," Siddons and Inchbald demonstrated that polite society was "not yet totally corrupt."[130] Wollstonecraft's philosophical "importance" could not excuse her private sins, nor could it "wash her clean" in the public eye.[131]

Siddons and Inchbald were moral exemplars for Britons who were pushed to similarly ostracize individuals who displayed qualities that smacked of new philosophy. *The Scientific Magazine* was unequivocal in its directive to readers: all Britons, whether "statesmen of the community" or "parents, anxious for the welfare of their children," had a clear duty to seek out and to expel Wollstonecraftian immorality and Godwinian reason.[132] The reviewer's language betrays a profound suspicion of unconventional relationships and an acute intolerance of social nonconformity. Like the authors of the medical treatises, pamphlets, and novels addressed in this chapter, reviewers used a powerfully persuasive rhetoric to condemn any sign of "a disposition to run counter to established practices and opinions."[133] The *Critical Review* urged Britons to take action against views that were "too much at variance with those which have been generally adopted."[134] These directives, which demarcated inappropriate practices and identified political illegitimacy, were never simply descriptive but rather were prescriptive.

We may be familiar with some of the reactionary anxieties and conservative sentiments expressed at the turn of the nineteenth century, yet we may have missed how the language of political reaction and moral reform became fused with medical discourses about sexual dysfunction, nerves and nervous disorders, and human dissection. In this era the fusion of the private and the public, the physiological and the political was used strategically to exclude reformers and radical thinkers from participating politically. Rather than directly address the arguments of Godwin's *Political Justice* (1793) or Wollstonecraft's *Vindications of the Rights of Men* (1790) or her *Vindications of the Rights of Woman* (1792), reactionaries needed only to represent the authors of these works as pathological, psychopathological, degenerate, or in Wollstonecraft's case, as susceptible to the "natural" biological weaknesses of her gender. Through the pillorying of their personal lives, the wider message transmitted to the public was this: democracy, materialism, modern medicine, and rationality made for a dangerous combination. This combination was all the more threatening when linked with the unfeeling and insensate body of an experimental philosopher *or* the sexually unpredictable, immoderately fertile, and overly nervous body of a woman radical.

4 Hygiene, Contamination, and Tom Paine's Toenails

> The reserve of reason ... like habitual cleanliness, is seldom seen in any great degree, unless the soul is active.
> MARY WOLLSTONECRAFT,
> *A Vindication of the Rights of Woman* (1792)

Perhaps no one was ever so blatant about unearthing the private sources of political corruption as the radical gentleman pamphleteer Charles Pigott. As we saw in the introduction to this book, he did not equivocate about his purpose for publishing scandalous material about the private lives of the upper orders. In his wildly scurrilous and very popular three-part *Jockey Club* and *Female Jockey Club*, he intended to reveal of what "superior materials" the aristocracy were "composed" in an effort to loosen their political hold.[1] These superior materials consisted largely of insatiable appetites for cards, horses, drinking, sex, and all other sources of debauchery. Pigott focused "the eyes of the multitude" on the connection between their own honest labors, the government's burdensome taxation policies, and aristocratic excesses.[2] His goals should not be confused, however, with the aims of members of radical groups like the London Corresponding Society (whose members tended to be of more humble origin); nor, as a debauchee himself, should Pigott be counted as part of the emerging "reform or ruin" movement of middle class moralists. Pigott was familiar with his subjects' lives because he moved in their circles and participated in some of the same activities. He was of an old landed family with the requisite credentials (including an Eton and Cambridge education); in his personal life he was, as his opponents liked to point out, as much a libertine as his targets. There is thus a paradox in Pigott's project: as Jon Mee puts it, "his Whiggish libertinism was both disavowed (in his attacks on upper-class immorality) and re-inscribed through a radical embrace of sexual 'freedom.'"[3]

We should not underestimate the power and scope of such narratives of politicized personal scandal. The number of sequels and editions, as well as the alarmed responses of conservatives, government officials, and other establishment figures—suggests that these pamphlets attracted a fairly wide audience. The court had serious fears about the dissemination of such "dangerous" writing. The Prince of Wales pronounced Pigott's *Jockey Club* "the most infamous & shocking libellous production" that had "ever disgraced the pen of man" and declared it as seditious as Thomas Paine's *Rights of Man*.[4] The papers of the wonderfully named John Reeves' Association for Preserving Liberty and Property against Republicans and Levellers contains alarmed letters from individuals of all classes who observed the buying and selling, and the reading aloud, of incendiary pamphlets in the streets. Among the letters sent to the Reeves headquarters at the Crown and Anchor tavern, and now held at the British Library, are reports about the distribution of Pigott's *Jockey Club* in particular. On 11 December 1792, an anxious correspondent wrote, "As the publication entitled the Jockey Club contains in my opinion a most scandalous Libel upon his Majesty I think it my *duty* to inform you that it continues to be publickly exhibited for Sale."[5] Another informant urged antirevolutionary associations to employ the same type of "medium" as Pigott had "to counteract the mischief" of scurrilous radical pamphlets.[6]

One Reevesite did just that. His anonymously authored *Answer to the Jockey Club* was quickly printed and distributed as "a good antidote to the poison of Pigot's [sic] infamous Books" that had "circulated throughout the Kingdom."[7] This proud "Member of the Jockey Club" attacked Pigott on the same grounds of immorality, arguing that the radical's own questionable affairs invalidated his allegations and brought his political motives sharply into question. This defender of his own (polite) class went on to describe how Pigott had himself "repudiated his wife" and "purchased the possession" of a certain Parisian lady's "charms with a forged draft" before abandoning her.[8]

Strikingly, in the *Answer to the Jockey Club*, Pigott's body and his questionable personal grooming habits are also targets. The defender of the status quo takes particular glee in informing readers about Pigott's struggle with lice infestations and his greasy, spotty complexion. While at Eton, Pigott's "particular neatness and attention to the furniture of his head" had earned him "the happy appellation of *Louse;* and at Cambridge, the beauty of a sallow face, enriched with variegated pimples, gained him the additional name of the *Ripe Whitlow*."[9] The author includes a poem, which had previously appeared in the *Morning Post* on 7 May 1792:

> Say, why does [Pigott] bear the Louse's name?
> His habits and his practice are the same.
> The natural Louse, by powerful instinct led,

> Finds peace and plenty in the school-boy's head.
> Louse—follows the same occupation,
> Lives on the heads of folks in higher station,
> Heads of the Jockey Club, and of the nation.[10]

Like the tiny parasite whose name he shares, Pigott is something of an atavistic creature here. He lacks civility; he has refused to adopt, or has left off, the rituals and routines associated with the care of the self in civilized society. He has reverted to living by animal instinct rather than being guided by discernment.

Pigott here is located within a genealogy of literary antiheroes who likewise suffer from bodily monstrosity. Quoting loosely from *Hamlet*, the anonymous author ranks Pigott with characters whose ill-formed bodies "were made by one of Nature's journeymen, that had not been an hour at the trade."[11] He goes on to compare Pigott's physical deformities to those of Laurence Sterne's Tristram Shandy, who suffers from a lack of vitality, a lack of a nose (lost to the physician's forceps at birth), a lack of a foreskin (lost to a falling window sash in childhood), and a lack of breath (the result of "skating against the wind in Flanders"). Ultimately, however, all of Tristram's physical defects result from the moment of his conception, when his mother became unfortunately distracted by an unwound clock. The newly conceived "homunculus" was destined to bear the unfortunate consequences of the first interruption of nature's work. Tristram is a victim of maternal impression: the diversion of the clock passes through the mother's imagination to mark the child's body, causing him a lifetime of health problems. Likewise cast "in the Shandean description," Charles Pigott traces a long trajectory back through his life's failures and bodily deformities to a flawed beginning: at his birth, the world had been similarly misaligned and nature had produced a monstrosity. At the moment Pigott was conceived, "the clock had not been wound up, the weights had not their proper draught, or the wheels their full velocity; so the homunculus was not electrified but affected, not at the birth, but at the origin. This is the best apology that can be made for a non-descript animal of the human form."[12]

In this view, Pigott's libelous attack on the British aristocracy, as well as his own propensity to cheat, betray, and steal, was connected to his bodily malformations. Pigott was a walking, talking, living example of the idea, so aptly expressed by the character of Tristram, that "a man's body and his mind . . . are exactly like a jerkin, and a jerkin's lining; rumple the one—you rumple the other."[13] Pigott's bodily habits were as degraded as his mind. His intentions, his beliefs, his philosophy, and his political principles were as unattractive as his stinking body, sallow complexion, and pocked skin.

The comparison of Pigott with Tristram Shandy conjures up the sense of both contagion and continuity. Disease and dysfunction never stay confined to one body. Physical dysfunction—a manifestation of intellectual weakness, political disloyalty, personal obsession, and philosophical inadequacy—is catching. In *Tristram*, bodily disorder is hereditary and transmittable: the father of the eponymous hero tends toward the "phthisisical" and suffers from sciatica; his uncle Toby is discharged from military service with a groin injury that leaves him sexually ineffective; and his brother Bobby, with his "wonderful slow parts," does not make it to adulthood. Tristram inherits physical weakness, which extends beyond family, rippling like waves of weakness throughout the community: Parson Yorick dies of much-feared consumption and each cursed body part of the servant Obadiah degrades until there is "no soundness in him"—and on and on it goes. Like Tristram, Pigott is not only the victim of a list of disorders but is the center of an ever-widening circle of disordered family members, servants, friends, and acquaintances.

The public exchange of reciprocal abuse between Pigott and his detractors demonstrates several important things: First, and most obvious, we can see it how adept loyalists became at appropriating and deflating radical strategies. Second, this kind of political propaganda was incredibly personal; it took aim at the most personal aspects of an individual's life. Pigott attacked inequality, government corruption, and the abuse of power by attacking people's sex lives, their addictions, and their personal appearance. The third characteristic of these exchanges has received less attention, although it was a particularly critical aspect of the era's political scandal: physical disease was connected to ideas about political contamination. Loyalists drew on medical information about hygiene and personal grooming habits in order to construct an image of radicals as physically monstrous, as mired in filth, as carriers of disease, and as sexually immoral. At the same time, they represented reformers and radicals as conduits through whom dangerous contaminants would be introduced into the body politic. Pigott may have been rendered monstrous by an accident of birth, but he had developed bodily deficiencies that, like his acts of class betrayal, were distinctly communicable. The contaminants at issue were political in nature—cosmopolitan liberalism, social equality, demands for individual liberties—but they acted very much like biological infections. Radical political ideas and demands for reform introduced instability and harm into an otherwise productive, ordered environment.

Roy Porter and George Rousseau once commented that "pathography may be the key to biography," and in many ways Pigott is an interesting case in point. The interconnectedness of body and mind meant that disease and disorders would greatly influence an individual's life and work. In the realm of politics, propagandists created a kind of politico-pathographic genre of scandal that identified intimate links between the individual's medical history and his political philosophy. Pigott's enemies made the story of his dirty body and his grubby personal habits the story of his public life.[14] He was not the only figure who was an object of pathography; in fact, the real story here is about Tom Paine. In the 1790s and the early decades of the nineteenth century, the narratives created about his diseases, alleged addictions, sexual proclivities, and personal hygiene had immeasurable effects on his career, the legacy of his political philosophy, and wider political culture.

As with Pigott, Paine was accused of dirty dealing. In the mid-1790s, propagandists made connections between the state of his body, his politics, and his debauched private life. Anti-Painites contended that his solitariness, his drunkenness, his dirtiness, his animalistic features, and his sexual deviance were all physical manifestations of his mutinous politics. Pointing to alleged reports of his slovenly dress, his pockmarked face, his boozy breath, his filthy sexual habits, and the stench of his unwashed body, loyalists argued that Paine's physicality revealed a lack of personal integrity and a disdain for moral decency and an honest day's work. His body bore testimony to the sins he had committed against a nation he had attempted to coax into seditious rebellion. Through the efforts of his political enemies, his allegedly diseased, alcoholic, sexually dysfunctional, pocked, and dirty body became the signifier of his true intentions.

A VERY PUBLIC VIVISECTION

In 1776, Paine could declare in *Common Sense* that "who the Author of this Production is, is wholly unnecessary to the Public, as the Object for Attention is the Doctrine itself, not the Man."[15] But by the end of the century, the question of "who" was a vital concern in British politics, so that the public came to believe "the Man" was very much part of "the Doctrine itself." In the years following publication of Paine's 1791 and 1792 *Rights of Man*, loyalists argued that the private lives of reformers clearly indicated just how much of a political threat they posed. This allegation became established almost as a principle, so that political contests often pushed the question of personality, personal morality, and private habits ahead of the question of political doctrine. The propaganda surrounding Paine's appearance, alleged lack of hygiene, sexual deviance, and alcoholism (the latter two having much to do with his "dirty" reputation) made his statement in *Common Sense* about the insignificance of the author's identity sound like wishful thinking indeed.

In 1792, the newly formed John Reeves' Association for Preserving Liberty and Property against Republicans and Levellers published a series of popular tracts aimed at countering the pernicious spread of Painite revolutionary clubs. In *A Bird in the Hand Is Worth Two in the Bush*, a worker renounces his newly formed radical ties because, having read the recently published *Life of Thomas Pain* (with its intentional misspelling), he now disdained any "association" with that notorious radical.[16] Popular loyalist propaganda did much to promote this image of contamination, of infection, of guilt by association. Britons were warned, as patriotic citizens, to make themselves knowledgeable about Paine's life in order to recognize the symptoms of his particular brand of disease and prevent its spread. Through his best-selling and hugely influential *Life of Thomas Pain*, the Scottish antiquarian and government propagandist George Chalmers initiated a public interrogation of Paine's private life that would continue for over two hundred years.[17] A quick survey of the political literature of 1792–93 reveals the degree to which Paine's biography immediately inspired many political commentators to urge their readers to familiarize themselves with those "truths" that lurked beneath the radical's public personae.

Chalmers's book—interestingly described by a late nineteenth-century biographer as "a vivisection of Paine"—and the anti-Painite propaganda that followed in its wake speaks to the same public that Paine addressed in the *Rights*. The populace needed to be apprised of "the truth" about the private affairs of an author who had become, for some, a political messiah.[18] Attacks on Paine's private life and his state of health were one way of dealing with the newly politicized members of the lower orders who were making a bid for citizenship status based on reason, rather than on traditional notions of custom and inheritance, political privilege and property ownership. The urgency of the times, and Paine's popularity, meant that even those who would otherwise avoid scandalmongering felt it necessary to address the unsavory rumors about Paine's personal habits. "Of the private history of Mr. Paine, I neither know any thing, [n]or wish to enquire," the member of Parliament Sir Brooke Boothby conceded, but since "these questions" were now pertinent, it was his duty to familiarize himself with Chalmers's biography.[19] The rather more plebeian "Citizens of Caledonia" published a 1792 New Year's address to Paine, in which they exercised their self-proclaimed "right to try a man as well as to judge of his book."[20] Such commentary was a harbinger and a consequence of the belief that an individual's political intentions and capabilities could be gauged by that person's habits, health, and sexual proclivities.

HYGIENE, DISEASE, AND SOCIAL ORDER

In her seminal work, *Purity and Danger*, the social anthropologist Mary Douglas situates attitudes and norms about the cleanliness of bodies, places, and spaces within a wider web of cultural meanings. She describes how dirt, contagion, and pollution are "analogies for expressing a general view of the social order."[21] This is as true for the "primitive" cultures that Douglas studies as it is for for nineteenth-century culture and our own. Attitudes about personal hygiene reflect larger negotiations about political questions and social relations. Appeals to nature are used to legitimize ideas about purity, nature, health, and goodness, and in an effort to fashion the individual into a good citizen, "the laws of nature are dragged in to sanction the moral code."[22] In other words, nature is used to reinforce practices of hygiene; those practices are then used to enforce codes of civility and communal values. In Europe at the turn of the nineteenth century, such appeals were made in service to combating the emergence of a historically specific political contagion: modern republicanism. In the 1790s, the process of solidifying cultural norms, maintaining political cohesiveness, and reinforcing normative moral and political values buttressed the nation against such dangerous contagions as Jacobinism, revolutionary fervor, antimonarchical sentiment, and British working-class radicalism.

Tom Paine's career reveals how intimately ideas about cleanliness and political culture became entwined. Literary critics and historians who have mapped the rise and fall (and subsequent rises and falls) of Paine's reputation and his politics have skimmed over the ways that antirevolutionaries, in their portrayals of Paine, appealed to public fears about disease and ideas about contamination. I argue that biographers and propagandists could make so much of Paine's supposed filthiness *only* because the rather loose standards of eighteenth-century personal hygiene were quickly giving way to a more fastidious emphasis on cleanliness. New knowledge was circulating about the impact of dirt, pollution, and foul air on the spread of both physical and moral disease. Physicians linked dirt and unclean habits with iniquity, apathy, social irresponsibility, irreligion, and political guile. Loyalists tapped into fears about revolution and the burgeoning emphasis on moral probity to forge a tripartite connection between bodily cleanliness, clean politics, and "clean living."

As a transatlantic figure, Paine's body was the special target of a rather lengthy list of both British and Anglo-American conservatives who were determined to turn Paine's fame into infamy and his popularity into ancient history. These antirevolutionaries portrayed Paine as physically monstrous, a representation that largely originated with George Chalmers's consistently reprinted 1791 biography and further diffused through the expatriate James Cheetham's 1809 American-published *Life of Paine* (printed in England in 1817). In the first flush of heady revolutionary fervor in the early 1790s, Cheetham had been a Painite, along with his radical brothers, collectively known as the three Jacobin infidels. He was affiliated both with the Constitutional Society and the Manchester Reformation Society. One of his own political enemies described him as a troublemaker who had run "with the *Rights of Man* in one hand, and *Age of Reason* in another . . . from tavern to tavern and from brothel to brothel, collecting and summoning together all that wickedness had rendered contemptible, drunkenness turned idle, and indolence made destitute."[23] When Cheetham was tried and acquitted on charges of conspiracy in 1794, he emigrated to New York, where he jumped back into politics as editor of the *American Citizen*. But after being unceremoniously ousted from the Republican Party, he announced his break with democratic politics and celebrated his apostasy with his venomous 1809 *Life of Thomas Paine*.

A dirty, diseased, alcohol-soaked Paine proliferated in word and image on both sides of the Atlantic. Even in private correspondence, he was described in the inflated language of vitriolic biographies. In an October 1805 letter to the scientist and physician Benjamin Waterhouse, the Federalist statesman John Adams raged against Paine's *Age of Reason*, but his most acerbic words were saved for the author himself:

> I am willing you should call this the Age of Frivolity as you do, and would not object if you had named it the Age of Folly, Vice, Frenzy, Brutality, Daemons, Buonaparte, Tom Paine, or the Age of the Burning Brand from Bottomless Pit, or anything but the Age of Reason. I know not whether any man in the world has had more influence on its inhabitants or affairs for the last thirty years than Tom Paine. There can be no severer satyr on the age. For such a mongrel between pig and puppy, begotten by a wild boar on a bitch wolf,

never before in any age of the world was suffered by the poltroonery of mankind, to run through such a career of mischief. Call it then the Age of Paine.[24]

Aside from this wonderfully over-the-top explosion of words, Adams gives an equally wonderful backhanded compliment about Paine's popularity and influence (although both were fading fast by this time). This passage presents Paine as something of a half-monster, half-animal, left behind in a distinctly uncivilized past while progress marches forward. He is an atavistic being, a hideous progeny who has gone out into the world to disseminate his foul doctrines and to prosper by way of an undeserved fame.

Adams's explosion of words uses language that dogged Paine from the early days of the French Revolution through the nineteenth century. In his *Rights of Englishmen: An Antidote to the Poison now Vending by the Transatlantic Republican Thomas Paine* (1791), the loyalist Reverend Isaac Hunt proposes that if said Englishmen were to peer into the looking glass of the ugly Tom Paine, they would "see all the prominent, dismal features, the scowling brow, the hard and brazen front of this dingy, ugly, voracious, boasted monster from America."[25] As a marker on the surface of the body, ugliness not only indicates that disease and dysfunction plague the organs within but also reveals the sickly political motivations and ambitions lurking in the mind. Deformed by his beliefs and his wasted life, Paine was monstrously animal-like and, in the language of countless pamphleteers, he was a filthy, drunken atheist. The intention is to tangibly demarcate Paine from "normal" God-fearing, family-loving Britons by making him appear a physical monstrosity who, more than simply lacking the cultural refinements of civilized society, is so filthy and unfamiliar as to appear subhuman. This characterization would make it difficult for readers to visualize him as one of their own and practically impossible for them to see him as a political hero.

The issue of cleanliness takes center stage both in Isaac Hunt's scurrilous pamphlet and in Cheetham's biography of Paine. Anecdotal material, such as the following remarkable passage, part of a letter allegedly written to Paine by his old friend and final carer, William Carver, was either made up by or reproduced by Cheetham:

> You appeared as if you had not shaved for a fortnight, and as to a shirt, it could not be said that you had one on; it was only the remains of one, and this likewise appeared not to have been off your back for a fortnight, and was nearly the colour of tanned leather, and you had the most disagreeable smell possible; just like that of our poor

beggars in England. Do you not recollect the pains I took to clean you? That I got a tub of warm water and soap, and washed you from head to foot, and this I had to do three times, before I could get you clean. . . . Have you forgotten the pains I took with you when you lay sick, wallowing in your own filth? . . . a friend of mine . . . assist[ed] me in removing and cleaning you. He told me he wondered how I could do it; for his part he would not like to do the same for ten dollars.[26]

Carver gives a blow-by-blow account of how he allegedly saved the ungrateful, drunken and disgusting Paine from languishing in a tavern by taking him in, only to witness the undignified state of the needy Paine's diseased and broken body. That Paine is described here, as he would be in many caricatures and satires, as wearing an almost nonexistent shirt is much more derogatory than it may at first appear to us. In *Fashioning the Frame: Boundaries, Dress and the Body*, Alexandra Warwick and Dani Cavallaro remind us that clothing is a "boundary" that "is meant to trace a neat line between self and other."[27] Any violation of this boundary places the naked subject, who is left exposed to outside contaminants, in a vulnerable position. However, in Cheetham's representation of Paine this is reversed: the public is vulnerable to the physically and politically contaminating Paine. Without clean and proper clothing, he exceeds personal boundaries. His dirty, monstrous body, like other monstrous bodies described by cultural theorist Margrit Shildrick, is seen "as dangerously contagious, capable of spreading its own confusion of identity."[28] Paine represents a confusion of identity: he was an outsider, an interloper without position, wealth, or connections, yet immensely influential. He politicized—or infected—whole nations of people who were likewise without position, wealth, or connections, inspiring them to demand enfranchisement and equal rights—demands that upset the social order and threatened the constitution.

In *Foul Bodies*, Kathleen Brown details the rising importance of the shirt in the first half of the eighteenth century. There were many features of the shirt's "peculiar, conflated relationship with the body itself," but one important cultural belief was "that civilized people covered their skins." There emerged, she explains, "a transatlantic sense of belonging to a community whose aesthetics and care of the body were captured by the laundered white shirt."[29] This shirt became the skin that expressed the person beneath: it expressed civility, modernity, honor, status, taste, manners, and sensibility. It was the sign of a disciplined person whose body was as refined as his judgment. But as is the case with all aspects of clothing and bodily regimen, much more information about identity is expressed through self-presentation and public interpretation. How one's body is clothed affects public perceptions about political trustworthiness and intellectual ability. The way bodies are presented has much to do with whose opinions are given credence.

The meanings attached to clothing and cleanliness form a particularly germane context to anti-Painite political scandal. The clothed body was a closed and contained body, but the shirtless body disseminated dirt, disease, and other less material substances. The portrayal of the shirtless Paine expressed fears about the propagation of his ideas. In violating the sartorial boundary between self and world, he indicated his unwillingness to respect social boundaries and moral limits. There was very little of the "drapery of life" between the body of Tom Paine, his American bar-room audience, and the poor beggars of England. With no such hindrances, his principles (like his foul body odor) were transmitted to and received by his audience as if by osmosis. The boundaries between him and the world were treacherously permeable. This permeability was most obvious in the unpretentious language of the *Rights of Man*. The straightforward writing of the man of humble beginnings and limited formal education had demonstrated how the aura of political privilege could be stripped away. Paine at least narrowed the gap between socially superior leaders and their challengers, and between politicians and the people.

In the 1790s and throughout the following decades, the sobriquet most often attached to Tom Paine's name was "filthy." But this word and the disgusting picture of his body presented in Carver's letters were not enough for propagandists like Cheetham, who insisted that any "description of Paine's filthiness" could only fall short of "the reality" since even imagination could not conjure "an object so offensive to sense."[30] The image of the dirty radical permeated anti-Jacobin literature in all its forms and tainted the reputations of other reformers by association, so that, for example, in his 1807 novel *George the Third*, Edward Mangin made reference to the "Jacobin toilette"—a newly adopted habit of personal grooming that counted such basic ingredients as soap as superfluous.[31] Indeed, Cheetham recalled anecdote after anecdote about a whole range of Paine's filthy habits. Taking pleasure in "nastiness," the radical "would eat his breakfast, if he could without washing himself."[32] He slept all day and drank grog all night until he fell off his chair onto a filthy, litter-strewn floor to sleep.[33] As time went on, his personal habits became worse. So, when in February 1808 he finally ran out of people who were willing to board him, he moved into a tavern that boasted a shoddy sixpenny show.

Left to his own devices in an environment that so obviously suited him, he was "drunk every day, he was neither washed nor shaved nor shirted for weeks."[34] In fact, Cheetham insists, "he was so indescribably and notoriously nasty, that he might well contend with the showman for the most numerous audience of curious spectators."[35] All attempts to intervene, even offers to pay for his baths, fell on deaf ears, since "his crust of filth seemed to give him comfort."[36]

Clearly, these representations were calculated to shock and disgust the reading public and to rouse them to join the anti-Painite countermovement. That these images had the power to disgust indicates the degree to which the issue of bodily cleanliness had by this time become an issue of public concern. Hygiene was a serious moral and medical matter. In 1762, Jeans-Jacques Rousseau insisted that "hygiene is the only useful part of medicine, and hygiene is rather a virtue than a science."[37] He went on, in *Émile*, to outline the importance of a lifetime habit of regular bathing and promoted the wearing of clean linen. In these same years, marked advances in epidemiology and interest in the relationship between an individual's private regimen and the state of the wider social environment intensified. As a result, there was an explosion of health advice manuals and studies on the environmental impact of personal cleanliness. New theories circulated about epidemics, largely due to observations and experiments performed by eighteenth-century prison and military doctors, who witnessed how rapidly disease spread among prisoners and enlisted men. Dr. John Pringle found that skin diseases—endemic in the overcrowded conditions of military camps—responded to ancient practices of bodily and sartorial hygiene, as well as the circulation of fresh air. Pringle's discoveries provided a major impetus for a "neoclassical revival of military hygiene."[38] In a somewhat ironic twist, the radical gentleman libertarian Charles Pigott was one of those individuals who contracted prison fever while incarcerated, awaiting trial for toasting the French Revolution with a reference to George III as a "German hog butcher." The indictment may have been thrown out, but the month spent in a damp prison meant the end for Pigott, who died shortly thereafter in 1794.

Crucially, a whole vocabulary of terms—such as *contagion, contamination, malignity, offensiveness*—proliferated in treatises on the spread of fever and smallpox and became part of common speech. Dr. John Armstrong's medicopoetic text, *The Art of Preserving Health: A Poem* (first published in 1744) indicates the degree to which discursive crossovers between medicine, literature, and politics were disseminated in literary forms. Armstrong describes how contagious materials festered in dirty dank corners and diffused through the air. Air was thought to be cleansing, bracing, and life-giving, but in the crowded and often squalid spaces of metropolitan cities, it became the rank carrier of disease. Invisible contaminants then entered the unsuspecting body:

> It is not air
> That from a thousand Lungs reeks back to thine,
> Sated with exhalations; rank and fell;
> The spoil of dunghills, and the putrid thaw
> Of nature; when from shape and texture she
> Relapses into fighting elements;————
> It is not air, but floats a nauseous mass
> Of all obscene, corrupt, offensive things.[39]

The inner organs of the body had a sympathetic relationship with the external environment, and in the newly urbanized, crowded modern world this environment had become fetid and polluted. Armstrong's passage appeared in British and American medical texts, including John Alderson's 1788 *Essay on the Nature and Origin of the Contagion of Fevers*. Alderson, a fellow of the Royal Medical Society of Edinburgh, argued that contagion had become most alarming at the end of the eighteenth century because of migration to cities and changes in human relations, which brought all kinds of people together in close proximity. The uncontrollable spread of disease had been a common problem in jailhouses and ships, but now cities had become like urban jails. "Multitudes who have no Crime to expiate, no Debt to discharge to the Public, no unrelenting Creditor to satisfy" lived in the same conditions as criminals and were thereby susceptible to the same diseases.[40]

Alderson and Armstrong were among a contingent of doctors who made claims about disease, modern life, industry, and political change based on a country versus city dichotomy. Alderson described a healthier past when "the Operations of Nature" had ensured that the body's effluvia had passed into the environment to decompose and become part of the organic cycle of life.[41] But now, "when the Human race" had relinquished "the Comforts of Independence" and had "crowded into Cities" in search of wealth, industry, and luxury, people had "breathed their own Destruction."[42] Armstrong's poem, which shared a similar diagnosis, gave this poetic advice to readers:

> Ye who amid this feverish world would wear
> A body free of pain, of cares a mind;
> Fly the rank city, shun its turbid air
> Breathe not the chaos of eternal smoke

And volatile corruption, from the dead,
The dying, sickening, and the living world.[43]

Both Alderson and Armstrong, as well as many other notable writers on the subject, exploited the nostalgic and well-established idea of rural life as the good life: the countryside remained as natural and unadulterated as God intended, while the city was a manifestation of human debauchery, selfish ambition, and unbridled commerce.

Medicopoetic writing on airborne contaminants and disease had much in common with other literary forms that extolled the virtues of a harmonious countryside. This conception of the English countryside was, to use Raymond Williams's expression, "a myth functioning as memory."[44] Medical texts on disease often promoted this myth in support of a conservative worldview and the established social order. Williams's observations about how the country and city became structuring symbols, which accounted for the economic and cultural changes associated with modernization, helps us understand how and why biographical political propaganda functioned so effectively in this period. This naturalized myth, which was embedded in medical writing, also helps us understand how the discourse surrounding cleanliness, impurity, and contamination could have been so effectively mobilized against Paine, so that it successfully silenced his politics. The various phenomena of modernization, including the rise of urban, artisanal Painite radicalism, were closely connected to the spread of disease. Mechanized labor and industry (and the resulting sedentary habits), along with progressive politics, newfangled philosophies, and modern morality, disrupted human ecology and endangered life.

In his 1992 book, *Explaining Epidemics,* Charles Rosenberg describes two early-modern models of understanding the spread of disease. Medical texts that warned of the dangers of an urban environment provide good examples of the "configuration" model. Advocates of this model, like Alderson and Armstrong, believed that changes to the "normal" and "health-maintaining" environment resulted in the rapid spread of disease.[45] By contrast, the "contamination" model, which Alderson and Armstrong also promoted, posited "the transmission of some morbid material from one individual to another."[46] Of course, these models appeared in different degrees and manifestations at different times, and as the examples above indicate, they were not mutually exclusive. Still, some late eighteenth-century and early nineteenth-century doctors leaned toward the contamination model, emphasizing the close reciprocity that existed between individuals. For them, lungs "impregnate the Atmosphere with . . . contagious Matter" that was then quickly inhaled by other sets of lungs.⁴⁷ This model of disease placed responsibility for the health of the wider community firmly with the individual.

Reflecting this emphasis on individual accountability in a codependent world, medical manuals counseled readers to live clean and upstanding lives. In his 1799 *Lectures on Diet and Regimen*, the physician A.F.M. Willich wrote that cleanliness did more than preserve "health"; it was also a vital "domestic virtue." He elaborated: "This domestic virtue ought to extend its influence to every object connected with the human frame; to the preparation and consumption of food and drink, to dress, habitation, household furniture, and all our physical wants; *in a word, cleanliness should not be confined merely to the interior domestic œconomy; it claims our attention in every place which we occupy, and wherein we breathe.*"⁴⁸ Clearly, this passage promotes a normative model of cleanliness, which applies to every sphere of material life, and it emphasizes in no uncertain terms the importance of hygiene in creating healthful and morally uplifting lives. Willich extends the parameters of hygiene into the public sphere, into the marketplace and convivial spaces. The emphasis is again on nasty environments as polluting air and on air as the conduit by which insidious materials enter one's body. But, the onus of disease prevention is manifestly on the individual. This is particularly so since, frighteningly, the very constitution of the self is changed through *invisible contact*. It made sense, then, that dirtiness became a violation of one's familial and communal responsibility. Dr. Bernhard Faust's *Catechism of Health*, for instance, counseled readers that cleanliness preserved one's virtue and cleared one's mind, as well as earned one "the esteem of others."⁴⁹ By the first decades of the nineteenth century, this discourse had become resolutely instructive about the effect cleanliness had on the wider social order.

In their influential work on the culture of contamination, Roy Porter and George Rousseau argue that "discourse about disease goes beyond recognizing the powers of pathogens: it may be freighted with associations like disorder and dirt which embody value judgments and emotive charges."⁵⁰ In fact, I would say that it is practically impossible to uncouple the language of disease from emotion and moral judgment. Perhaps the most obvious example of how dirt became associated with vice and social deviance is William Clayton's mid-nineteenth-century pamphlet, *Lecture on Dirt Delivered to the Harrow Young Men's Society*. Although it appeared some decades after Paine's biographies, it demonstrates how much the medical-moral stress on cleanliness had evolved. Clayton defines dirt as a sign of the most sinful of natures. Since "DIRT IS POISON!" he shrills, it follows that unclean households are responsible for poisoning the air and thus other people around them.[51] Dirt, discontent, and the fumes of alcohol sully the air and contaminate urban dwellers. "Dirt," Clayton argues, "is the chief hinderer of God's work in our bodies" as well as "the chief cause of our bodily discomfort and ailments, and even of premature death."[52] Cleanliness is not just next to godliness: it is godliness. We must seek out pure air, in both a material and a moral sense, in order to cleanse the body—the dwelling house of God—and to keep the brain and the soul functioning as he intended. Dirt is a sign of personal corruption and a potentially devastating source of social, moral, and physical infection. Individuals who do not attend "with peculiar care to the means which God has provided for freeing our bodies" from "internal dirt" are "extremely culpable."[53] "The dirty man cares for nobody," Clayton admonishes, and "slinks away from respectable people."[54]

This is disciplinary discourse. No one wants be a deadly carrier of infection or a dirty threat to innocent others. Doctors at the time urged governments to take charge of sanitation and to enforce personal hygiene practices. Willich wrote, for instance, about how the ancient Jews transmitted important rituals and regimens to the Egyptians, Greeks, and Romans, so that those who "were pronounced unclean" were also pronounced "unfit to hold any intercourse or communion with others, until they had performed the appointed ablutions."[55] He approved wholeheartedly of the way members of the community and various religious bodies took charge of enforcing bathing habits in ancient cultures. So important were practices involving the care of the self that the Spartans refused to trust bathing "to the caprice of individuals'; rather they considered it "a public institution" to be managed by the state.[56] Willich was urging social order enforced from the top down, but his stance was also part of new methods of governmentality—to use Foucault's expression—that evolved in much more nuanced ways. In the case of the rise of hygiene, the middle classes in particular became enmeshed in processes of self-discipline. Manuals like Willich's encouraged readers to demonstrate personal virtue, domestic economy, and social responsibility by keeping clean.

Both the configuration model of disease (unhealthy environments produce illness) and the contamination model (individuals spread infection) provide a framework for understanding the rhetorical thrust of Willich's arguments and other medical and political writing on hygiene. The message of these tracts was that altering the existing social order or upsetting the normal balance of communities produced conditions favorable to the spread of disease. In addition, the idea of a solitary person being responsible for the "morbid Excretion of Effluvium from the Body" into the wider world where it caused disease and death was a powerful image, which acted as a potent paradigm for political propagandists of all kinds.[57] In turn, all of these connected ideas about disease, hygiene, and contagion provide a context for understanding the effectiveness of propaganda against Paine and his politics. Anti-Painite representations effectively made use of both models of disease, which curbed his influence and destroyed his career. Paine's call for liberty and equality altered the social landscape, for uppity laborers and pushy mechanics refused to stay in their place. From Paine's mouth and hand, the effluvium of republicanism and revolution entered the wider world; his call for rights and liberties caught the people's imagination, and their enthusiasm spread like an uncontrolled fever.

At the same time, the configuration model of disease helps us understand how dangerous the Painite revolutionary clubs were thought to be, as they mushroomed in villages and towns across the nation and, in particular, attracted artisanal urbanites in centers like London, Manchester, and Edinburgh. The spread of associations such as the London Corresponding Society was described in remarkably similar terms as the spread of jail fever and smallpox.[58] Anti-Painites emphasized the reciprocal relationship between radical politics and bodily impurity. They cast republicanism as a parasitical political philosophy that vampirically drained its adherents of their vitality. The image of the unsuspecting populace being contaminated and its lifeblood forever altered is not far off from representations of dirt as contamination. In his polemic against dirt, William Clayton insisted that "dirt is not a part of our nature: it is a parasite thriving on our heart's blood, like a vampire [that] sucks away the life, without the poor patient's knowing anything about it."[59] In similar ways, biographers insisted that Paine's own parasitical nature was written on his body, much as Bram Stoker's Dracula would be identified by his pointed canine teeth, hairy palms, and long, sharpened fingernails. Isaac Hunt remarked on the "length and strength" of Paine's fingernails and toenails and on "the sharpness of his *nails and teeth*."[60] These features indicated that, having given his body and soul over to republicanism, Paine had himself become a feeder. He was an atavistic being, whose nails indicated that he was a throwback to a less civilized age or, at the very least, was left over from a less fastidious age, an age before the world understood about contagion and disease.

Literary scholarship has unearthed the relationship between the trope of the vampire and the types of political and medical representations we have seen here. Eve Sedgwick has written about how the self is often presented in gothic literature as "a vesicle of life substance" that is "separated from the surrounding reality by a thin membrane."[61] When "the protective membrane" that surrounds the self is ruptured—by, for instance, the penetrating teeth of the vampire—that self is threatened with "dissolution through an uncontrolled influx of excitation."[62] This image of reciprocity between self and outside world, and self and other, is useful for understanding the literary and visual construction of Paine. The existence of this cultural trope also gives us a sense of how menacing Paine would have appeared to a public that had witnessed the horrors of revolutionary excess across the Channel *and* had also experienced the daily horrors of disease (puerperal fever, smallpox, consumption, etc.).

PAINE'S STIGMATA

Paine's nails were his stigmata. Sociologists Erving Goffman and Gerhard Falk have shown how common physical signifiers allow communities to maintain a sense of cohesion.[63] Corporeal markings—whether deemed appropriate or inappropriate—are visual cues that federate individuals and stigmatize others. The act of stigmatizing unites the majority group who define themselves against the stigmatized outsider. Common identities are established through the ritualized disciplining of individuals who express nonstandard or deviant ideas and behaviors. Stigmatized individuals are differentiated from the "normals," to use Goffman's term, since "by definition . . . we believe the person with a stigma is not quite human."[64] This perceived lack of humanity has classical origins: for the ancients, the stigma identified the bearer as a traitor whose traitorous qualities tainted those with whom he or she had contact.

Biographers identified a remarkable variety of stigmatizing phenomena on Paine's body. The radical's political and personal sins were inscribed on his face and body in the same way that Old Testament villains bore the mark of their transgressions. Stories circulated about how a Presbyterian immigrant to America, Grant Thorburn, had tried to convert Paine. In his memoirs, Thorburn described how the irreligious radical had fallen into squalor, so that "he was the most disgusting human being you could meet in the street. Through the effect of intemperance his countenance was bloated beyond description—he looked as if God had stamped his face with the mark of Cain."[65] Making a similar comparison, Charles Harrington Elliot pointed out that there was more than a "strange coincidence in sound and character" between "Paine" and "Cain."[66] As in the embittered biblical fratricide, in which Cain bore the mark of his crime, the body of the modern-day radical testified to his misdeeds, so virtuous folk could recognize him for what he was.

Paine's biographers also cast him as the exiled Old Testament king Nebuchadnezzar, who the Bible describes as having hair "like eagles' feathers" and "nails like birds' claws."[67] Although Nebuchadnezzar is a biblical character, he is represented, like Paine, as an atavistic body that refused to be scrubbed, groomed, dressed, and modernized. Both Halford and Cheetham described how genteel people who came into contact with Paine were horrified to see that his toenails had "'exceeded half an inch in length' and grew, bird-like around his toes 'nearly as far under as they extended on top.'"[68] We have already seen how Paine's nails were given as evidence of his animalism and his vampirism, but in light of a growing emphasis on personal hygiene, his toenails were a slightly different type of stigmata. In the late eighteenth and early nineteenth centuries, the newly disciplined and socially aspirational body, with its significant markers of bodily restraint—trimmed hair, fresh breath, clean linen—clashed against the filthy and corrupted bodies of past generations and non-Europeans.

In his 1792 caricature, *Tom Paine's Nightly Pest* (figure 4.1), James Gillray portrays the filthy Paine covered only by a coat, asleep on a rickety bedstead, his head on a pile of straw barely held together by torn cloth. Paine's jutting toenails match those of the starving and regressive sansculottes, portrayed elsewhere in Gillray's canon (see, for instance, the 1792 print *French Liberty/British Slavery*). The message of *Nightly Pest* is that Paine's liberty and equality would halt productivity and bring an end to real justice—and cause all Britons to regress to the same state of filth and poverty as he had.

There is something very significant about the way that satirists and biographers fastened on this particular and most incidental of body parts. At the end of the eighteenth century, the ostensibly unimportant nail became the focus of doctors who outlined their proper care. "Long nails, especially as they were in fashion some years ago," Dr. Willich wrote in his *Lectures on Diet and Regimen*, "disfigure the hands, and prevent the feet from expanding properly."[69] Times had changed, and for an increasingly health-conscious public, shorter, neater, cleaner nails were de rigueur. Paine's biographers employed the methodology of medical writers, diagnosing and prescribing proper care for each body part rather than

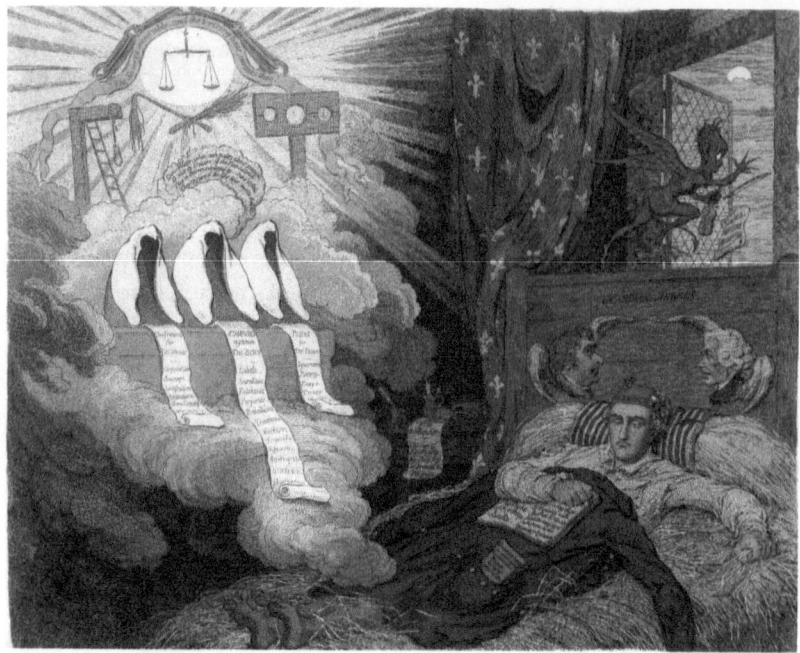

Figure 4.1 James Gillray, *Tom Paine's Nightly Pest* (1792 © Trustees of the British Museum, London)

the body as a whole. In their dissection of Paine's living body, his toenails became part of a campaign to map moral deviance and to locate nefarious political ambitions on the body's surface. His political opponents insisted that the public should use his pathological physicality to recognize his philosophies as outmoded, corrupt, and dangerous. There is, in all the scurrilous biographies, an effort to physically demarcate political incapacity in a way reminiscent of physiognomical or phrenological efforts to identify criminality and deviance. Anti-Painite biographers read political motives on the body in the way that physiognomists conceived of the body as a text upon which one could read character, motive, and intelligence.

In fact, like physiognomists, Paine's biographers insisted that his dysfunction could be read in his face. In his *Life of Thomas Pain*, Chalmers informed readers that in Paine's youth, even before he had been so horribly scarred by revolutionary politics, he had "always appeared to female eyes a dozen years older than he was, owing to the hardness of his features, or to the scars of disease."[70] This may be an implicit suggestion that

Paine had suffered from smallpox (as at least one scholar has recently claimed). Like Gillray's visual image of a pocked Paine, Chalmers's reference to the scars of disease exploited deep cultural fears about contamination. It also expressed the aim—of scientists and laypeople—to render the body transparent or, more precisely, to accurately identify character, intelligence, motives, and criminal tendencies from bodily clues.

In the eighteenth century, smallpox was a horribly contagious disease that quickly covered the entire surface of a healthy body in terrible rashes and suppurating, stinking pustules. Those few who survived the disease were stigmatized by permanent scars—marks of human vulnerability—that once would have been filled with putrefying blisters, reminding observers of a living body already in a state of advanced decomposition. For these reasons, the disease was a particularly traumatic illness, psychologically and socially. Victims were often so horrendously scarred that they were almost unrecognizable to acquaintances. They were not only shunned socially but often looked alien even to themselves. The sense was that one could never fully recover from the cruel disease that, as the seventeenth-century physician Martin Lluelyn wrote, "strove to deface" and, in the words of the poet Henry Jones, left "deep degrading Spots."[71] There is a body of seventeenth- and eighteenth-century therapeutic poetry that expresses the alienating anguish of permanent physical change. In "Beauty's Enemy," Henry Bold describes how the faces of smallpox victims were so disfigured that "the Soul would hardly, own / The Body, at the Resurrection!"[72] This is a frightening image of misrecognition and estrangement. Smallpox so disfigured the face—the site of recognition, communication, and personal identity—that in effect the survivor had his or her personal identity erased. In the case of Paine, his facial scars signal the loss of an original self, which was tied to his birthplace, his loyal and God-fearing family, his past, his home, his nation. His scars are reminders that he rejected all to become a wandering, rootless citizen of the world.

Paine's pockmarks also signal disruption and disorder. David Shuttleton makes the point that smallpox "presented a particularly intensified site of disruption, where the stabilizing distinction between the governable body cultural and the disruptive body natural breaks down."[73] Shuttleton's "governable body cultural," which invokes Foucault's docile body, might be identified as the loyal, upstanding average Briton. But Paine's pockmarks signify his refusal or inability to fit this mold: he is uncultured, unruly, and animalistic; he displays a "disruptive body natural." This is *not* the naturally cooperative and innocent body of Rousseau's noble savage, but a body that might be described by Thomas Hobbes: an anarchistic, inherently selfish product of an indifferent state of nature. With its bodily odors, its layer of dirt, and its animalistic sexual urges (about which we will see more), Paine's body is a frightening reminder of how easily humanity could revert to a pre-enlightened, precivilized state. The fear that this type of bestial body had the potential to cause political disorder gained "a fresh intensity" in the 1790s, as Shuttleton notes, because of both the tumultuous political climate and the development of inoculation.[74] Edward Jenner's use of a cowpox serum, obtained from afflicted animals, was deeply disconcerting to his contemporaries. James Gillray's cartoon *The Cow Pock; or, The Wonderful Effects of the New Inoculation!* presents a benign-looking Jenner inoculating innocent Britons who display a distinctly frightening set of side effects. Not only do they become animal-human hybrids with cow-like features, but they also pass on their deformities to the next generation of beasts. Of course, Tom Paine was giving birth to a beastliness all his own.

Funnily enough, Paine was actually represented as having given birth. Chalmers cast him as a monstrous mother—in a portrayal reminiscent of those monstrous mothers whose imaginations allegedly "impressed," or marked, their children in utero (see chapter 1 for more on maternal marking). Chalmers described how Paine was implanted with the anarchistic desires of fraudulent forefathers like Rousseau and had become pregnant with illusory political theories. These ambitions and desires had maternally imprinted the writing Paine produced. After "a few months labour" and with the assistance of publisher J. S. Jordan and a group of London democrats (whom Chalmers described as "men-midwives"), Paine delivered the *Rights of Man*. This "mutilated brat" was presented to an unsuspecting public on 13 March 1791.[75] In their rush to deliver this political progeny, Paine and his posse of democratic schemers had abandoned any concern about its welfare. "Determined to deprive the child of its virility, rather than so hopeful an infant should be with-held from the world," their haste had resulted in mutations in the form of grammatical errors.[76] According to Chalmers, the poor writing of Paine's pamphlet attested to its lack of potency, a characteristic that could be traced back through its family tree. This is an entirely different way of stigmatizing Paine, who appears as a serious threat to emerging notions of what Julia Kristeva refers to as "the self's clean and proper body."[77] The clean and proper body is typically a closed, male, rational body; while dirty bodies, leaky bodies, fat bodies, and pregnant bodies are classified as improper. It would seem a stretch to associate Paine with the abject pregnant body, but that is precisely what Chalmers did.

THE DISEASE OF INTEMPERANCE

Paine's drink of choice was brandy. It was an unfortunate one. Although brandy had been a medicinal drink in classical times, in the 1790s, physicians saw it as personally damaging and socially dangerous. The 1794 translation of Bernhard Faust's *Catechism of Health* suggests that brandy, which was "fiery, and destroys like fire," was in a different category from all other liquors.[78] Its effects were material and spiritual, bodily and political, and the result was the same in every American and European nation. Faust claims: "In proportion to the quantity of brandy consumed, were the evils which health, strength, reason, virtue, industry, prosperity, domestic and matrimonial felicity, the education of children, humanity and the life of man had to encounter."[79] This highly didactic passage demonstrates how abstract notions of disease were yoked both with the scrutiny of private habits and with much wider values attached to emerging models of national, familial, and individual identity. Faust pits brandy drinking against a list of Enlightenment principles as well as the values associated with the modern nuclear family. In this medicomoralizing discourse, brandy represents a refusal to be governed by reason, to subscribe to accepted definitions of virtue, and to take a full part in commercial enterprise. Most of all, drinking brandy signals one's refusal to fit into conventional, conservative models of private life: brandy is hostile to marriage, domesticity, and the raising of virtuous, industrious children.

Stopping just short of blaming the drink for the fall of humanity, Faust employs nostalgia to promote his vision of health for the modern era. Like other medical writers we have encountered in this chapter—Willich, Clayton, Alderson, and Armstrong—Faust also contrasts a Rousseauvian vision of the healthy, clean good old days with the degradation and immorality of the present:

> Our forefathers in former times, who had no idea of brandy, were quite different people from what we are; they were much more healthy and strong. Brandy, whether drunk by itself, or at meals, cannot be converted into blood, flesh, or bone; consequently, it cannot give health or strength, nor does it promote digestion: it only makes one unhealthy, stupid, lazy, and weak ... brandy deprives all who addict themselves to the immoderate and daily use of it—of health, reason, and virtue. It impels us to quit our house and home, to abandon our wives and children, and entails on its wretched votaries, misery and disease, which may descend to the third and fourth generation.[80]

It seems, then, that brandy acts upon the human body and psyche in the same way as dirt, disease, and even, as we have seen, masturbation. Like all of these things, brandy contaminates one's body, renders one unproductive, changes one's character, endangers one's family, and thus imperils the nation as a whole. Moreover, Faust's pinpointing of brandy as the cause of some unspecified "disease" that a father passes on through his offspring is a warning of the dangerous generational persistence of the sins of the father. Contaminants do not confine themselves to the existing generation: once introduced, they spread down through the ages.

These types of warnings about alcohol provide a necessary context to visual and verbal representations of Paine's alleged intemperance. Disease, disorder, and alcoholism are inscribed on his face in James Gillray's 1793 caricature *Fashion before Ease; or, A Good Constitution Sacrificed, for a Fantastik Form* (figure 4.2). Making reference to Paine's early career as a stay maker, the cartoon shows him heaving roughly on the laces of a handsome Britannia, his foot placed unceremoniously on her backside as he tries to squeeze her healthily voluptuous figure into a French form. His hard-set expression demonstrates that his brand of politics is as uncivilized and noxious as his personal habits and his body contrasts sharply with the healthy state of Britannia. His scrawny legs and his grotesquely pocked and reddened face attest to disease, hard drinking, and a lack of care of the self. As this image indicates, Paine's stinking body and unclean habits were directly related to *both* his intemperance and his politics.

Cheetham and John S. Harford, another Paine biographer, give very similar descriptions of the sick, stinking, putrid state of the radical's body when he was incarcerated in France in 1794. Ignoring the deplorable conditions of his damp jail cell and the resulting jail fever (which saved Paine from the guillotine), they insist that the rankness of his body was owed to very heavy drinking.[81] Cheetham recalls how "a medical man of great eminence, who rendered him professional service in France," had testified that Paine's "body was in a state of putrefaction, probably occasioned by drinking brandy, and that so offensive was the stench that issued from it, he could hardly be approached."[82] The reader would likely feel visceral repulsion at this description rather than sympathy. Cheetham's moralizing medical discourse links intemperance with revolutionary politics, so that following the chronology of Paine's life was following a trajectory of political anarchy and escalating physical deformity, both of which were exacerbated by his drunkenness. Cheetham traces the entwined nature of Paine's decline: "It does not however appear, that he constantly

Hygiene, Contamination, and Tom Paine's Toenails / 153

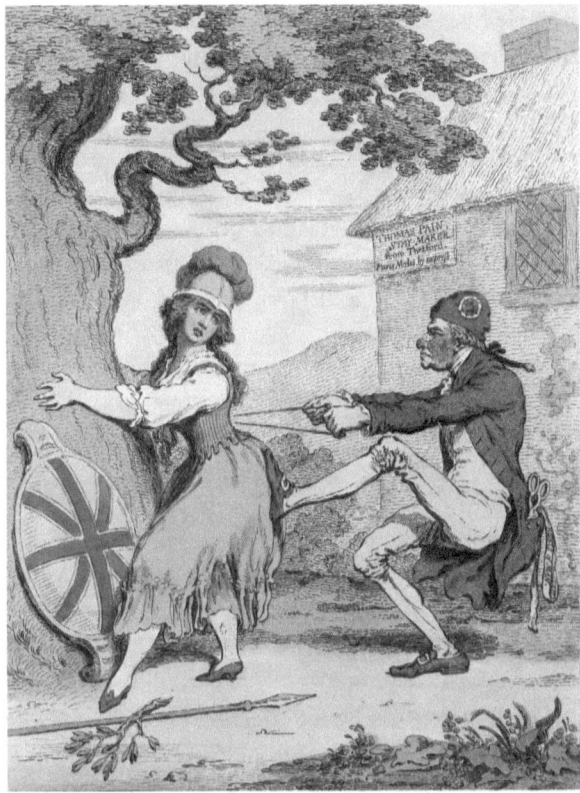

Figure 4.2 James Gillray, *Fashion before Ease; or, A Good Constitution Sacrificed, for a Fantastik Form* (1793 © Trustees of the British Museum, London)

drank to excess before he left America, in 1787: he was poor. His habitual drunkenness seems to have commenced with the delirium of the French Revolution. The practice gained upon him in London. 'Reason had been let loose.' Wildness naturally followed. A commotion of thoughts is necessarily succeeded by a commotion in action. In France, after he was elected to a seat in the Convention, by whose committee he was immured, his intemperance seems to have increased with the increase of French violence."[83] As this passage indicates, revolution caused drunkenness and was itself a type of delirious inebriety. Among the French populace, the fervor for republicanism had given rise to mob violence; likewise, Paine's abiding faith in reason and his growing loyalty to the cause of republicanism was equaled by a dangerous enthusiasm for brandy.

In Harford's 1819 biography, Paine is long-nailed, ragged, starving, and animalistic. He lives his life "in holes and corners" like a wild creature, where he takes in a filthy diet fit for swine and a daily amount of brandy which "would have quickly killed any ordinary man."[84] Harford's biography articulates the same aims and follows in the same tradition as Cheetham's (and also repeats many passages verbatim). The anecdotes about Paine's drinking are deeply damaging because, like all good scandalmongers, Cheetham and Harford provide eyewitness accounts and give details that, in their specificity, have an aura of authenticity. Cheetham describes how a faithful farrier named William Carver had generously opened his doors to Paine, even though the latter insisted on drinking "his quart of brandy a day." From Carver's, Paine then moved to the house of the bachelor portrait-painter Mr. Jarvis, where he "had fits of intoxication, and when these came on he would sit up at night tippling until he fell off his chair."[85] On one occasion, when Jarvis left him to his bottle until four in the morning, Paine passed out on the floor. When Jarvis attempted to help him up, Paine complained of "vertigo" and launched into a discussion of the mind-body problem: "My corporeal functions have ceased, he said, and yet my mind is strong. My body is inert, but my intellect is vigorous."[86] This seems a rather curious plea, and one wonders what the tactical reason for including it was, since biographers portrayed Paine's political philosophy and his material body as one. Paine's insistence that his intellect was untouched by his bodily disorders conveys a sort of Cartesian dualism, which his biographers did not seem eager to advocate.

SEXUAL DYSFUNCTION AND BIOLOGICAL-MORAL RESPONSIBILITY

Paine's lack of personal hygiene, his diseased body, and his addictions were also linked to his allegedly dysfunctional sexuality. His sexual abstinence in marriage, his preference for bachelorhood, his aversion to having children, and his penchant for sexual violence correlated to his failure to conform to emerging models of hygiene and normative familial models. In addition, Paine's opponents argued that his dangerous politics were a direct manifestation of his sexual deviance.

Along with Chalmers and Cheetham, a host of other political writers delved into Paine's shadowy past; they argued that his disastrous marriages provided clear evidence of biological and temperamental deficiencies and political unsuitability.[87] No one had ever been able to confirm, for instance, whether Paine's first wife, Mary Lambert, had died as a result of a miscarriage brought on by his "ill usage" or whether she was alive and hiding out from her husband in "extreme obscurity."[88] Biographers insisted that when Paine then married Elizabeth Ollive at Lewes, Sussex, the widowed or still-married Paine had falsely claimed bachelor status on his 1771 marriage record.[89] With relish, propagandists probed into the most intimate details of Paine's relationship with Elizabeth, focusing on his alleged sexual inadequacies—particularly his failure to consummate this three-and-a-half year marriage—in order to demonstrate how sharply his domestic life contrasted with the virtuous and honest lives of average Britons.

Cheetham tells a bizarre story about Paine's abstinence or impotence. The same Mr. Carver who, as we have seen, Paine roomed with in America near the end of Paine's life, had apparently also been a schoolmate of Elizabeth Ollive in Sussex some decades earlier. While in England, Carver had become well-acquainted with the "extraordinary fact" that "from some cause which Paine would not explain, and which is yet ascertained, he never . . . had *sexual intercourse with his wife*."[90] Moreover, Cheetham informs readers that "this almost incredible circumstance" became a point of neighborhood discussion.[91] His account is worth transcribing:

> Despised by the women, jeered by the men, and charged with a want of virility, Paine submitted . . . to a professional scrutiny. He was examined by Doctors Turner, Ridge, and Manning, who pronounced that there was not natural defect. On Doctor Turner's inquiring into the cause of his abstinence, Paine answered, that was no body's business but his own; that he had cause for it, but that he would not name it to any one. It appears that he accompanied his wife from the altar, but that, though they lived in the same house for three years after their marriage, they had from the day of their nuptials separate beds, and never cohabited together.[92]

So Paine's private life was made public on three levels: his alleged sexual dysfunction made him the subject of local Lewes gossip; it earned him the indignity of an examination by physicians; and it was fodder for readers on both sides of the Atlantic. The community acted as a normative standard of such relations, a moral barometer against which Paine was judged as lacking "the ordinary sensibilities of an ordinary man."[93] Such judgments were intended to circumscribe Painite influence while promoting a normative model of marital sexual relations intimately tied to maintaining the social and political status quo.

That Paine's abstinence earned him a physical examination by a team of doctors indicates the degree to which sexual behavior and desire had become the purview of medicine. Previously accepted models of sexuality were no longer seen as one's personal business or as part of everyday life. As Foucault has detailed in his seminal work on the history of sexuality, medicine entered the bedroom in this period and set about defining normal sexual function and censuring behaviors newly identified as dysfunctional, unnatural, or immoral.[94] That Doctors Turner, Ridge, and Manning pronounced Paine physiologically normal but sexually abnormal was more damaging than if he had had a clear physical disability. Such a prognosis indicated that his abnormality resulted from moral and *philosophical* deviance—the latter of which may seem an odd categorization, but in the eighteenth-century mind-set it was not. In fact, reactionaries argued that Paine's intentional abstinence was a symptom of self-serving political ambitions and a thirst for fame. Using a hybrid discourse that collapsed the private, the political, and the medical, Chalmers speculated in his biography that Paine's *"malicious impotence"* was due either "to natural imbecility or to *philosophical indifference*."[95] Similarly, in his pamphlet *The Republican Refuted*, Charles Harrington Elliot described how Paine had an "artificial, not *constitutional* insensibility to the charms of *bridal* youth and beauty."[96] This amalgamated language appeared, too, in more popular print forms, which effectively reduced important debates about rights and constitutions to nudge nudge, wink wink jokes about Paine's sex life. One broadside, which offered a brief synopsis of Paine's life "put in Metre," declared its intention:

> To judge of zeal,
> For public weal,
> Men's private lives we scan;
> Enough thy life
> Had plagued thy wife,
> Denied *her Rights in Man!*[97]

Such politically connotative language skillfully collapsed Paine's grossly unnatural desires (or, in this case, his lack of natural ones) with the abstract or bodiless quality of his political ideology.

Charles Harrington Elliot's pamphlet is particularly significant for the discomfort it expresses about nonreproductive sexual practices and about the choice not to have children. Elliot takes Chalmers's *Life of Thomas Pain* as his starting point but focuses still more "intimately" on the theme of Paine's unnaturalness. Elliot describes how, on one occasion, under the influence of "beer, gin, and tobacco," the "tyrant" Paine went so far as to deflower his innocent and beautiful wife by forcing the family cat "where the reader must guess, for indignant modesty cannot be more explicit."[98] Elliot's rhetoric of sensibility—his indignant modesty—distances his civilized self from the distinctly atavistic, sociopathic Paine. Of course, Elliot did not have the benefit of the psychoanalytic vocabulary Freud would provide a century later, but he depicted what we would now identify as sociopathic symptoms or indicators of antisocial personality disorder.

Paine's sexual perversity is either related to or results from his lack of that apparently most basic of human instincts—the desire to procreate. Elliot informs readers that Paine confessed to prostitutes (he preferred them to his alluring and virtuous wife) that since he had "married for *convenience only*, his wife's breeding would be subversive of that prudent object. And as for the tender emotions of nature, he had long since learned to keep them in due subjection."[99] Paine's refusal to have children and to perpetuate his family name (no matter how humble), bewilders Elliot, who sees this as indicative of a sexual monstrosity beyond the pale of normal biological function. Paine not only defied the laws of nature, he turned his back on the most fundamental of social duties. In other words, Elliot claims that Paine abnegated his "biologico-moral" responsibilities. We have seen how these responsibilities were defined and endorsed for women, but evolving models of masculinity also emphasized the importance of marriage, procreation, domestic duty, and fatherhood. Late eighteenth-century masculinities are related to the emergence, earlier in the period, of what Lawrence Stone described some years ago as the "closed, domesticated nuclear family" and to what Ruth Perry has more recently—and critically—termed "the privatized marriage."[100] As historians and literary scholars have demonstrated, as the century wore on, British models of masculinity became much more closely aligned with domesticity, paternity, and the demonstration of familial qualities. These emphases were in large part motivated by political anxieties produced by the events of the French Revolution.[101]

Indeed, the political angle to sexual dysfunction is potent. Elliot fulfilled his own political duty by informing readers of the links between Paine's sexual barbarism and his treasonous intentions. A man who, "with a predetermined, unyielding resolution" and "*in stern despite of nature*, met all the unveiled charms of the bridal bed without enjoyment" was a man who had been formed by "monster-making nature"—the same monster-making nature, Elliot argued, that had produced traitors and regicides such as Guy Fox and François Ravaillac (the assassin of Henry IV).[102] Political and personal deviances are conflated, so that Paine is both an anomaly of nature and a conspirator. His genealogy, which included more recent subversives than Fox and Ravaillac, was sketched out by William Cobbett. In the days before he defected to the Painite cause, Cobbett warned his British and American readers that the progenitor of Paine's ideological family tree was Jean-Jacques Rousseau, a man whose politics and sex life were equally notorious. Rousseau had seduced men's wives and daughters until he had made a "philosophical" marriage that produced bastard children; then he had played the "philosophical father" and sent them all off to the foundling house.[103] Along the way, Rousseau had admitted in his *Confessions* to having practically "committed incest" with the much older Madame de Warens; in turn, "mamma" had expressed her "most tender affection for her adopted son *Rousseau*" by taking him "to bed with her!"[104] Rousseau's life, self-confessedly filled with personal entanglements and dubious sexual proclivities, could not be divorced from his advocacy of such principles as the primacy of the general will or of equality.

For all his alleged impotence, Paine followed in Rousseau's licentious tradition. He approached decent women with a "French familiarity," seduced wives, debauched young virgins of reputable families, insulted polite English ladies, and frequented common prostitutes. There was a distinct lack of respectful moral boundaries in Paine's circle, so that he even seduced the wife of his Parisian friend, host and political ally Nicolas de Bonneville. Using the language of liberty, Paine lured Madame de Bonneville from her husband, convincing her to immigrate to America, taking their children with her. She may have been willing to perform those "secret services" that only women in her "position" were willing to "perform," Cobbett reasoned, but it was Paine who had committed the far greater crime by breaking up a family.[105] Alongside popular medical manuals outlining normal sexual function, Paine appeared a pathological deviant; against the widely circulating discourses of domesticity, he looked like a sexual predator. As personal probity became ever more closely aligned with marriage and family, with domestic comfort and familial virtues, Paine's dirty bachelorhood seemed profoundly immoral. At the hands of his scribbling enemies, he became a social and political pariah.

Compared to the increasingly standardized notion of normality, then, Paine's body was disordered, abnormal, excessive, and monstrous. His dirtiness was an atavistic or regressive signifier and his drinking was a sign of modern corruption; his sexual transgressions signaled his preoccupation with the unclean "lower" regions of the body; his refusal

Hygiene, Contamination, and Tom Paine's Toenails / 159

to procreate revealed the depth of his unnaturalness; his intemperance indicated how far humanity had strayed from a Rousseauvian-style noble innocence. How remote was the polluted modern body from its former natural robustness! As the language of these biographies makes clear, the loss of bodily integrity was proportionately linked to a loss of moral and political integrity. Indeed, material and moral expressions were often indistinguishable: words such as *filthy, odious, tainted,* and *polluted* were heard as much in sermons as read in health treatises and the the types of political propaganda discussed here.

DECLINE, DEATH, AND SHAME

The interconnectedness of ideas about cleanliness, contamination, sexual dysfunction, and politics is perhaps most clearly articulated in descriptions of Paine's last days. There are two remarkable and interrelated passages from Cheetham's biography, the first of which, although lengthy, is worth close consideration. It is taken from a letter allegedly written by the physician, Dr. Manley, who attended the dying Paine in 1809:

> I observed that his feet were oedematous, and his abdomen beginning to be distended with water, which, with several other circumstances equally unequivocal, indicated dropsy, and that of the worst description, as I soon found it pervaded every part of his body. . . . About this time he became very sore, the water which he passed when in bed excoriating the parts to which it applied. . . . And here let me be permitted to observe, (lest blame might attach to those whose business it was to pay particular attention to his cleanliness of person) that it was absolutely impossible to effect that purpose. Cleanliness appeared to make no part of his comfort; he seemed to have a singular aversion to soap and water; he would never ask to be washed, and when he was he would always make objections; and it was not unusual to wash and dress him clean, very much against his inclination. In this deplorable state, with confirmed dropsy, attended with frequent cough, vomiting and hiccough, he continued growing from bad to worse, till the morning of the 8th June, when he died. Though I may remark, that during the last three weeks of his life, his situation was such, that his decease was confidently expected every day, his ulcers having assumed a gangrenous appearance, being excessively foetid, and discoloured blisters having taken place on the soles of his feet, without any ostensible cause, which baffled the usual attempts to arrest their progress: and when we consider his former habits, his advanced age, the feebleness of his constitution, his constant practice of using ardent spirits, ad libitum, till the commencement of his last illness, so

far from wondering that he died so soon, we are constrained to ask, how did he live so long?[106]

An interesting comparison can be drawn between Dr. Manley's public dissection of Paine and the way conservatives like Richard Polwhele used Mary Wollstonecraft's death from puerperal fever to remind the public of the diseases specific to women, insisting that such specificity indicated women's natural role as childbearers. In a similar fashion, Manley/Cheetham use an image of Paine's fluid-filled, urine-soaked, and offensively leaky body, with its weeping pustules and layer of filth, to remind readers of men's capacity to slip back into barbarism. Their propensity to do so, in this view, is countered by civilized modes of living, which include bodily cleanliness, self-restraint, temperance, and sexual moderation.

It is also significant that Manley insists that the putrid, diseased Paine wallows in squalor, despite the attention of carers who fulfill their moral obligation to clean, clothe, and nurse him. This connection between domestic care and cleanliness is highlighted in a second, subsequent passage from Cheetham's biography. This particular passage reports how, as Paine watched his sad life ebb away, he lost the defiance that had gained him so much popularity some years before: "No one could recommend matrimony with greater force than Paine. By habit he was totally indifferent to his person. Cleanliness, without which there can be no comfort, he entirely disregarded. In his old age, when the affectionate attentions of a wife are inestimable, he had no house, no home; no one to help or to comfort him."[107]

This is more than just a lesson about the importance of marriage, or more accurately the possession of a wife who performed care-taking duties. This is Paine allegedly articulating his own desire for a "normal" domestic life with a nursing wife who, as a moral touchstone, would have saved him from his descent into brutishness. Physically and mentally shattered, poor and friendless, he allegedly gave up raving against the system and came to respect the long-standing institutions and customs he had fought to change. Recognizing his mistakes, he realized that domesticity and marriage were conducive to a person's happiness, that religion was good for the soul, that king and court were good for the spirit of the nation, and that a hierarchical social system was a necessary part of human relations. If Paine had possessed a wife whose duty it was to scrub his linen and bathe his body, he would not have ended life pissing himself in a filthy bed.

SHAME AND GOVERNMENTALITY

These two passages demonstrate how Paine's biographers fought ideological battles without ever discussing political ideologies. They launched their attack through representations of his body, which conflicted with emerging ideas about the importance of hygiene, cleanliness, and what we would now call heteronormative sexual practices. As a result, Paine was ever more marginalized—and so was his political philosophy. The type of medicalized scandal we have seen here, which penetrated freely into traditionally private space, was not a sign of increased liberty of the press; rather, it was a strategic instrument of political one-upmanship. Biographers like Cheetham and Chalmers used every rhetorical device at their disposal to set Paine at a distance from an ordered, rational, productive, and moral society. His solitariness, his drunkenness, his dirtiness, his animal features, and his monstrosity were manifestations of pathology. They were also a result of his sins against the family and the nation. Such representations indicate the flexibility of this type of highly personalized propaganda. The monstrous Tom Paine was as coldly impotent as William Godwin, then, but whereas Godwin funneled his enthusiasm into a rational philosophy, Paine funneled his into offensive acts of (ultimately unfulfilling) sexual violence. As was the case with Godwin and Wollstonecraft, portrayals of Paine's sexual appetites were deeply contradictory.

Helpfully, Foucault uses the word *governmentality* to refer to something akin to *the conduct of conduct* or *the government of one's self and others* in the modern world. Ideas about proper and improper ways of acting circulate in society and are negotiated and contested, yet the individual internalizes established ideas under great social and cultural pressure.[108] Indeed, in the late eighteenth and early nineteenth centuries, the term *government* appears in political, medical, and moral writing, which detail proper household management, urge sexual restraint, and advocate self-control. Foucault, along with Norbert Elias and a host of others, have given us a whole vocabulary to capture the ways that emerging regimes of body care and self-management coincided with the professionalization of medicine. The post-Enlightenment stress on social regulation produced a climate of therapeutic and moral self-regulation. In this era, "constraints through others from a variety of angles were converted into self-restraints," Elias argues, and he notes that "the regulation of the whole instinctual and affective life" was accomplished ever more widely and evenly through "steady self-control."[109] As a result, "the more animalistic human activities were progressively thrust behind the scenes of people's communal social life and invested with feelings of shame."[110]

If shame was a disciplinary mechanism, then print was the medium through which it operated most efficiently. Part of the changing apparatus of social control—whether it had an identifiable source or not—must include political material like these Paine biographies. Paine's political enemies used medicine and morality to recruit readers to take an active part in a public rejection of Paine and his contaminating politics. A subject's pathology, dysfunction, or unnaturalness need not be thoroughly explained or evidenced, but simply generally delineated. Images of physical monstrosity, which morphed cleanly into representations of political monstrosity, exploited anxieties about contamination and degeneration to establish a *cordon sanitaire* around Paine. Patriotic citizens had a duty to be wary of the signs of political virulence, domestic turmoil, and physical monstrosity; they must, as Isaac Hunt put it, "be guarded against [Paine's] baneful, abominable, infectious, and corrupting breath, enemy to life and matter, and every institution and character, wise, sacred and illustrious.[111] If Britons loved their country, they had to "mark out" and "point out" the radical element that threatened their king-esteeming, God-fearing, family-loving way of life.

Further, the act of "naming and shaming" political troublemakers also operated *self-reflexively*. Readers were prompted to examine and to adjust their *own* responses to the monstrosity they confronted on the page. Cobbett made this point emphatically when he insisted that Paine's treatment of his wife should "excite the indignation and resentment of every virtuous married woman" and rouse "the detestation of every honourable man."[112] If the reader did not feel indignant at Paine's filthiness, his sexual dysfunction, his homelessness, and his politics, then by extension that reader lacked virtue, knowledge, and discernment—which posed a serious risk to the rest of the population and jeopardized the health of the nation. Individuals could not remain apathetic about their own physical, moral, and political failings. There was an immense pressure to conform to a deeply gendered normative code of morality, to demonstrate cleanliness and restraint, and to practice a conservative politics. Paine's destitution and isolation, his misfortunes, his loneliness, the deplorable state of his body, and the torment of his mind were warnings to would-be radicals—and endorsements for quiet, virtuous living. Immorality, manifested in either political or private life, would not be tolerated in political leaders, or political upstarts, or in the people themselves. It was incumbent upon *all* members of society to contribute to the maintenance of civil order by clean living.

THE DURABILITY OF THE PAINE MYTHOLOGY

Of course, we can never know for certain what effects representations have on a political figure's life and work; however, we might surmise about possible effects on political culture. We know that Paine was a hero of the American Revolution and recipient of immense praise for *Common Sense* and *Rights of Man*. Then, in the mid-1790s, he became the object of great public animosity, and by the early nineteenth-century his writing was out of favor. He found it impossible to have the third part of *The Age of Reason* published in America until 1807. Some of his stellar decline must be due in part to reactionary propaganda that had forever twisted the "truth" about the events of his life, his health and habits, and his politics. The images perpetrated by James Cheetham continuously reappeared and were recast in subsequent generations so that attempts at vindicating Paine were more than difficult.

In his 1893 biography of Paine, Moncure Daniel Conway despairs at "how many good, and even liberal, people" have accepted what he calls "the Paine mythology." He points to Leslie Stephen's representation of Paine in his 1876 *History of English Thought in the Eighteenth Century*. In this major contribution to political philosophy, Stephen perpetrates "the old effigy of Paine elaborately constructed by Oldys [Chalmers] and Cheetham," but as Conway admits, he could hardly be blamed, since the London Library where he had researched the volume only carried those distinctly negative biographies.[113] The case was similar on the other side of the Atlantic, where Theodore Roosevelt's 1888 reference to Paine as a "filthy little atheist" was repeated consistently.[114] Even in Howard Fast's popular work *Citizen Tom Paine* (1943), a fictionalized attempt to defend Paine's politics, the radical appears as dirty, brandy-soaked, and unshaven; he is a "graceless staymaker, whose hands always had dirt under their nails."[115] Fast's citizen Paine is still cast in the mold of Chalmers's or Cheetham's Paine. Filthy and diseased, he is a man forced into a bathtub by soap-advocating, benevolent individuals. Fast imagines an unlikely scene in which the poet William Blake finds Paine—"drunk and howling foul songs"—and takes him home, where he "gave him a bath."[116] Paine is an ill-mannered parvenu in a world reserved for educated politicians whose gentlemanliness and mutuality are immediately indicated by their cultivated speech.

These myths are also alive and well on the scholarly front, although they are sometimes perpetrated involuntarily. In recent decades, introductions to editions of Paine's work have included the same famously negative quotes from Paine's nineteenth-century political enemies. Although sympathetic to Paine and advocates of his work, editors Gregory Claeys, Philip Foner, Michael Foot, and Thomas Kramnick all describe how Paine was referred to as, among other things, a "loathsome reptile," a "demi-human archbeast," and "an object of disgust, of abhorrence, of absolute loathing to every decent man."[117] This is reportage and it provides important historical context, yet these types of representations continue to receive attention, to the detriment of Paine's reputation and work. To this day, Paine and his ideas do not receive due consideration. The Paine mythology has influenced decisions about whether or not he should be commemorated as a figure of importance. In towns across America, park commissions have consistently voted against erecting statues of Paine, and for years the American Hall of Fame showed no interest in including him in its hallowed halls. Dirty Tom Paine continues to be seen as an advocate of lawlessness, social insubordination, and moral nihilism.

Scholars as diverse as Julia Kristeva, Judith Halberstam, Arnold Davidson, Margrit Shildrick, and others have argued that what we define as monstrous is invariably a reflection of our own deepest anxieties. And there are as many monsters as there are anxieties. Fears about the precariousness of civilization, criminality, sexuality, human "nature," racial difference, disease, and our own destructive impulses give birth to society's leviathans. Tom Paine is a reflection of the fear that progressive change will reveal the arbitrariness of power and the frailty of social hierarchies. For those desperate to maintain the political status quo, he is a monstrous embodiment of the possibility of a universalist, liberalist commitment to rights that spans the globe. He is a homeless monster whose rootless cosmopolitanism cannot be tamed by partial affections to family, community, nation, or the "weaker" sex. He represents the fear that the barbarians are forever at the gates. Indeed, he *is* one of those barbarians and, according to the myth, a debauched, diseased, and particularly filthy one. However, the real fear is that the form of "barbarism" he embodies is distinctly modern and manifestly liberal.

PART III

Royal Pathologies

5 Gout vs. *Goût*

Taste, Community, and the Monarchy

> It is a common Saying, That every Man past Forty,
> is either a *Fool* or a *Physician*.
>
> GEORGE CHEYNE,
> *An Essay of Health and Long Life* (1724)

Early in the second decade of the nineteenth century, Napoleon Bonaparte conquered territories and forged new alliances, while the exiled king of France was gout-ridden and wheelchair-bound. Britain's Prince Regent had offered Louis XVIII allowances and right of asylum—a generosity that was likely motivated by more than political solidarity. Tellingly, each of them had at different times employed the famous French restaurateur and pastry chef Antoine Beauvilliers to create lavish and groaning tables of delicacies, which they consumed with gusto. In contrast to Napoleon's vitality, the two obese, indolent, and physically shattered monarchs suffered desperately from the usual symptoms of gout: inflammation, swelling, fever, and intense pain in the foot and knee joints.

Gout was understood to be a disease that attacked gentlemen of a certain age, with certain kinds of appetites. A disease rarely seen among the laboring classes, gout had pride of place in a category of ailments that Roy Porter and George Rousseau describe as "high-life disorders in an age of pleasure."[1] Throughout the eighteenth century, there was debate as to the origins of the disease and about whether gout attacked those with "hearty and hale constitutions" or those who had ruined their constitutions with high living. For all the disagreement among doctors, they generally concurred that "the Gout most commonly seizes such Old men, as have lived the best part of their Lives tenderly and delicately, allowing themselves freely Banquets, Wine, and other spirituous Liquors, and at length by reason of the Sloth that always attends Old-Age, have quite omitted such Exercises as young Men are wont to use."[2]

This assessment, first made by Thomas Sydenham in his 1683 *Treatise on the Gout*, was reprinted and remained relatively current throughout the eighteenth century and into the next. In other translations of this

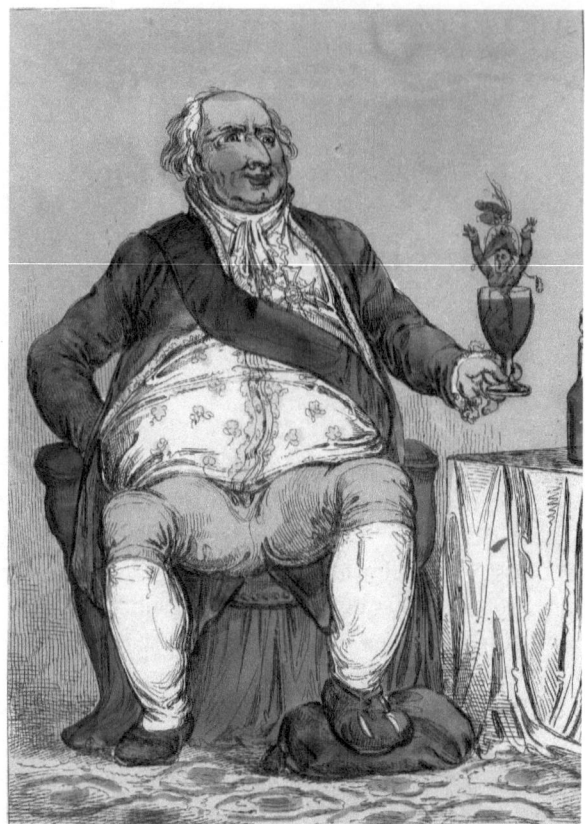

Figure 5.1 William Heath, *A Pleasent Draught for Louis* (1814 © Trustees of the British Museum, London)

treatise and in subsequent works by physicians such as George Cheyne and William Cadogan, words like *voluptuous*, *luxurious*, and *easeful* captured the habits of goutish well-to-do men. These eighteenth-century doctors became famous for treating a disease that was, in its positive interpretation, a sign of civilization and refinement and, in its more negative sense, the by-product of artificiality, excess, and corrupting luxury. By the early nineteenth century, gout had become enmeshed in a web of political and moral associations. Gout was allied with luxury, excess, and unbridled consumption. It was caught up with questions about how individual taste and desire should be reconciled with communal responsibility. Gout's location between nature (was one born with gout?) and

Gout vs. Goût / 169

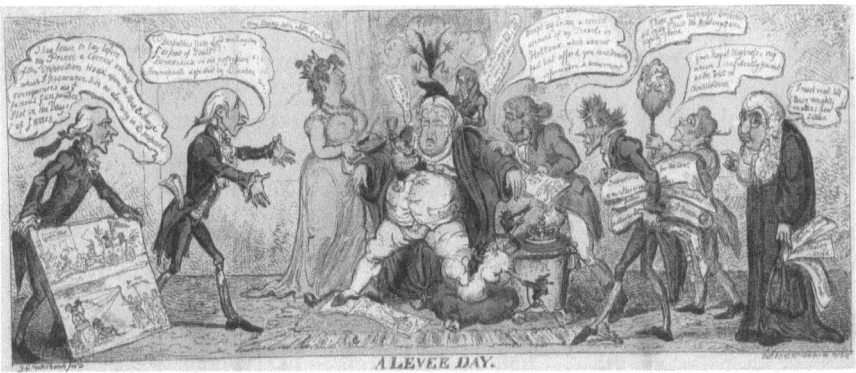

Figure 5.2 George Cruikshank, *A Levee Day* (1814 © Trustees of the British Museum, London)

culture (did one acquire gout as a result of personal habit?) meant that it became a focus of a range of debates about nature versus culture.

Two prints, both published in 1814, flesh out the politics of this disease. The first (likely the work of William Heath) celebrates Louis XVIII's triumphant return to the French throne (figure 5.1).[3] At first glance, Louis appears to be the model of triumph: his pose and smile are assured, his body clothed in royal style, his form seated as if upon a throne, his size huge compared to the newly defeated lilliputian Napoleon. Yet this image of assurance is imperiled by the gouty leg, propped up on a pillow to ease the pain of the joints, the foot encased in a shoe that has been split to allow for the uncontrollably swelling flesh. Louis's throne, like the monarchy in general, is threatened by a similar sense of excess: the shoe fails to contain the overabundance, the chair is overburdened by his bulk, and the mass of expanding softness at his waist strains his shirt buttons and escapes from his coat. This is a body that refuses to be kept in check. Louis may be about to consume Napoleon, but the glass of wine in which the latter flails is *more* irresistible. That wine is also responsible for demolishing Louis's health in the first place.

There are noteworthy parallels between Heath's image and another print that appeared the same year. George Cruikshank's *A Levee Day* (1814) (figure 5.2) is an ironic interpretation of Samuel Johnson's oft-quoted phrase that "he who does not mind his belly will hardly mind anything else." The Prince Regent sits upon a chair almost identical to Louis's, oblivious to everything but the demons of excessive living that torture him: vapors, dropsy, and colic. The cures (rich turtle soup) served by his latest mistress, Lady Hertford, and by the fat imp ("Punch") balancing on his protruding stomach are ironically indicative of the cause of his disease. The two figures on the left, Lord Sidmouth and Lord Liverpool, inform the regent of Napoleon's defeat through the medium of a caricature. In the inset image, a carriage is topped by a flag announcing the "Death of Buonaparte," yet the prince is so incapacitated by his gouty body that he is incapable of acknowledging, let alone reacting, to political news. His tailor and the wigmaker—with their bills—are first in the queue before the court recorder, who bears a list of persons condemned to death. There is a specific political message here: it was common knowledge that the regent, who had final decision as to reprieve or execution, did not perform this most consequential of tasks with any consistency. Instead, his stomach overrides any sense of duty and obligation, sympathy or compassion—and the papers that protrude from Judge Silvester's bag indicate clearly that the desperate, hungry people who have committed crimes of necessity, including thefts of basic foodstuffs much less exotic than turtle soup, are left to their fates.

These images give us a sense of how the goutish body became politicized in meaningful ways. In their cultural history of gout, Roy Porter and George Rousseau make the point that "the idioms of politics and those of bodily physiology were of a piece."[4] Gout became emblematic of a monarchy increasingly out of step with the tenor of the times. In a political campaign that elicited the participation of reactionaries and reformers, parliamentarians and journalists, aristocrats and the middling sort, gout was used against a declining court culture associated with excess and extravagance. The Prince Regent's health became a measuring stick by which the state of the crown and the moral course of the nation were measured. George's gout provided material evidence of his personal failings: his excessiveness, poor taste, unreasonableness, and debauchery. It also indicated his political incapacity and by extension the incapacities of the monarchy more generally; in fact, gout was used to support all kinds of arguments about why monarchical power should be circumscribed. Goutish George became the unwitting impetus behind a campaign to decrease monarchical intervention in day-to-day political decision making. His corpulent body and its concomitant disorders were used to encourage the transfer of public trust from the monarchy to a Tory government.

By the end of George's life, the monarchy had much less overt political authority, less intervention in day-to-day politics, but much more to do with reflecting the moral values of the nation. The royal family was expected to act as an exemplar of national character, to demonstrate domestic harmony and familial values—something that George, whether in his incarnation as Prince of Wales, as Prince Regent, or as King George IV, failed spectacularly to do. As a result, he was fashioned into a figurehead for a privileged segment of society that, in the years following the French Revolution, had consistently abnegated its duty by displaying qualities that were seen as distinctly un-English.

But he was caught in an even wider and increasingly dominant conflict between, on the one hand, privilege, prerogative, and excess and, on the other hand, an emerging middle-class emphasis on restraint, moderation, and stability in public and private life. The growing prominence of restraint appeared, too, in medical writing on eating and drinking. By the end of the eighteenth century, as Alan Bewell rightly points out, *diet* was "a central term in an emerging biopolitics of health."[5] As this Foucauldian-inflected comment indicates, the emphasis on restraint in dietary matters reflected a similar emphasis in questions of morality and politics. The rhetoric that circulated about the regent's body—its corpulence, its goutiness, its intemperance—was a product of new cultural alliances between moral and political excess, between bodily disease and ideas about national pathology, between aesthetic taste and eating habits, and between individual health and the health of the community. As a result of these new pairings, the prince became the object of public attention and a mechanism through which new connections between taste and health—and the constellation of ideas about moral and political uprightness that circulated through them—were promoted to an audience of average citizens. Examples of George's bodily excesses were used to support the emergence of a new modern model of masculinity, which was about self-discipline, bodily restraint, political sobriety, and devotion to family. For the new public man (a man of taste, polite sociability, and political responsibility), bodily restraint was contiguous with the demonstration of love of country *and* love of home.

THE MEDICOPOLITICAL CONTEXT OF GOUT

Roy Porter and George Rousseau identify two competing medical models of gout in the eighteenth century, both of which had important political repercussions. Those who subscribed to the "constitutional" model of the disease posited that gout was inherited. Symptomatic outbreaks should be seen in a positive light, they suggested, as evidence that the body was reacting in a natural way to overconsumption. In other words, painfully swollen joints were signs that the body was righting itself by excising pollutants and restoring balance. As the term *constitutional* might indicate, there is a political angle to this model of gout. In fact, the language of medical manuals, and even personal correspondence on this subject, resonates powerfully with political debate in the age of revolutions. The letters of Edward Gibbon, member of Parliament and author of *The History of the Decline and Fall of the Roman Empire*, for example, provide a politicized pathography of life with gout. In 1775, Gibbon personified gout as a figure who had "not asserted his rights" unduly but had "exercised them in a very gentle manner," so that Gibbon was "rather benefited than injured by his [gout's] transient visit."[6] Some years later, he contrasted a happy period of relief from his symptoms with a temporary decline in the cooperative spirit of Parliament. While "the body Gibbon" was restored to "a perfect state of health and spirits," unfortunately the "state of public affairs" had descended into "Anarchy."[7]

This constitutional model of gout, like Gibbon's politics, is conservative. Gibbon shared Edmund Burke's view of the constitution as an organic entity that reflected a nation's slow and careful development; in similar fashion, gout was indicative of the body adjusting organically to its environment. Gout was a reminder of the responsibilities that came with one's aristocratic pedigree: as an educated man of the polite classes, one bore the weight of a thoughtful and thus sedentary life. The goutish constitution, like the nation's constitution, was organic, deep rooted, a vital part of one's identity. The resonances between this constitutional model of disease and a conservative understanding of politics and nationhood were amplified in the 1790s. In his 1789 *Advice to Gouty Persons*, Richard Kentish anticipated the language of Burke's *Reflections on the Revolution*, advising readers that gout was their "hereditary right" and as such they should keep their "tenure" secure upon their "patrimony."[8]

The etiology and the philosophical underpinnings of the constitutional model of gout were challenged, however, by reform-minded physicians who instead posited a "diseases of civilization" paradigm. In fact, if supporters of the constitutional model anticipated or echoed the conservative, reactionary Burke of the 1790s, then early advocates of the diseases of civilization model were Thomas Paine's associates. The political ideas circulating in the American revolutionary era influenced medical writing and in particular this second model of the disease. Physicians like William Cadogan argued that gout was *not* hereditary but rather resulted from what we would now term lifestyle. In his 1771 *Dissertation on the Gout*, he prescribed a treatment that included moral and therapeutic purification and a complete "reform" of one's habits.[9] While his more conservative-minded opponents insisted that gout should be accepted as the way things were, Cadogan placed himself firmly on the nurture side of the nature-nurture debate in this case. (By way of a caveat, I would also point out that competing models of gout were not always mutually exclusive: as one example, the Scottish physician William Grant initially situated gout within the disease of civilization model, but as gout became endemic and resisted cure he described it as hereditary.)

In *A Successful Method of Treating the Gout by Blistering* (1779), the physician William Stevenson used much stronger terms in his polemic against society's abiding respect for "every thing that is hereditary." Straying some way from solely medical topics, he railed against the weight of custom, which crushed liberty, reason, and progress. Humans, he argued, were bound by history, heredity, and convention. Britons had an absurd, sycophantic veneration of the past; as he explains:

> Hence our dignified estimation of hereditary blood, imbued with which every action is honourable, selling our country, after having first sold our conscience; debauching other men's wives and daughters, and defrauding tradesmen of their bills.—Hence our foibles, defects, oddities, whims, prejudices, and prepossessions, are held to be a sacred part of our sacred selves . . . because they belonged in kind to our fathers or mothers, perhaps, to progenitors higher up, till we arrive at the first parent of all, who, we are told, "got a son in his own image." . . . The gout, we strangely consider as being derived to us from hereditary tenure, and a part of our fathers' or grandfathers' last will and testament.[10]

Stevenson's medical pamphlet, written during and clearly informed by the debate surrounding the American Revolutionary War, reflects the arguments Tom Paine made for independence in his 1776 *Common Sense*. Stevenson's rejection of genealogy sounds like the colonists' assertion of their right to live free of the paternal tyranny exercised by the parent nation.[11] The American colonists did not feel an unquestioning loyalty to the king nor did they revere the time-honored traditions that upheld his position.

Arguments against medical hereditarianism were bound up with arguments against hereditary succession. Radical medical treatises rejected the tenacious hold of customs, traditions, and practices that had become a great encumbrance on a progressive generation. Political reformers urged government reforms that reflected the current generation's own interests and values; similarly, physicians like Stevenson suggests that gout-ridden sufferers should break free from an attitude of resignation and inevitability. Aristocrats who inherited their elevated social and political positions, but who proved themselves incapable of refraining from gorging and guzzling, were equally incapable of exercising discrimination and rationality in the fulfillment of public duties. In foregoing their paternal responsibilities, these individuals also rescinded their paternal authority and its attendant privileges. Stevenson's medical arguments accorded with the influential political arguments Paine subsequently made in *Rights of Man* (1791) for the abolition of hereditary branches of government.[12] Although in a different context, the question of individual entitlement that Paine addressed is much like Stevenson's; both are against tyranny, privilege, and the exercise of arbitrary power.

Porter and Rousseau insist that "the gout debate is unintelligible unless its politics are foregrounded." This is even more the case after 1789, they argue, when "the polarization of [medical] positions mirrored the political polarization of the times," which saw "Old Corruption assailed by reformers, aristocracy threatened by liberalism."[13] Reform-minded doctors like Thomas Beddoes, physician and friend to Samuel Taylor Coleridge, used a political terminology galvanized by the ideals of the French Revolution. In his three-volume *Hygeia; or, Essays Moral and Medical* (1802), Beddoes characterized the constitutional, hereditary model of gout as "reactionary" and drew analogies between political and corporeal pathology to urge reform in medicine, in politics, and in the private lives of individuals. This superstitious and irrational theory, Beddoes argues, was employed by those who saw a certain way of life threatened. In fact, "in attempting to speak of this disorder, one feels as if on *tabooed* ground," he complained, since "the prejudices of the darkest ages cling as fast as ever to the idea of gout."[14] Like Stevenson's, Beddoes's statements are reminiscent of Tom Paine's arguments for self-governance and for generational renewal, countering a Burkean political conservatism that clings to custom, continuity, and hereditary distinction. For the most part, such diseases were not bequeathed, Beddoes insists, rather "*our chronic maladies are of our own creating.* . . . Our taste must be corrected."[15] Gout was less a matter of genetics (to use an anachronism) and more like "many other maladies which persons, blindly eager for sensual pleasure, bring upon themselves."[16]

As Beddoes's comments indicate, clear moral implications follow from his emphasis on the effects of environment or lifestyle (another anachronism). The medical status and etiology of gout were subject to much politically inflected debate, but imperatives about eating practices and other personal habits stemmed from the diseases of civilization model in particular. Still, whichever model doctors subscribed to, there was a general consensus about excessive consumption and a lack of physical exercise as strong contributing factors, if not causes. Since advocates of both the constitutional and the civilization model of disease believed that class-bound practices, as well as habits of thinking and of being-in-the-world, inscribed themselves on the body, then it followed that individuals had a duty to live virtuous, clean, temperate lives.

As early as the 1720s, George Cheyne insisted that "the *Rich*, the *Lazy*, the Voluptuous, who suffer most by the gout" could put the cause of their suffering down to two evils: "*Wealth* and *Vice*."[17] Likewise, William Buchan identified "*excess* and *idleness*" as the culprits, for which he prescribed a regimen of "*universal temperance*" and exercise that involved "labour, sweat, and toil."[18] Many of these prescriptive medical guides sound very much like Jean-Jacques Rousseau's writings on regimen, education, and ethics and his theories on human nature. Like Rousseau, physician Robert Campbell turned to hypothetical nature as a normative guide in a world disfigured by commerce and luxury. In his 1747 vocational manual for London tradesmen, Campbell blamed civilization for pathologizing natural man. In a refined society, "Vice and Immorality" and "Luxury and Laziness" grew in prevalence until "Men became Slaves to their own Appetites" and thereby subject to "new Diseases" and "unheard of Distempers, both chronick and acute."[19]

In 1792, this point was underscored by another physician who insisted that since there was an "intimate connection between the body and mind, and the sympathy of its organs with one another," then it followed that intemperance and gluttony produced "diseases of body and mind" and caused gout to be "so common among corpulent people."[20] In *A Treatise on the Gout*, published that same year, the Edinburgh physician Thomas Jeans gave a further boost to the mind-body connection. He insisted, quite simply, that the disease was a physical sign of a love of vice, artificiality, and luxury.[21] As such, readers were held morally and medically responsible for the onset of their disease, as well as for their cures. The message was that health required individuals to rein in their desires, control their imaginations, change their habits, and reform their lives. Stevenson gave perhaps the most unequivocal version of this message. "Before people can be cured of the Gout, they must be cured of their *vices*," he wrote. "Intemperance, voluptuousness, and gluttony, by which both mind and body are unqualified for exercise, are the parents of Gout, as well as of every other disorder. Prevent the one, and you prevent the other."[22]

The antidualistic diagnoses and cures offered by Stevenson, Beddoes, Jeans, and others reveal much about changing medical-moral emphases in this period. By linking immorality with excessive eating, these eighteenth-century physicians began to medicalize the appetite. Physicians forged sympathetic relationships between physiology, pathology, habit, and personal character and in so doing, gestured toward a constellation of emerging moral concerns. What one consumed directly correlated to one's own moral standing, a fact to which the body bore observable testimony, but individual diet and taste were also implicated in the well-being of the body politic. Intemperance and gluttony—which produced swollen stomachs and grossly inflamed joints—had much wider social and political implications. Indifferent and lethargic aristocrats and sheltered courtiers who spent their lives reveling in luxury were out of step with a strengthening middle-class emphasis on industry, transparency, and communality. At the end of the century, excess and apathy were seen as threatening to a society already under threat from war, political disaffection, and revolutionary fervor.

TEMPERANCE

James Gillray's 1792 paired images of the contrasting styles of monarchical consumption, *Temperance Enjoying a Frugal Meal* and *A Voluptuary under the Horrors of Digestion*, are among his best-known works. Scholars have detailed the various ways these images contrast the thriftiness and frugality (or miserliness) of King George III and Queen Charlotte against their gorging, excessive son, the Prince of Wales. Gillray's images reveal much about the way monarchs were being called to public account for their personal lives in new ways in the 1790s. Yet I am most interested in how eating practices in particular became conflated with moral failure and political irresponsibility. In these images, the temperate body is juxtaposed against the excessive body in order to define both as manifestations, not simply of political ineptitude, but of an ineptitude borne out of a particular brand of immorality inseparable from practices of consumption.

The many details in *Temperance Enjoying a Frugal Meal* (figure 5.3) signal the restraint exercised by the miserly George III and the avaricious Charlotte: the shabbiness of the king's chair, the pictureless frames, and more tellingly, the parsimonious meal of unsugared tea, boiled eggs, salad, and water.[23] Relative to the meanness of their diet is the abundance of their private funds, stockpiled at public expense (as the "Table

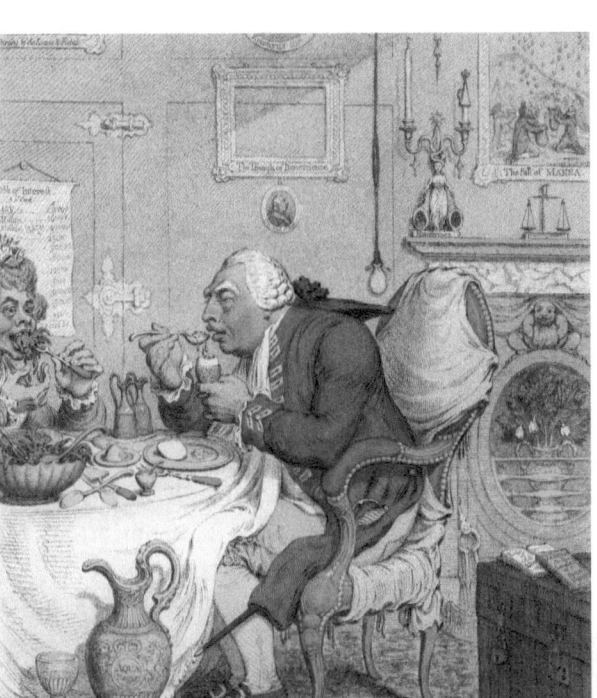

Figure 5.3   James Gillray, *Temperance Enjoying a Frugal Meal* (1792 © Trustees of the British Museum, London)

of Interest" behind the queen's back indicates). Scholars have argued that like much of the satirizing of George III, Gillray's picture lacks the intensity of attacks on the Bourbons or the English princes. Marilyn Morris observes that while the French used "exposé to chip away at the mystique of monarchy," British satirists of George III used comic lampooning.[24] But whereas Britons may have expressed, to use Richard Godfrey's perceptive phrase, a "perverse affection" for George and Charlotte, they did not feel similarly toward their sons.[25] For the Princes of Wales, in particular, scandal often took the form of outright mutinous attack. This synopsis is probably right, yet I want to tease out the more nuanced meanings behind the comical representations of the king's extreme temperance.

In Gillray's *Temperance*, the royal reading material is *Essay on the Dearness of Provisions* and *Dr Cheyne on the Benefits of a Spare Diet*. These are made-up titles that reference George Cheyne's popular treatise *The*

Natural Method of Cureing the Diseases of the Body, and the Disorders of the Mind Depending on the Body, in which he famously advocated a temperate diet consisting of only vegetables and milk. In Gillray's caricature, then, the king and queen are linked negatively with the scarcity faced by the poor, yet also positively, since they exercise the type of dietary restraint and personal self-command that reflected political responsibility. Radicals, however, interpreted the royals' temperance as an extreme and biologically unnatural form of restraint that was connected to other unnatural forms of bodily restraint. In his 1795 *Political Dictionary*, the radical libertine Charles Pigott connected the king's alimentary austerity with both his notoriously spendthrift household and his political incapacity. He compared George with King Nebuchadnezzar: both were beastly kings who "ate grass and potatoes"; as such, "it would greatly conduce to the welfare of his people" if George "was turned out to grass before the meeting of every session of Parliament."[26] Rather bizarrely, Pigott's representation of the king has something in common with representations of Tom Paine, who as we saw in the previous chapter was also compared to the bestial Nebuchadnezzar. Of course, comparing George to the biblical king was an attempt to undermine George's political authority and challenge his right to rule by uncovering his private foibles, frailties, and fallibilities, but Pigott also portrayed George's extreme temperance as both a failure of character *and* biology. The argument, not unlike that used against Paine, was that the king's personal habits reflected a regressive tendency, something of a reversion to a precivilized state of human nature.

Also like Paine—but not to the same degree—George III was tarred with sexual abnormality. The king's dietary restraint was closely related to aberrant personal and political policies surrounding royal marriage and the sexual practices of the court. The king upheld the idea that royal marriages were distinctly public acts, and he enshrined this principle in legislation. The Royal Marriages Act of 1772 was intended to keep the royal family from "irretrievable ruin" or from the type of public dishonor that encouraged antimonarchists.[27] More specifically, the act compelled the Prince of Wales and his siblings to marry Protestant sovereigns approved by the king, thereby avoiding the types of mistakes made by George III's unscrupulous brother, the Duke of Cumberland. In 1771, the duke had married a commoner with a questionable moral and political past (allegedly including a sexual liaison with the king's son, the Prince of Wales).[28] But reformers lambasted the legislation as draconian. It was, they argued, a father's attempt to stunt the natural desires of his children by insisting on their sexual abstinence; it was a legalized form of repression, which gave rise to perverse, destructive sexual habits. The father had effectively made it impossible for his sons to find a legitimate outlet for their natural sexual drives, ensuring they would not conduct themselves in a responsible, manly way.

When George III's mental state deteriorated in 1788, almost certainly as a result of the hereditary disease porphyria, the leader of the Whigs, Charles James Fox, argued that the Prince of Wales should take over as sovereign. The Tories, under Prime Minister William Pitt, insisted that Parliament had the right to decide who would be regent. During the ensuing Regency crisis (before the king recovered in 1789), the debate around the Royal Marriages Act intensified. George III's Whig challengers suggested that the act was an early sign of his mental incapacity. Driving his sons to seek reckless passionate encounters as an outlet for their natural sexual energies was evidence that the mad king had lost all control over his household. On these grounds, supporters of the Regency defended the Prince of Wales's secret 1786 marriage to the twice-widowed Catholic Mrs. Fitzherbert. On the surface, they argued, the morganatic marriage might appear as an act of the prince's selfish insolence against his father and an insult to the nation's laws. Yet what could one expect? It was a very natural reaction to an unnatural forced celibacy.[29]

In *A Letter to a Friend on the Reported Marriage of His Royal Highness the Prince of Wales* (1787), the radical John Horne Tooke described the Royal Marriages Act as an "unnatural act of parliament" and a "political superstition" that demonstrated the despotic nature of both the king's interventionist political policies and his equally problematic familial prohibitions.[30] There was something startlingly inhumane and thoroughly unnatural about a father who would use legal statute to insist on his son's celibacy. It was, Tooke insisted, analogous to prohibiting a child from eating or from using his eyesight.[31] What normal person would "degrade his children to something worse than castration, to the unmanly state and abject condition of a Friar . . . to compel them by an unnatural law, *without any fixed period*, to a life of forced celibacy, until . . . like the pope, [he] shall be pleased to grant a dispensation to restore them to the dignity of manhood, and reinvest them with the natural rights of an animal"?[32] In light of what is known about the prince's notorious sexual affairs, characterizing him as a celibate friar may seem a bit ridiculous; nevertheless, Tooke's blame of the "popish" king makes George III appear grossly unnatural, superstitious, and despotic. There are connections between Tooke's charge and that leveled by figures like Denis Diderot, who condemned religious sexual repression as unnatural in *The Nun* (1760), and the Marquis de Sade, who linked religious celibacy to excessive and violent sexuality.

Charles Pigott's 1794 *Female Jockey Club* had similar things to say about the carefully confined lives of England's six princesses. Pigott argued that though "physical enjoyments are essential to us all," the king and queen very deliberately set about preventing their daughters from experiencing them.[33] In their attempts to keep the princesses chastely hidden from male attention, George and Charlotte sacrificed "the loveliest part of the creation to the sterile solitude of celibacy, as if *Royalty* were incompatible with *Nature*."[34] Enforced celibacy was a sign that Britain's first family had strayed "so far wide from nature's rules" as to willingly adopt the "most immoral and unnatural sanction[s]."[35] As in Tooke's writing, biology, politics, and morality are inseparable in Pigott's political considerations. True to his libertarian roots, he rankled at prohibitions on bodily pleasure, yet his accusations about the grossly distorted nature of monarchical lives also seem calculated to appeal to a growing middle-class emphasis on nature as the measure of morality and decency.

As was the case with George III's sons, the daughters' forced celibacy gave rise to sexually dysfunctional behavior. In fact, a princess was rendered doubly unnatural because, as part of court privilege, she was first lavished with "foreign luxuries" and a "diet" that enflamed her "naturally sanguine temperament" before being forced into spinsterhood or a passionless marriage.[36] Custom and ritual may have been markers of refinement and civility, but according to Pigott such markers could never and should never supersede natural biological function. Arranged marriages "pledged" complete strangers "to copulation" and to acts of the "grossest sensuality."[37] "To thwart *nature*" was to invite "fatal" consequences and to initiate the most "desperate excesses," including incest. If a sister, "raging with the fire of nature," was "checked in her course" she might even find her way "to a brother's arms," where she could then satisfy "her ardent invincible passion."[38] Casting himself as a sort of political and moral physician, Pigott expressed outrage at the gullibility of Britons who bought into the king's moral façade, which made a mockery of natural, healthy impulses. Like a physician, Pigott proposed the cure: the overabundance of temperance in the royal household, which in turn led to an overabundance of sexual excess, should be treated with a course of "purgation."[39]

As is commonly known, bleeding and purging were prescribed for a pack of pathologies in this era. Many doctors, including George Cheyne, William Buchan, William Cadogan, and John Abernethy, advised patients to eliminate all bodily pollutants in this way. They advised fellow physicians to restrain their overweight, alcohol-sodden, and gout-ridden patients and to insist they leave off drinking and other "unnatural" practices. Not without a touch of wonderful irony, William Stevenson warned gout sufferers, "You must leave your crapulary debauch, your bottles, your w[hores]; nay more, you must leave your affected, hypocritical self, for your best resemblance, the *childhood of Nature*."[40] This provides important context for Pigott's prescription of purification. Although Pigott was a libertarian, antimonarchical radical, there is an underlying conservatism in the connections he makes between politics, sexual dysfunction, and the affective family unit. Like the prescriptions of moralizing physicians, his appeal to nature was distinctly normative: he defined and advocated "natural" sexual expression while defining unnatural sexual relations. He exploited society's anxieties about the effects of excessive sensuality in his own cautions about imposing limits on sex. The message, ultimately, was that the best thing for a princess was to live as normally as possible by finding a decent man, getting married, having a family, and settling down into a quiet domestic life.

"THE PRINCE OF WHALES":
SENSUS COMMUNIS AND THE PROBLEM OF EXCESS

The corpulent, intemperate, and excessive Prince of Wales was *the* consumer par excellence of the 1790s, and his style of consumption was deeply out of step with emerging moral, medical, and political values. In both his public and private lives, George embodied recklessness, promiscuity, disloyalty, irresponsibility, and lack of restraint—all of which were in evidence on a body marked by moral failure. His heavy imbibing and voracious feeding were linked with sexual intemperance, an addiction to horses and gambling, and an unrestrained penchant for jewelry, military uniforms, and sartorial enhancements. His excesses were reported in newspapers, pamphlets, and contemporary biographies. Like other propagandists who urged the prince's reform, William Augustus Miles, a one-time supporter of William Pitt, used a type of personal but politicized vocabulary that situated individual action within the larger political landscape. Miles insisted that the prince should be "restrained, within the limits of Sobriety and Reason," and that he should be reminded of his duty to exercise "the virtue of self-denial."[41] According to many observers, one of the areas of the prince's life that was most in need of restraint was his eating habits.

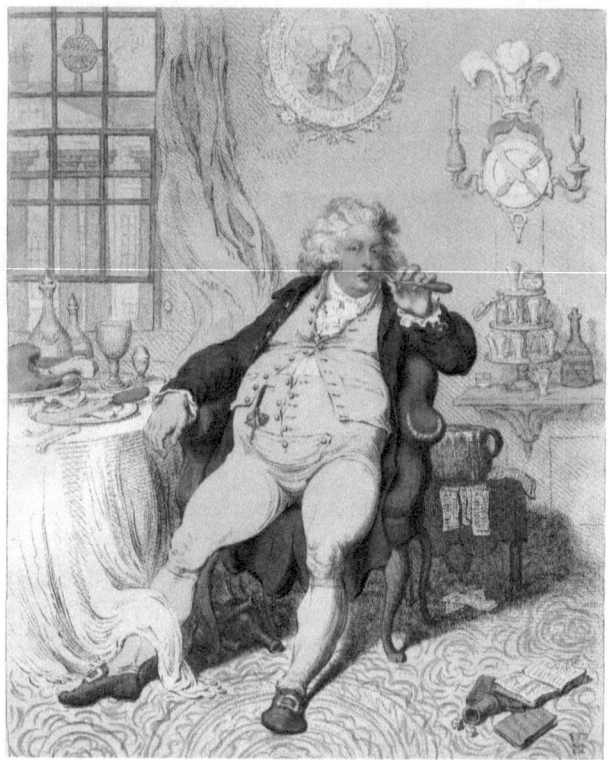

Figure 5.4   James Gillray, *A Voluptuary under the Horrors of Digestion* (1792 © Trustees of the British Museum, London)

Like its companion piece discussed above, Gillray's 1792 *Voluptuary under the Horrors of Digestion* (figure 5.4) has received attention in studies on diet and in political histories. However, I want to focus more specifically on the political implications of Gillray's image of eating and excess. *Voluptuary* is an image of a public figure whose particular mode of consumption was out of step with then-current events and modern values and wholly severed from the lives of his subjects. So obviously indifferent to the condition of his own body, how could the prince sympathize with the plight of humble subjects affected by war and scarcity? In the politically exigent atmosphere of the 1790s and in light of mounting pressure on public figures to demonstrate personal probity, Gillray presented an individual whose excesses marked him as unfit for public office. Coming from an era in which private virtue became so closely aligned with civic virtue, this image reminds us that in the public imagination personal taste is linked to political events like famine, war, and revolution.

Eating has always been bound up with notions of sociability and regional and national identity; yet, in the early nineteenth century, eating became a particular focus of philosophers who wrote about dining practices, of gastronomes who published treatises on tasteful tables, and of doctors who emphasized the relation between consumption and health. Eating became more strongly connected to a whole realm of other things: aesthetics, ethics, politics. In fact, in the first decades of the nineteenth century, food consumption was discussed as much in philosophical and political terms as biological ones. *Moderation* was a key bridging term, linking the material (eating) and the social (civic responsibility). In Gillray's *Voluptuary*, the prince's voracious eating and drinking are associated with gout, venereal disease, and vice: the prince suffers from a too-full stomach and, as the advertisement for Leake's patent pills on the floor indicates, from syphilis. He adopts the typical posture of gout sufferers, and the tablecloth wraps around his leg in anticipation of the binding that will encase his swollen limbs. Gout and venereal disease were considered gentleman's diseases, but by the end of the century they were also thought to be symptomatic of an indifference toward and a lack of understanding about the wider community. Gout and venereal disease became symptoms of a selfishness that sought its pleasures in the dark or, as Gillray's image indicates, alone at one's groaning table, cozened away from the difficulties of the wider world.[42]

The prince's solitary dining reflects his disconnection from political reality and from family, community, and nation. His remoteness is part of a regression that recalls Thomas Hobbes's description of natural man. George may be surrounded by the trappings of wealth in Gillray's image, but the overflowing chamber pot, the voraciously chomped joint, the discarded bones, and the two-pronged iron fork (with which he picks his teeth) are also signifiers of precivilized life. In her discussion of this image, Denise Gigante calls attention to the significance of that outdated fork, which had been replaced earlier in the century by the more civilized four-tined fork. She notes that in Gillray's *Temperance Enjoying a Frugal Meal*, the king and queen also use a two-tined fork, but in that context it seems old-fashioned and homely; in contrast, the prince's two-pronged utensil is uncivil and degenerate. In fact, the atavistic prince is worse than Hobbesian man in a state of nature, for he has had every privilege of civilization yet still indulges in primitive practices.[43]

Immanuel Kant's writing on eating and communal dining helps us understand what is at stake in the image of the voluptuary prince. In his 1798 collected lectures, *Anthropology from a Pragmatic Point of View*, Kant tackles, among other things, the relationship between material phenomena, ethics, and aesthetics. Kant is concerned with the progress of culture, the reciprocities of citizenship, and the individual's obligation to him or herself and to others. Of course, Kant's arguments were unlikely to have had much direct influence on British perceptions of the eating habits of the Prince of Wales, but his articulation of ideas about communality express wider emerging attitudes in Britain and Europe. He raises topics near and dear to the hearts of cosmopolitan British radicals when he outlines what it is to be a citizen of the world. Kant's cosmopolite is an enlightened individual whose sovereignty is not compromised by considering the tastes and views of others; instead, his or her compassion and understanding is expanded by contact with others.

On the one hand, eating is the most banal act. We are all biologically required to eat, and while our food choices may seem an expression of individuality, they are largely determined by the human history that precedes us. Our taste buds are moderated by a lineage of cultural practices and our judgments about cuisine are bound up with established tastes. Eating is an axiological enterprise; that is, it always involves value judgments about taste, landscape, and regionalism. On the other hand, Kant contends that eating should reach a higher level—a level of sociability worthy of enlightened cosmopolites. The model of enlightened eating is the dinner party, for "there is no situation in which sensibility and understanding unite in one enjoyment . . . as a good meal in good company."[44] The host may demonstrate his taste (for Kant this is a distinctly male enterprise) by choosing a variety of appealing food and drink, but consumables that appeal to the senses and are universally enjoyed remain secondary. Food is only "the vehicle for supporting the company" and encouraging "reciprocal and common conversation," in which guests share information, establish common values, and set aesthetic and moral standards.

The royal family, as represented by Gillray, can have no part in this type of commensurate dining: the king and queen may form a small party, but their clearly spare conversation mirrors their frugal meal of water, salad, and soft-boiled eggs. However, as a solitary diner, their *Voluptuary* son is that much worse. According to Kant, "eating alone (*solipsimus convictorii*)" is deeply "unhealthy" and unethical for the philosopher or thinking man.[45] The solitary diner who gorges, or as Kant puts it, indulges in "solitary *feasting*," is even more removed from ethical sociability. For the secret greedy gobbler, eating becomes "fatiguing work rather than a stimulating play of thoughts," whereas "a table companion with alternative ideas" would "have offered stimulation through new material."[46] Admittedly, Kant's solitary diner is still a contemplative individual who gets lost in his own thoughts—and this may seem a far cry from Gillray's prince, whose empty expression, chaotic table, and stuffed and motionless body signal anything but a thoughtful life. Yet Kant's description of what critic Peter Melville helpfully terms a "pathology of self-fixated ingestion" helps us grasp why Gillray's popular image of the companionless George incited and continues to incite not only the mirth of viewers but feelings of repulsion and distrust.[47]

Significantly, Kant defines the "conversation" of the communal dinner table as "reason applied to taste"—an equation that gastronomers and connoisseurs would develop further in the coming decades.[48] The prince, with his painful, debilitated, straining body, is clearly a man without reason. Fat dulls. The highly successful surgeon William Wadd, who would become one of the surgeons to George IV in 1821, makes this point in his treatise, *Comments on Corpulency* (1829): "If the Goddess of Wisdom were to grow fat, even she would become stupid."[49] Affairs of state could not be trusted to a man whose digestion used up the immense amounts of energy required for sharp-minded political activity. In Gillray's image, the prince's glassy and uncomprehending eyes indicate a refusal to engage with the world. In fact, the word *self-consuming*—a word Kant uses to describe the solitary feaster—captures the expanding body of Gillray's voluptuary prince. Paradoxically, the prince grows in size but his mind and body are eaten away by venereal disease, gout, and various forms of devouring pleasures. He could be the model for the deplorable figure of mindless excess—"the spoiled human being"—that Kant describes as so satiated with *"overindulgence"* that he has reached "that disgusting state that makes life itself a burden."[50]

I want to return to the issue of communality and its relation to eating, as it is an important one. Kant's communal table is the material embodiment of shared ideals; the sense of security and equality in this environment encourages the exercise of collective judgment. Kant's point, as Peter Melville explains, is that "acts of incorporation are cooperative—both aesthetically managed and ethically motivated."[51] The combination of aesthetics and ethics gestures toward an important Kantian concept: *sensus communis*. Kant adopts this term in the *Critique of Judgment* (1790) to refer to a shared sensibility or a wider understanding about what it means for a community to flourish. He uses the term to raise the question of how rational, autonomous individuals might cohere into peaceful, cooperative communities. The ligaments that hold a people together are shared ideas about beauty, agreement about what constitutes tasteful art and good literature, as well as shared practices surrounding food.

But England's debilitated voluptuary not only fails to contribute to *sensus communis*, he actively destroys it. In the words of the pamphleteer William Augustus Miles, the Prince of Wales had more than a "share . . . in relaxing those ligaments which unite and bind men together."[52] Throughout his reign as heir apparent, as regent, and finally as king, he was charged with poor taste, excessiveness, selfishness, and a blatant disregard for the welfare of others. George's voracious and uninhibited appetites—sexual and gastric—consumed any trace of fellow feeling. If he wanted someone else's wife, Miles writes, he would destroy her and her family to have her. As George hankered after ever more exotic and expensive delicacies, he drained the public coffers, thereby turning Britons who loved their country into Britons who resented their country. He was in danger of producing disaffected citizens like those across the Channel who were waging war against their own nation, its government, and its crown.

RATIONALITY AND THE NEW MAN OF TASTE

Throughout his canon, Kant is at pains to define "taste" and to distinguish it from what it is not. In the *Anthropology*, he aligns reason with taste in sociable conversation; he also defines *"The art of good living"* as extending hospitality and "living with taste."[53] It was difficult to act with "moderation" and "sobriety" in the most privileged circles of society, where overindulgence jeopardized good taste.[54] Kant makes a fine distinction between two forms of excess among the rich: *"Luxury (luxus)* is the excess, in a community, of social high living *with taste* (which is thus contrary to the welfare of the community). Excess *without taste*, however, is public *debauchery (luxuries)*.—If we take the effects of both on the community's welfare into consideration, then luxury is a *dispensable expenditure* which makes the community *poor*, while debauchery is one that makes it *ill*."[55] Although indulging in luxury necessarily monopolizes wealth, if individuals were to choose tasteful entertainments and pleasures, they could positively affect the cultural life of communities. High living with taste can refine and advance the arts and sciences.

In contrast, tasteless and excessive indulgence in luxuries is debauchery, which, Kant argues, "gorges" and gives rise to "disgust" among those with taste.[56] A lack of self-control in the face of physical pleasure—eating, drinking, sex—results in perceptible harms to the perpetrator and cripples the entire social body. Debauchery feeds off the community until that community becomes weak, withdrawn, and passive. Significantly, Kant's distinctions have a more pragmatic than purely philosophical application. Tracing distinctions about taste and eating reflects wider public perceptions about tasteful (and thus laudable) behaviors versus blindly excessive (and therefore improper) behaviors. The aim of the *Anthropology*, after all, is to reveal information about how the individual exists and can better exist in communities.

So how *did* one live tastefully? Who *was* the model of tasteful consumption at the turn of the nineteenth century? What *specifically* did the art of good or ethical living look like? These questions were addressed and at least partially answered by a new culturally influential figure: the gourmand or gastronome (also termed gastronomists or gastronomers). This group of culinary aesthetes flourished in the early nineteenth century, in the Paris of the Directory. As restaurants also appeared and grew in popularity during this time, they produced guides and reviews that explained how, where, and what to eat. The gastronome became an identifiable figure, following in a similar tradition as the art or music connoisseur. Crucially, he also used a medicopolitical vocabulary not unlike that employed by physicians and political propagandists, among others. The writing about haute cuisine in these decades is filled with bridging terms like *rationality*, *nature*, and *reason*, which promoted certain political views, social values, and ideas about health and disease. Gastronomical writers promoted their values as part of a wider exchange of ideas in the democratizing public sphere: while some of them set culinary standards for the wealthy, they also reached a much wider audience through publication. Other gastronomes, a little more like today's TV chefs, were keen to spread their opinions about dining, hospitality, taste, and good living to a growing middle-class audience. Whoever their intended reader, gastronomers "disseminate[d] knowledge of elite standards beyond the elite," so that, as Stephen Mennell points out, they performed the dual function "of articulating elite standards and of democratizing taste."[57] This is echoed by Denise Gigante's statement that gastronomes "participated in a democratization of taste by publishing the codes of good living."[58]

The widening of public interest in gastronomical culture, as described by Gigante and Mennell, and the linking of aesthetic, ethical, and medical subjects in gastronomical guides had ramifications for the public perception of George, who became regent in 1810 and king in 1820. The branding of him as an enemy of good taste—in spite of the fact that he prided himself on having the best chefs, demonstrating a flair for fashion, and stunning people with his grand architectural schemes—placed him at variance with the new man of taste. Like Kant's *Anthropology,* the gastronomical manuals of the early 1800s made phenomenological links between eating practices, sensual experience, and the formation of the human subject. Gastronomy, or the art and science of eating, was defined by the most famous nineteenth century gastronome, Jean-Anthelme Brillat-Savarin, as "the rational knowledge of all that relates to man as an eater."[59] Gastronomes embodied a new ideology of taste and promoted a whole catalog of updated eating rituals. Importantly, they advocated four main qualities (which seemed to be absent from the regent's life): communalism, refinement, rationality, and healthfulness. I want now to expand on these four values in order to more fully chart the cultural changes under way in these decades.

First, gastronomes consistently emphasized the point that eating was as much a sociocultural and political act as it was a biological one. Of course, "the arts and pleasures of the table had always involved a political dimension as a social force of community," as Denise Gigante observes, yet "nineteenth-century gastronomers literalized this tradition."[60] Besides writing about forks and fish courses, gastronomical writing extended an eighteenth-century philosophical tradition that included Kant, Burke, and David Hume. In this tradition, taste and aesthetics were a vital and inseparable part of the process of defining communal and national identities. The early food critic and restaurant writer Alexandre Balthazar Laurent Grimod de la Reynière's tremendously successful 1803 *Almanach des gourmands* (which was followed by seven further almanacs, from 1804 to 1812) should be seen as an important extension of this philosophical tradition. Each almanac featured the deliberations of a panel of food judges, or *jury de gustateurs,* who evaluated produce, foodstuffs, and dishes, paying careful attention to their geographical and anthropological genealogy. Grimod defined gourmands as distinctly cosmopolitan figures. Food sophisticates should be geographers of taste, with an acute sense of place, an understanding of local produce, and a sensitivity to regional differences. They should know, for instance, that "excellent smoked beef shall be synonymous with Hamburg; cod, with Ostende; freshly salted young herring and Holland," and one should think of Naples "at the mere mention of macaroni . . . likewise Genoa and crystallized lemon, Bologna and sausage . . . Florence and chocolate."[61] And the list goes on . . .

This sense of being connected to the world by consuming the food of one's neighbors is related to a second characteristic of gourmands: refinement. Like other writers in this genre, Grimod insisted that temperance, discrimination, and precision were needed to cultivate the "exceptionally delicate palate" of the gastronome. This emphasis is a significant feature of the "civilizing of appetite" that was under way in this era, a process that, according to Stephen Mennell, was the cultural outcome of wider availability and increased choice of ingredients and dishes.[62] Even among the wealthiest eaters, there was a turn away from "quantitative consumption for the expression of social superiority" to considering "the qualitative possibilities" of food and drink.[63] Traditional aristocratic and courtly eating practices were often based on quantity and excess; but, quite simply, it became gauche to express one's standing through extreme overindulgence. As Mennell puts it, "The courtly ethos was antithetical to that of bourgeois economic rationality; lavish consumption was too closely part of the courtier's social identity for him to economise like a good bourgeois."[64] Mennell is referring mostly to France here, but *middle class* can easily replace *bourgeois*, and the statement then applies equally to Britain. In the gastronomical guide *Apacian Morsels*, Gabriel Hummelberger includes a long critique of the egregious gluttony and shockingly excessive household accounts of historical kings, aristocrats, and religious leaders, including one particular pope's gratuitous taste for peacock. "Such as indulge the gratification of any appetite to excess, are far below the brutes," Hummelberger declares, but then quickly adds that neither should we deny the pleasures of the flesh or be miserly or sparing. Our economic and social circumstances should determine the level of our self-indulgence: "to debar ourselves of any enjoyment within the bounds of innocence and reason, is 'to live like Nature's bastards, not her sons.'"[65] Polite diners demonstrated their distinction by making refined, cultured choices.

Indeed, refinement is the means of reconciling a seeming contradiction between this new food culture, with its elaborate menus and elegant dishes, and the simultaneous emergence of the (largely) middle-class emphasis on self-control, moderation, and restraint. Indeed, this was an era in which reams of religious and moral tracts advocating moderation in all things appeared alongside epicurean guides detailing the proper preparation of calf's head in aspic and specifying which utensils, from an astonishing array, one should eat it with. Medical manuals promoting temperance and strict dietary regimens were sold alongside almanacs extolling the virtues of the *mayonnaise de volaille* served at Le Grand

Véfour in Paris's Palais Royale. In actuality, gastronomes shared a cluster of values with otherwise disparate groups, among them political reactionaries, moralists, Evangelicals, and Malthusian economists. In various ways, each of these groups was keen to usher out eighteenth-century excess in favor of a much more rational and self-disciplined way of life, which these proponents saw as politically necessary. They promoted a reasonable and socially responsible moderation at table, in the bedroom, in social circles, and in public life.

As this last sentence indicates, refinement and good taste were connected to a third emphasis: rationality. The gourmand was foremost, as Gigante puts it, a "'rational epicure,' no mere unthinking eater or glutton driven by physical compulsion."[66] The new man of taste curbed the appetite in order to become more thoughtful about his choices. In fact, the term *rationality* appears everywhere in this new genre of food writing. In his 1820 gastronomical poem *Tabella Cibaria: The Bill of Fare*, the author and amateur artist Ange Denis Macquin draws a clear distinction between the indelicacy of the glutton and the "rational pleasure" of the gourmand. While the former gorges and appreciates nothing, the latter "seeks for peculiar delicacy and distinct flavour in the various dishes presented to the judgment and enjoyment of his discerning palate."[67] The linking of palate (associated with taste and judgment) with the function and health of the organs of the body is another aspect of the epicurean man of reason. In his axiomatic guide to dining, *Physiologie du Goût* (first published in 1825), the great icon of food connoisseurship, Brillat-Savarin, differentiated between gluttons and gourmands. He joined a chorus of gourmands who described the latter as "rational" and "opposed to excess" and the former as dyspeptic individuals who suffered from indigestion and intoxication, and who were "incapable of either eating or drinking."[68]

Likewise, in his *Essays, Moral, Philosophical, and Stomachical, on the Important Science of Good-Living* (1822), the English gourmand Lancelot Sturgeon distinguished carefully between a glutton and an epicure with the following explication:

> Gluttony is, in fact, a mere effort of the appetite, of which the coarsest bolter of bacon in all Hampshire may equally boast with the most distinguished consumer of turtle in a Corporation; while Epicurism is the result of "that choicest gift of Heaven," a refined and discriminating taste: this is the peculiar attribute of the palate, that [a large appetite] of the stomach. It is the happy combination of both these enviable qualities that constitutes the truly estimable character, the real epicure. He is not only endowed with a capacious stomach and an

insatiable appetite, but with a delicate susceptibility in the organs of degustation.[69]

As these comments indicate, digestion and medical disorders such as indigestion and dyspepsia were related to cultural expressions of civility, sensibility, and discrimination. The physical and the intellectual, the material and the metaphysical, the medical and the aesthetic were collapsed in gastronomical writing.

Sturgeon's remarks call up the fourth quality claimed by the gastronome: that of health. The "art" of gastronomy could not be separated from the "science" of digestion. One of the greatest explicators of the medical aspects of nineteenth century gastronomy was the eccentric Warren Street eye doctor and gastronome William Kitchiner. In his tremendously successful publication, *The Cook's Oracle* (1817), he defines "the cardinal virtues of Cookery" as "CLEANLINESS, FRUGALITY, NOURISHMENT AND PALATEABLENESS."[70] He intends to address only those "who make nourishment the Chief end of Eating, and do not desire to provoke Appetite beyond the powers and necessities of Nature." He easily reconciles medicine and art, health and pleasure; therapies for ailments are offered alongside discourses on aesthetic or philosophical concerns. According to Kitchiner, the gastronome should embark on taste excursions to any realm of pleasure available to him and should stop only when his desires threaten to compromise the body. Such a man follows "the purest Epicurean principles of indulging the Palate as far as it can be done without injury or offense to the Stomach, and forbidding nothing but what is unfriendly to Health."[71] Eating should be as aesthetically pleasing a cultural experience as possible, yet ultimately nature defines what is proper for our diets, while matters of health curtail our pleasure in consuming. We may go so far as to desire that dining be a purely cerebral, or even a metaphysical act—an act unbounded by the demands of the body—but as he explains in a motto that pays close tribute to Samuel Johnson, "the *energy of our* BRAINS *is sadly dependent on the behaviour of our* BOWELS."[72] One of the positive sides to this equation is that eating is a means of personal improvement. Intelligence, character, and aesthetic sense can be vastly improved by feeding the bowels in a tasteful and rational way.

Kitchiner was participating in ongoing medical debates about the role of digestion and its operation with respect to other physiological systems. As we have seen earlier, links between immorality and excessive eating had been forged in medical manuals a hundred years before the emergence of gastronomy. I want to pause and return to physicians such as George Cheyne, William Cullen, and William Buchan, who offered diagnoses and prescriptions in popular treatises packaged as public education. The eighteenth-century health movement, as C. J. Laurence pointed out some time ago, produced "a profusion of literature aimed at the individual, in the Utopian hope that widespread education would improve the health of the community in general."[73] Reform of the individual body through diet, exercise, and cleanliness was part of individual moral reform, and both physical and moral improvement were vital for the health of the nation as a whole. The emphasis on disciplined eating and drinking, prevention of disease, and personal responsibility contributed to the modern medicalization of the appetite. Importantly, doctors like Cheyne, Cullen, and Buchan also promoted the idea that possessing knowledge about anatomy and medicine was itself a measure of taste. The individual who neglected learning about medicine, Cullen argued, "has but a sorry claim either to taste or learning."[74] In other words, there was a similar move toward democratization in both medicine and gastronomy: the former emphasized public health and individual well-being, while the latter brought about a democratization of taste.

Democracy, epicureanism, and discipline also indicate a classical context to the emergence of gastronomy and its relation to the science of dietetics. Motivated by the belief that domestic medicine would reform the morals and bodies of the populace, Buchan and Cheyne were among those who revived an ancient interest in care of the body and a concomitant concern with hygiene. In fact, the classical world figures in important ways in the nature versus culture debate that was so dominant in the eighteenth and nineteenth centuries. Cheyne looked to ancient Greece as a national model for the challenges faced by modern, urban, increasingly cerebral Europeans who, as a symptom of their advanced state of civilization, suffered from diseases like gout, disorders like obesity, and nervous conditions like melancholy and hypochondria. In the hearty and hale days of ancient Briton, people had the capacity to resist disease and did not need the services of physicians. In *The English Malady*, Cheyne describes how "the ancient *Greeks*, while they lived in their Simplicity and Virtue were Healthy, Strong and Valiant: But afterwards, in Proportion as they advanced in Learning, and the Knowledge of the Sciences, and distinguished themselves from other Nations by their Politeness and Refinement they sunk into *Effeminacy, Luxury,* and *Diseases*, and began to study *Physick*, to remedy those Evils which their Luxury and Laziness had brought upon them."[75] The Greeks of the ancient world were to be admired, then, for their invention of the idea of public medicine, gymnastics, games, baths, and hygiene. Yet they only did so in order to combat the bodily weaknesses and ailments caused by sedentary study and their love of luxury. The modern world had no choice but to do the same.

The connection between ancient physic, eighteenth-century health manuals, and nineteenth-century gastronomy lies in the fusion of aesthetics and medicine, with moderation and discipline as the key mediating values between the two. In fact, the ancient concept of "hygeia"—cultivating the perfect body and obtaining a pleasurable life through a perfection of one's regimen and the surrounding environment—shares common aims with Cheynean dietetics and modern gastronomy. Michel Foucault's two books on ancient sexual ethics, *The Use of Pleasure* and *The Care of the Self* reveal some of these shared aims and draw connections between, among other things, classical and modern bodily regimens and ideas about proper, self-disciplined bodies. In a section on dietetics, part of his larger study of how the ancient world dealt with bodily appetites and sexual practices, Foucault shows us that in the long history of the formation of the subject, at certain times and for certain reasons there have evolved codes of personal ethics that place great stress on discipline and moderation. Dietetics and exercise were significant components of the development of what he terms an "aesthetics of the self."

In his reading of Plato's *Republic* and *Timaeus*, Foucault traces an ideology about the ill effects of culture on the body that is remarkably similar to Cheyne and other modern medical writers. Foucault paraphrases Plato's claim that, according to Homer's accounts of earlier times, people had very little use for dietary regimens because "the manner in which they nourished themselves and exercised their bodies, was in accord with nature." However, "when men had forsaken the rough, healthy life of former times," society then had to counter the effects of culture. One of the ways it did so was to create dietary and exercise regimens; as a result, "dietetics came into existence as a kind of medicine for soft times; it was designed for mismanaged lives."[76] In many ways, Foucault's reading of Plato's interpretation of Homer captures the underlying principle of the medical angle to the art of modern gastronomy. Foucault concludes that dietary regimen became part of how one's life was managed—and how one managed one's own life. Systems of regulating diet "enabled a set of rules to be affixed to conduct" and allowed for behaviors to be "indexed to a nature which had to be preserved and to which it was right to conform." In other words, "regimen was a whole art of living."[77] Readers internalized the guidance offered by gastronomical and medical guides. There is in both classical and modern writing on this subject a nostalgic looking to a more natural past as a guide to what the body can be and how far it has strayed. Yet, bodies in the present day always require the assistance of progressive medicine and newly developed dietary regimens. The aesthetics of eating, ideas about the body beautiful, and ways of living a good life are distinctly contemporary—in whatever age.

Indeed, efforts to reconcile a nostalgia for a healthy past with the seduction of modern luxuries similarly motivated nineteenth-century dietetics. In his 1801 *Practical Treatise on Diet*, William Nisbet observes in a now familiar refrain that "artificial life" had come to prevail everywhere, "from the palace to the cottage," and that "the evils" attendant on said "artificial life may be considered as the great foundation of medicine."[78] In the mixed-up modern world, diseases of civilization like gout "had become a Proteus" so that both men and women suffered from what had once been gender-specific diseases; in fact, men were now so weak as to suffer from, of all things, hysteria.[79] But for all his denunciation of the trappings of culture and their effects on health, Nisbet had to admit that a return to a natural, authentic, and simpler way of life was impossible. In "modern times," he wrote, "the simple state of nature is now in every vestige unknown."[80] Primal nature did not exist; doctors and philosophers could not legitimize their diagnoses and treatments by referring to something that was nonexistent. Nisbet's conclusion, like Rousseau's, was to necessarily accept modernity but to make efforts to identify the vestiges of nature that were left. The traces of the natural past should guide our eating practices.

The vestiges of nature could be found in the material body. New knowledge about the internal functioning of the body provided guidance for damaged, mixed-up, and enervated moderns. The physician-gastronome William Kitchiner's arguments recall the surgeon John Hunter's privileging of the stomach as the regulative center of the whole bodily enterprise. In his *Principles of Surgery*, Hunter placed the stomach above the brain as necessary for animal life: "An animal can exist without any senses, brain, or nervous system, without limbs, heart, or circulation, in short, without anything but a stomach."[81] He conceived of the stomach as most sympathetic with the mind and of digestion as a process of converting food "into part of ourselves"—anticipating the gastronome's emphasis on food as shaping not only the body but also less tangible things like character and intelligence.[82] Although Hunter is generally considered a vitalist, his views were influenced by the skeptical tradition of British empiricism, through John Locke and David Hume, as well as by Enlightenment models of the body as machine, outlined most notably by the French anatomists and physiologists Julian Offrey de La Mettrie, Marie François Xavier Bichat, and the naturalist Georges Cuvier. Hunter's mechanistic views about the functions of the body's organs reconciled with a belief that, ultimately, there was an overarching living principle or vital element distinct from the material body and its functions.

Kitchiner uses similar analogies to describe the body as a watch, a machine made of the most intricate parts and yet run by the most simple of mechanisms. In his *Art of Invigorating and Prolonging Life, by Food, Clothes, Air, Exercise, Wine, Sleep, &c. and Peptic Precepts*, Kitchiner compares the stomach to the watch's "regulator" and equates food to "the Key by which the machine is wound up."[83] In this view, what and how we eat directly determines our mental alertness and the functioning of the body as a whole. Humans are responsible for maintaining their own physiological and mental balance by quite simply adjusting what enters the stomach and how it gets there. For this reason, Kitchiner is very precise about the mechanical processes of ingestion and digestion. He reminds readers that "the sagacious *Gourmand* is ever mindful of another motto— 'Masticate, Denticate, Chump, Grind, and Swallow.'"[84] In a testament to good taste and an Enlightenment faith in precision and categorization, Kitchiner calculates precisely the optimum number of bites that must be applied to each type of food so that the diner can obtain the greatest epicurean pleasure *and* the greatest health benefit: "the mean number of Munches, that solid meat requires, to prepare it for its journey down *the Red Lane*," ranges "from 30 to 40, (according to the tenderness of the meat)."[85] In such a way, Kitchiner's medicogastronomical program might be termed a utilitarian approach to eating, combining as it does pleasure and happiness with rationality and economy.

Kitchiner is concerned, too, with the effect of digestion on human emotion, and sympathy in particular. He addresses Kantian concerns about how food and dining practices tap into feelings of compassion and understanding, thereby attaching individuals to their communities. One of Kitchiner's peptic precepts is that the stomach is the organ most connected to emotion: it is, he writes, "the centre of Sympathy."[86] He equates the physiological sensitivity of the stomach, compared with other body organs, with the emotional receptivity of sensitive people. In fact, he speaks about the stomach as if it was *itself* sensate, as if it had its own feelings and moods: "If either the Body or the Mind be fatigued,—the Stomach invariably sympathizes;—if the most robust do any thing too much, the Stomach is soon affronted."[87] This image of the stomach as a sympathetic entity is echoed by the noted gatekeeper of taste, Gabriel Hummelberger. In his 1829 *Apacian Morsels*, which offers a "veritable science of the mouth," Hummelberger insists that the stomach "certainly possesses the most exquisite sympathy, and is feelingly alive" to any "injuries" we might do to it. Treating the stomach like "either a pudding-bag intended to be filled, or like a pair of saddle-bags, built for stowage, and to be crammed as full as it can hold," will cause it to complain resentfully.[88] The sensitive stomach should be neither a victim of excess nor a sufferer of restriction; rather, it should be treated as if one's happiness depended on it.

The dual emphasis on sympathy and refined restraint recalls that nebulous "thing" that acts as a socially cohesive force, *sensus communis*. Without a doubt, ideas about community and ethics took on new meaning in the context of gastronomy, as did the relationship of those things to individual eating practices. As Hummelberger observes, sounding much like Kant, "the table is the only chain which connects every branch of society."[89] Hummelberger also emphasizes that diners must be rational, autonomous individuals who imbibe the opinions and ideas of others as they eat with them. This feast of sociability is a model of the type of communal sharing and patriotic feeling that connects otherwise disparate and socially divided people. The qualities of the gastronome—cosmopolitan, communal, refined, rational, and healthy—are all part of expressing one's good taste. They are also part of living as good and as beautiful a life as one can. The enlightened gourmand is principled and philosophical; he understands his body's physiology and cares about his health, as much as he cares about appearances and aesthetics. As such, he carefully identifies the finest foods and consumes them thoughtfully, reasonably, and communally. He is the legitimate citizen of a civilized nation.

Based on these assertions, then, the frugal King George III and the parsimonious Queen Charlotte were not rational, tasteful, sociable diners; still, as we know, the real threat to good taste and sensus communis was the regent. Unable to care for himself, dulling his wits with wine, deadening his brain with obscene amounts of meat, using the utensils of an uncivilized "bolter of bacon," and detaching himself from others with his greedy excesses, the Prince Regent existed apart from the people. Where the nation's king was expected to sit at the head of the table as the genial and generous host who communed with his subjects, George instead closeted himself away to indulge in unseemly feasts. This is the image of a tasteless man, devoid of the capacity to exercise reason in his personal choices; as such, it seemed impossible for him to act appropriately as head of state. He could not be trusted to act on behalf of Britons, whose views and concerns he would not hear, did not understand, and could not sympathize with. Books, pamphlets, caricatures, and especially regional and national newspapers are full of reportage, editorials, images, and letters from the public that record the negative reaction he received from all corners of society and in all circumstances. Consequently, the regent and later King George IV occupies a crucial place in the history of constitutional evolution. As we will see further in the next chapter, the legitimacy of the throne was sorely tested during his reign, and the political role of the monarch became a much more symbolic one. With a king who did not have public support, it made sense that real executive powers should reside securely with the people's valid representatives in the government.

6 Hottentot Buttocks, "Strange Chinese Shapes," and George IV's Oriental Appetites

> But stay the curious appetite, and taste
> With caution Fruits you never tried before
> JOHN ARMSTRONG,
> *The Art of Preserving Health* (1744)

In 1770, Edmund Burke observed that the independence-seeking inhabitants of the American colonies—once Britons themselves—had become alienated from their parent nation. He represented the breaking of faith between America and England in the following terms: "When men imagine that their food is only a cover for poison, and when they neither love nor trust the hand that serves it, it is not the name of roast beef of Old England that will persuade them to sit down to the table that is spread for them."[1] Significantly, Burke expressed political estrangement through differences in culinary tastes. Loyalty, patriotism, and regional and national identities, as we know from the last chapter, were closely bound up with food. The analogy between food choices and patriotic feeling captures precisely the growing distrust and suspicion the colonized felt toward their colonizers, as well as the growing cultural distance between the two nations. Roast beef may have been John Bull's favored dish, but it was not Uncle Sam's. American identities had cohered around a geographically specific cuisine; in large part, Americans had ceased to view roast beef as part of their communal table, indicating how far the kinship between nations had deteriorated.

How dominantly roast beef symbolized Englishness is evidenced throughout print culture, but one particular American article, published in the 1876–77 *Harper's New Monthly Magazine* gives a revealing retrospective: "In England, during the early times, the food served upon the table was simply a gigantic forerunner of the taste of the English at present. They were always a race of meat-eaters. Wild boars and huge bullocks were roasted whole at their mediæval feasts. An ancient ballad-singer asserted the invincibility of the Britons so long as they were 'fed upon beef,' and according to present appearances their invincibility will not be subverted for a long time to come, if beef is, in reality, the basis of England's strength."[2] Race, taste, and character are inseparable. English character—pugnacious, robust, and indomitable—has a material basis in meat eating, particularly beef. That character, which defines and unites a race, has stayed steady because the nation's tastes (slightly adapted for the modern world) have stayed steady.

Food has played an integral role in shaping the course of human history. It has also had a hand in fashioning national, regional, and individual identities. Onno Oerlemans uses the term "symbolic osmosis" to express the idea "that characteristics associated with a type of food would, in one way or another, be passed on to those who consumed that food," while Beatrice Fink describes this phenomenon as "phagic determinism."[3] This principle is perhaps best encapsulated by the gastronome Jean-Anthelme Brillat-Savarin's famous 1825 phrase, "Tell me what you eat, and I will tell you what you are." Although this aphorism expresses materialist ideas about the sympathetic relationship between body and mind, food and health, matter and immaterial thought, Fink problematizes the easy materialist cause and effect relation it suggests. As she points out, Brillat-Savarin's saying is the fourth of twenty in the "prolegomenon" of his *Physiologie du Goût* (1826). The third one, just before it—"The destiny of nations is dependent upon the manner in which they feed themselves"—calls attention to the sociocultural aspects of the food = self equation.[4] Still, the fact remains that food is a determiner of identity, whether on an individual or a collective level. Questions of national identity and patriotic feeling in the nineteenth century could not be separated from the politics of *both* personal and collective consumption. One of the questions citizens of this era asked was, if one became what one ate, then how did consuming foreign food (and other commodities) alter one's constitution?

Brillat-Savarin's mottoes express principles previously outlined in eighteenth-century medical writing. George Cheyne's *Natural Method of Cureing Diseases of the Body* (1742) had discussed similarly antidualist ideas. A pioneer of what would become the mantra of health-conscious writers in succeeding generations, Cheyne emphasized the connection between habits of consumption, physical and mental health, and what we would now term quality of life. At one point, he used the vegetarian, teetotaler Isaac Newton as an exemplar of temperance and self-control, attributing the scientist's intellectual acumen to his diet of bread and water. Newton's facility for "just and close thinking" was owed to his "superiority of parts," which were in turn enhanced by his "extreme

Temperance and *Abstinence*."[5] Eating "the *lightest* and the *least* food," Cheyne deduced, made possible "the clear, ready and pleasant exercise of the *intellectual* faculties."[6] To echo a theme from the last chapter, controlling ingestion could do so much more than simply control one's body shape. In this chapter, however, I want to look specifically at how national identity and the issue of racial difference became important themes in writing about diet and representations of politically privileged eaters. This chapter explores the relationship between the body, ideas of foreignness, medical understandings of disease and epidemic, and political culture. The intensifying medical attention on dietetics and the global spread of disease influenced how the regent's obese body and his tastes for all things foreign were represented as threatening to national identity, to the health of the body politic, and to distinctively English ideas of morality.

CONSUMING TASTES: IDENTITY, HEALTH, AND FOREIGNNESS

The diet Cheyne recommended in *The Natural Method* and in his earlier *English Malady* (1733) was a quintessentially English one that addressed a quintessentially English set of symptoms. His recommended intake of vegetables, milk, and no more than a half pound of "Flesh Meat" per day was a far cry from the English roast beef diet described in the *Harper's* retrospective. The new English regimen, as promoted by Cheyne and others, was a distinctly modern one that rejected the nostalgic, medievalist vision of "huge bullocks" as the culinary source of England's strength. In the modern commercial, industrial Britain, feasting on huge bullocks was a source of weakness, which rendered gentlemen gout ridden, dull witted, apathetic, and lazy. The British diet needed to be expunged of the excesses associated with both a heroic chivalric past *and* the wealthy, mercantilist present, with its global trade of foodstuffs and cuisines. In doing so, the new English diet would counter the ill effects of modern civilization, including melancholy, hypochondria, gout, drunkenness, and especially, obesity.

Cheyne was not alone. In the eighteenth century, poets, artists, and physicians emphasized the idea that eating indigenous foods, prepared in traditional, native ways, would produce a regional identity that was authentic and honorable. In his study of disease and colonialism in the Romantic era, Alan Bewell explains that diet demarcates cultural differences between nations. He points to William Hogarth's *Beer Street* as an image that equates drinking local beer with strength, health, and liberty; in contrast, Hogarth's partner print *Gin Lane* portrays foreign drink (gin originated in Holland) as rendering the British constitution weak, diseased, and vice ridden.[7] As another example, Bewell points to passages in Tobias Smollett's *Humphrey Clinker* as quintessential statements about what constituted English-style eating in the eighteenth century. The character Matt Bramble expresses this nostalgic vision of a rural, healthy, clean, and self-sufficient way of producing local food in the countryside:

> I drink the virgin lymph, pure and crystalline as it gushes from the rock, or the sparkling beveridge, home-brewed ... my bread is sweet and nourishing, made from my own wheat, ground in my own mill, and baked in my own oven, my table is, in a great measure, furnished from my own ground; my five-year old mutton, fed on the fragrant herbage of the mountains ... my poultry from the barn-door, that never knew confinement ... my own garden yields in plenty and perfection; the produce of the natural soil, prepared by moderate cultivation. The same soil affords all the different fruits which England may call her own.[8]

Clearly, this is an idealized image of the English countryside, which portrays ecologically sound methods of production and consumption. The people who live in this world have strong bodies and sound minds, they respect the landscape, and their healthy productivity drives both the local and national economies. Bramble articulates a romanticized vision of village life, in which people are deeply rooted in a native soil that yields bread, mutton, eggs, and indigenous apples.

This vision of a healthy, organic, cohesive England has an immediately identifiable culinary identity, with its own unique rituals of communal dining. Such an image contrasts sharply with the alimentary identity of George IV. In the years of his reign as regent and as king, biographers, pamphleteers, and journalists questioned his exotic tastes; by the time of his death in 1830, his reputation as a lover of Eastern delicacies, which had adulterated his constitution and the nation's, was cemented. Looking back from 1830, the biographer Robert Huish recalls how, from the age that George reached his majority until the day of his death, his appetites resembled that of an Oriental tyrant rather than an honest Englishman. It is not insignificant, Huish recalls, that in celebration of George being made Prince of Wales on 12 August 1783, "a large turtle, of the enormous size of four hundred weight, was killed ... being a present sent to the Prince from the East Indies."[9] George's taste for turtle must be understood in the context of late eighteenth-century ideas about the relationship between eating and the self. To an observing public, George's intake of exotic foods "phagically determined" his character so that he resembled an Eastern sultan or a Turkish tyrant. Far from reflecting his Englishness, his culinary tastes demonstrated a supposedly "Oriental" love of opulence, overindulgence, and domination—qualities that clearly threatened national cohesion and individual liberties. This early taste for turtle set a pattern of eating behavior that would never sit well with his subjects.

George's intake of exotic foods paralleled his consumption of other luxurious foreign goods. This taste for foreignness was conflated with his vast appetite for women, clothing, and expensive architectural projects and was interpreted in public prints as indicating a lack of discrimination and loyalty. By the turn of the nineteenth century, he was fully ensconced in an Orientalized world he had created in the heart of Brighton but that seemed to have very little to do with the region or with England in general. Images proliferated of a voraciously consuming monarch who had adopted a model of Turkish tyranny. In 1812, a pamphleteer claiming the name of the earlier pseudonymous writer "Junius" ranked George with "the Cadis, Bashaws, the Vizier, the Divan, and the Grand Sultan himself."[10] In his dealings with women and in particular with his legitimate wife Princess Caroline, George had acted the domestic tyrant. When he launched the secret inquiry into his wife's private affairs—the 1806 "Delicate Investigation"—he felt no compunction about exploiting his political connections. Corrupting the law with impunity better suited "a country like Turkey," according to this Junius.[11] But Britain was stuck with its very own Oriental sultan.

Robert Huish equated such sexual behavior with profoundly antipatriotic sentiment. He accused George of a xenophobia that was not directed at foreigners, as one might expect, but rather at his own people. Huish recalled how "the bacchanalian orgies" the regent held at his renovated-in-the-Oriental-style London residence Carlton House had been "of a most extraordinary description, and might be said to resemble more the interior of a Turkish seraglio, than the abode of a British Prince. . . . The dances which were exhibited for the amusement of the companions of the Prince were performed by females, whose sole aim and study appeared to have been, like the dancing girls of the East, to perfect themselves in voluptuousness of attitude, and in a shameless exposure of their person, to the unrestrained gaze of the libidinous voluptuary."[12] In Huish's description of the regent's private life, Oriental architecture, foreign goods, sensuality, and Eastern entertainments commingle in a very un-English scene. There is, in this passage, a distinctly threatening politics of visuality at work: the regent's libidinous gaze is only as uninhibited as the public's gaze is absent. In the style of the French monarchy—but in stark contrast to King George III and Queen Charlotte—the prince cossets himself away behind protecting walls where, free from the disciplinary gaze of the public, he can participate in an orgy of licentiousness.

BODIES AND BUILDINGS:
FOREIGN FLESH AND ALIEN ARCHITECTURE

I want to tease out the significance of architecture a bit more here. The public perception of the Prince Regent's Orientalized residences is significant and not unrelated to how medical discourse affected political culture. If the newspapers and caricatures that circulated in the first three decades of the nineteenth century are anything to go by, George IV's tastes—alimentary, architectural, and sexual—were closely entwined in the public mind. Moreover, these interrelated tastes were in conflict with the emerging medical and moral emphasis on restraint and the political significance attached to transparency. As we will see, the public interpreted George's consumption of exotic food, of grand Oriental architecture, and of other men's wives as all part of the morally perverse and politically dangerous world he had created behind the walls of his residences.

Once declared regent in 1811, George had the funds to hire architect John Nash to create an extraordinarily fantastical Indo-Chinese masterpiece (or monstrosity, depending on your view). The Brighton Pavilion boasted an astonishing collection of chinoiserie. The immense Robert Jones–designed Banqueting Room was filled with metal palms, blown glass, and crystal dragon chandeliers. Lacking a cohesive theoretical structure, the Regency style was an eclectic mix that included everything from neo-Gothic to neoclassical to Indo-Oriental. Several contemporary visitors noted this architectural eclecticism. In a letter of 27 October 1820, Princess Lieven searched for words to explain the Pavilion: "How can one describe such a piece of architecture? The style is a mixture of Moorish, Tartar, Gothic, and Chinese and all in stone and iron. It is a whim which has already cost £700,000, and it is still not fit to live in."[13] The Comtesse de Boigne described an earlier form of the building as "the most heterogeneous magnificence [that] had been gathered at vast expense from the four quarters of the globe and piled beneath the eight or ten cupolas of this ugly and eccentric palace, the several parts of which displayed not the slightest architectural unity."[14]

Even favorable comments represented the Pavilion as something out of "The Thousand and One Nights."[15] Lady Bessborough's partially sympathetic rationalizing of the prince's Oriental taste could not hide her distaste for the "strange Chinese shapes ... in outré and false taste" that filled his home. She rationalized George's vulgarity as a defense mechanism: throughout society "there was such an outcry against French things" that he became "afraid of his furniture being accused of jacobinism."[16] In the suspicious, hostile postrevolutionary environment of the 1810s, flagrant architectural discord and rooms full of Louis XV furniture could be interpreted as reflective of a dangerous politics. The regent may have been the farthest thing from a Jacobin, but his "false" taste for strange Chinese shapes also communicated hostility to England and Englishness.

The Pavilion was the perfect setting for Oriental-style feasting on wine, women, and exotic food (including mulligatawny, which was purportedly introduced to England by one of the regent's chefs). At the beginning of 1817, the famous French chef Marie-Antoine Carême—previously employed by Napoleon, the Rothschilds, Talleyrand, and the Russian tsar—took over the mind-bogglingly extensive kitchens. The unrivaled "King's Kitchen" had a three-room confectionary for lavish desserts, two rooms for pastries, and an icehouse that supplied sorbets and ice cream. And that was just the sweet courses. Carême planned and executed extravagant dinners, the details of which were often reported in the newspapers. The British public learned, for instance, that on 18 January 1817 the French chef oversaw an incredibly elaborate banquet in honor of the visiting Grand Duke Nicholas of Russia, which included an unprecedented 127 dishes, including a four-foot-high marzipan Turkish mosque.

Just as contemporary observers thought of George's eating habits as indicative of his character, they conceived of his buildings as speaking volumes about his abilities and priorities. In fact, the idea that buildings are texts that communicate values and ideas has a long history. Cultural-anthropological scholarship has helpfully revealed some of the connective infrastructure between architecture, food, and politics. In the twentieth century, thinkers as diverse as the anthropologists Mary Douglas and Claude Lévi-Strauss, the semiotician Roland Barthes, and the sociologist Pierre Bourdieu have adopted a broadly phenomenological approach to reading cultural phenomena. Douglas's seminal work describes how to "decipher" a meal; Lévi-Strauss addresses the structural grammar of food; Barthes decodes the culturally specific language of French foodstuffs; Bourdieu explores how class ideologies underpin food choices and dining habits in French society. In similar fashion, architects and their critics—past and present—conceive of buildings as texts with grammars. A diverse group, from John Ruskin and A. W. N. Pugin in the nineteenth century to the spatial theorists Gaston Bachelard and Henri Lefebvre in the twentieth, have interrogated the narrative or discursive quality of architecture.[17]

Spatial arrangements as well as design elements and motifs, including decoration, detailing, arches, and planes, effectively communicate a complex web of messages. From these, individuals can intuit a nation's customs, ideologies, and historic evolutions. According to Victorian architects like Pugin, who deplored the Brighton Pavilion and all that its style represented, the measure of a building's aesthetic beauty and cultural legitimacy was its ability to communicate a nation's heritage, identity, and religion. For this reason, Pugin and a host of others revived neo-Gothic styles in particular, which were seen as part of a Christian English tradition, expressive of English craftsmanship, history, and values. In this view, architecture and design should not only suit the building's purpose but also impart a sense of a nation's shared beliefs and values. Architecture and society exist symbiotically: built structures, like food, contribute to a society's salvation or play a role in its brutalization.

These two strands of cultural criticism—anthropological and architectural—help us understand the kinds of things that were at stake in the scandalizing and Orientalizing of the regent. These semiotic ideas were already in circulation in the early decades of the nineteenth century. George's body, his eating habits, and his buildings were all read like texts, which seemed to signify a personal immorality inseparable from political corruption and ineptitude. Satirical images made these points visually. To the popular satirist William Hone, George appeared as "an old fat MANDARIN," who sat in his "CHINA SHOP like a large Joss." Hone's satirical poem *The Joss and His Folly*—published in 1820, the year the regent became king—is illustrated by two George Cruikshank caricatures. In the first (figure 6.1), which precedes the poem, the rotund and Orientalized George sits atop an ornate Chinese teapot, which has the Brighton Pavilion etched on its side. Hugely triangular (or pear-shaped), George forms the pot's lid. He and his Chinese castle are surrounded by Oriental servants and objects, making up "the queerest of all the queer sights," in Hone's words.[18]

In the next image (figure 6.2), George has become the teapot; his body has morphed into the building/objects/food he consumes: he is what he eats. Evoking the characterization of Oriental people as enigmatic and given to hiding their thoughts behind indecipherable faces, George is por-

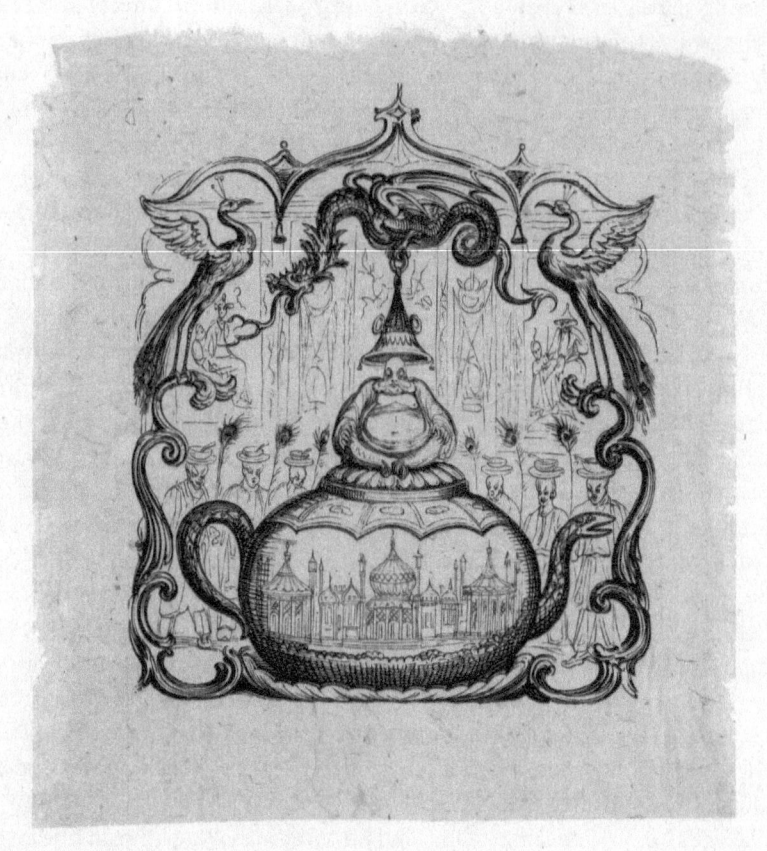

Figure 6.1 George Cruikshank, "The Folly at Brighton," from William Hone, *The Joss and His Folly* (1820 © Trustees of the British Museum)

trayed as doubly opaque here. His countenance is hidden beneath expressionless features as well as extra layers of fat. The image also invokes a tradition of viewing rotund faces as opaque or impenetrable. For instance, the eighteenth-century German scientist and aphorist Georg Lichtenberg claimed that people with "plump faces" could "laugh under their fat, so that the greatest physiognomist shall fail to notice it," while "poor slender creatures" had their "souls seated immediately beneath the epidermis" and were therefore forced to "ever speak a language which can tell no lies."[19] In the visually centered post-Enlightenment world, much weight was placed on the ability to recognize whether an individual was virtuous or vice ridden, healthy or diseased, honest or corrupt. In an age that

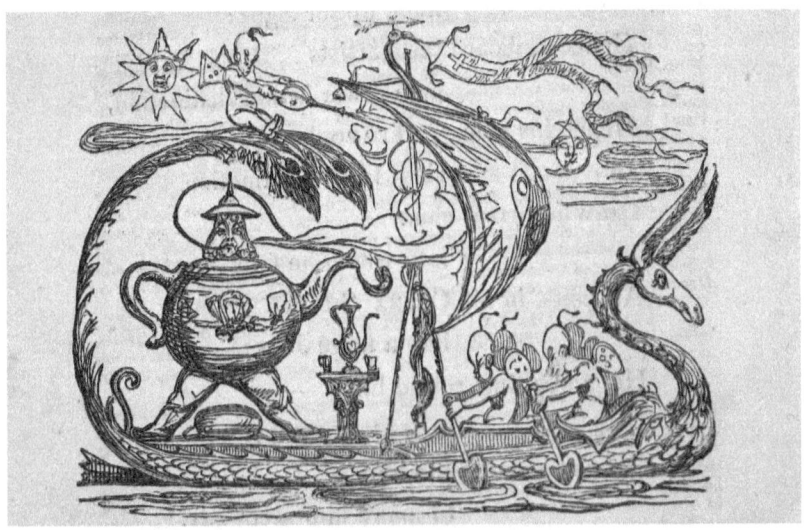

Figure 6.2   George Cruikshank, "A living teapot stands," from William Hone, *The Joss and His Folly* (1820, photo by Corinna Wagner).

emphasized transparency as a means to unimpeded perception, George's body presented a problem. It signaled his deceitfulness and his desire to operate behind the scenes, where, for instance, he agitated for increased allowances to support his extravagant and illicit tastes, instigated court cases against his legitimate wife, and indulged in numerous affairs with married women.

George Cruikshank's caricature *The Court at Brighton a la Chinese!!* (1816) (figure 6.3) is one of the most effective images of Britain's Orientalized Prince Regent. For Cruikshank, the Pavilion's design, the activities it housed, and the personal and political character of the regent communicated similar things. In this picture, the obese Orientalized George commands delegates to get "fresh patterns of Chinese deformities to finish the decoration of the Pavilion." The regent's current lover, the married Lady Hertford, sits on his right, where she makes the sign of the cuckold over her husband's bald head. That Lord Hertford is only too obliging to offer up his wife in exchange for his position as Lord Chamberlain further emphasizes the moral mayhem of George's court. In other words, the same sense of disorder defines as much his eating and drinking habits as his sexual practices, his architectural projects, and his politics.

Revealingly, the material objects in Cruikshank's scene are traded in

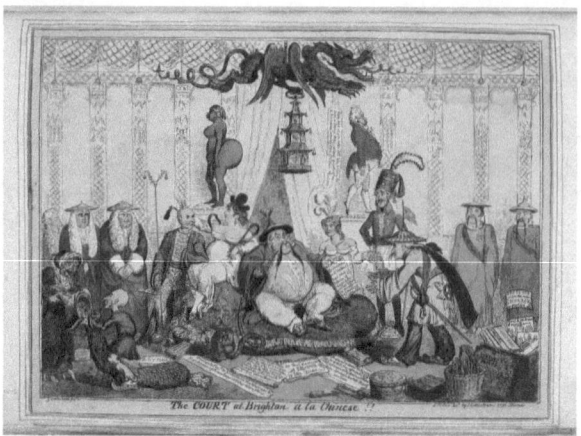

Figure 6.3 George Cruikshank, *The Court at Brighton a la Chinese!!* (1816 © Trustees of the British Museum, London)

private, indicating furtive cross-cultural contamination. In and around the chest in the right foreground are "Presents for the Emperor of China," including two portraits of the regent and some "Curious Prints"; volumes of the pornographic novel *Fanny Hill*; "Pretty books" and guides on "The Art of making Punch"; bottles of "Cordials"; and "Wigs & Whiskers" along with curling tongs and a hairbrush. These objects signify a global circulation of luxury goods that contradict ideas about English modesty, simplicity, and fair dealing. Each of these objects represents the worst of the nation's culture: pornography, alcohol, frivolous reading material, and the tools of the trade for the emasculated dandies and French hairdressers who served vacuous aristocratic women on the make. These goods are exchanged in a symbolic economy: they signal licentiousness, intemperance, vanity, vulgarity, and general bad taste. The point is that the world's most powerful and enlightened nation both imported and exported the types of items that signified and produced its own impending decline.

Cruikshank's caricature of the Orientalized regent also depicts a sexualized instance of the circulation of human foreign "goods." Princess Charlotte, George's only legitimate child requests that her "Papa" command one of his subordinates "to bring me over a China Man instead of getting me a Husband among our German Cousins!" This is a more problematic image of cross-cultural contact at Brighton. That the female heir to the throne would desire and demand a Chinese husband indicates a shocking dissolution of distinctions, between European and Oriental, primitive and civilized, natural and unnatural as well as between male and female roles. Perhaps the most disturbing instance of categorical breakdown, however, is indicated by George's own body. Forever altered through foreign contact, he is at once a Grand Mogul, a Chinese emperor, and a Hottentot Venus—character types that represent unchecked sensuality, irrationality, primitiveness, and unimpeded despotic power. The viewer's eye is particularly drawn to the two statues flanking the royal divan. They are mirror images: one is a lifelike representation of Sarah Baartman, or the Hottentot Venus (as she became known), which has been inscribed "Regency Taste!!!!!." The other, bizarrely, is the regent cast in Baartman's form as the "British Adonis." This conflation of gendered, racialized bodies and the amalgamation of cultural identity—English and Hottentot—is worth considering in more detail.

A subject of titillation for journalists, novelists, and scientists, Baartman was exhibited at the Egyptian Hall of Piccadilly Circus in London after 1810 and in Paris after 1814.[20] In the latter city, she was under the guardianship of the comparative anatomists and zoologists Georges Cuvier and Henri de Blainville. In their studies of the living Baartman and in their postmortem report of her dissection, Cuvier and Blainville compared her to an orangutan. Her steatopygous (protruding) buttocks and what they called her "Hottentot apron" (enlarged labia) were equated with animal sexuality and mental debility. Hottentot women were alleged to have elongated labia, a condition given the Latin term *sinus pudoris* (alternately and tellingly translated as "veil of shame" or "drape of decency"). The enlarged labia became a defining characteristic that separated defective and overly sexualized African women from their "normal" European counterparts (Voltaire considered the Hottentot apron a sign that Africans were of a different species).[21] Contemporary medical reports and anthropological studies suggested that Baartman's body was deformed by a biology that signaled her proximity to the apes.

The historian of science Londa Schiebinger observes that by the time of Baartman's appearance in Europe, focus on the allegedly enlarged "Hottentot genitalia had grown into a grotesque voyeurism," from which anatomists and naturalists "were not immune."[22] Biologist Anne Fausto-Sterling also identifies the sexualized quality of the scientist's gaze; for her, the intense scientific interest in sexual and physiological difference betrays anxieties about infection by "savage" others and at the same time fears about European desires for those savage others.[23] Further, Baartman is an object of anxiety because she embodies a range of conflated identities, which transgress boundaries of self and various others. While her

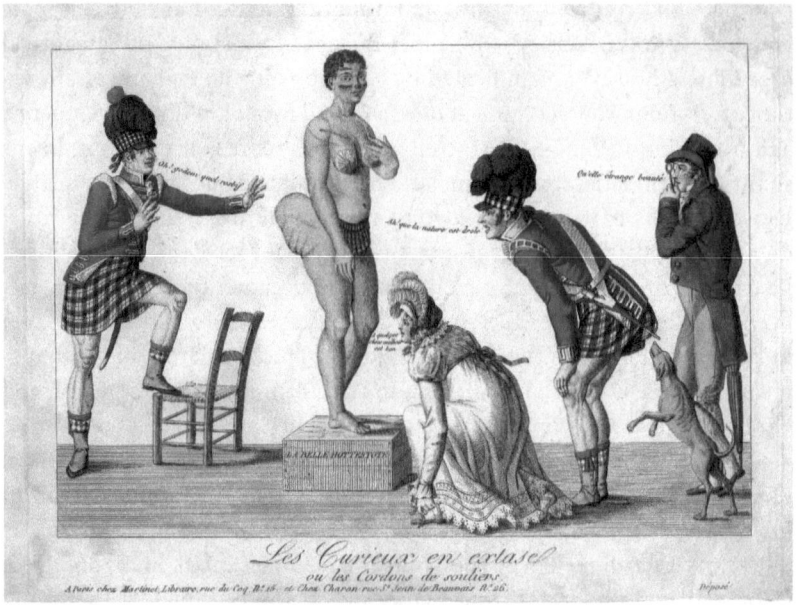

Figure 6.4 Louis François Charon, *Les curieux en extase* (1815 © Trustees of the British Museum, London)

anatomy defines her as female, she displays allegedly masculine traits like sexual aggression, physical strength, and intemperance. In other words, she is simultaneously a female-male hybrid, a human-animal, a scientific subject and a sexual object. As such, she is at once loathed, feared, and desired.

The French caricature *Les curieux en extase* (figure 6.4) demonstrates how the Hottentot Venus was seen to instigate voyeurism or scopophilia (sexually pleasurable looking) and provide the occasion for a blurring of "natural" distinctions. Cultural fears and individual pleasures overlap in the comments of the two British military men pictured, one of whom is mesmerized by Baartman's huge bottom and the other of whom is keen to get a glimpse of her "Hottentot apron." The man on the left cries "Oh! God Damn what roast beef!" in reference to her buttocks, while the other answers, "Ah! how comical is nature." Roast beef—the symbol of Englishness—is here transplanted onto those body parts most associated with sexual, moral, and racial difference. This image is informed by the principle that, just as a nation's architecture and food expressed the long, organic development of a distinct cultural identity, so too did inhabitants' bodies develop from a particular ethnic stock and specific environment. In other words, what was natural for one nation was not natural for another. Moreover, all things were not equal: one nation's "nature" could be far more advanced than that of another. Accordingly, less advanced nations were a source of disdain, amused titillation—and profound anxiety.

There are revealing parallels between the representation of Baartman as embodying a dangerous intermingling of biological and cultural difference and the representation of the regent's mixed identity. The chaotic nature of George's tastes and behaviors—his Oriental buildings, his foreign food, his dandyism, and his notoriously unconventional sexual tastes (for much older married women)—signaled the kinds of violent confusions associated with revolutionary France. He may have avoided the taint of Jacobinism by shunning French furniture at his Brighton Pavilion, but the appearance of Orientalized, animalistic, overly sexualized, and despotic figures in the regent's court (and the way he seemed to physically morph into them) was a similar indication of the world turned upside down. In Cruikshank's caricature of the Brighton court, George's body—with his inflated chest and exaggerated buttocks—is similarly deformed by habits that align him with the animalism of Baartman. It is as if his embrace of artificiality and foreign luxuries has taken him so far from nature that he, rather paradoxically, regresses to a precivilized state of nature. This state of nature however, has little to do with the Rousseauvian noble savage and more to do with Hobbes's selfish, unchecked, appetite-driven natural man.

These last two images of Baartman (figures 6.3 and 6.4) hint at another context in which the world was out of kilter. While eighteenth-century medical writers most often pinpointed an African origin for diseases like pox or syphilis, they also argued that the advanced state of culture in England was to blame for such diseases. They contrasted the cultural regression of civilized Europe with the hardier, natural state of precivilized peoples. As we saw in the previous chapter, doctors targeted regressive luxury and identified artificiality as a key contributor to gout and other such diseases of civilization. In his mid-eighteenth-century *Dissertation on the Gout*, William Cadogan, for example, argued that fussy, overly prepared dishes and overcooked meats contributed to a range of digestive problems in English people, in contrast to cannibals and Tatars, who remained "amazingly strong and vigorous" and "free from our diseases."[24] There are connections here to the argument, also discussed in the previous chapter, that in a state of nature human bodies are stronger and more resistant to disease than modern bodies, weakened by luxury and learning. But there is also a surprising reversal of the civilized-uncivilized binary, which often characterizes the West versus East opposition in this era. The refined English have pathological, weak bodies while the cannibal and the Turk triumph in glowing health.

CONTAGIOUS APPETITES, FOREIGN CONTAMINANTS, AND THE GLOBAL CIRCULATION OF DISEASE

As Cadogan's text indicates, in this period consuming nonnative foods and goods was a form of artifice linked to pathology and there was often a distinctly racial and gendered angle to the medical tenet that nature should be protected from the corrupting influence of artifice. Using rather disconcerting imagery, Cadogan genders and personifies nature, whom he describes as being raped by an equally personified culture. In the horrible irony of the slaver-enslaved relationship, violated nature comes to love the hand that feeds her: "Nature, *like a true female*, cries out at the first violence, but submits in time, is reconciled, and grows fond of the ravisher."[25] Cadogan's representation of an acquiescent female nature also appears in literature. For instance, in *Visions of the Daughters of Albion* (1792), William Blake's subjected slaves are broken and eventually become "obedient" to their captors until "their daughters worship terrors and obey the violent."[26] Likewise, according to the dictates of social convention, subjugated women sacrifice their natural desires and offer themselves up in exploitive, loveless marriages; even the female figure who seems to defy convention willingly submits to what she perceives as male sexual needs in order to please.

Among other things, such images are about the dangers of submission to authority and blind compliance with prevailing ideologies. There are connections between Blake's vision and Cadogan's dystopian vision of modern society, in which nature becomes subsumed by culture. In this society, humans who revel in luxury and artificiality are no longer able to differentiate between the false and the real, or between the natural and the unnatural. To stave off such a descent into a chaotic and distinctly unhealthy world, says Cadogan, it was incumbent upon "philosophers to distinguish between the real wants of nature and the artificial calls of habit" and it was the responsibility of ordinary people to make every effort "to break the enchantment of bad customs."[27]

Enchantment and artificiality were the allied enemies of nature and nation. Modern luxuries jeopardized the health of the nation; likewise, foreign contaminants threatened the English constitution. In this era, Britain's efforts to establish and protect its boundaries—whether militaristic, biological, or cultural—were attempts to preserve its physical borders as much as its identity. Literary scholars have noted that ideas about the circulation of disease provided a frame for writers to express fears about the increased global circulation of goods, values, and people. There is, as Susan Sontag puts it, a "link between imagining disease and imagining foreignness."[28] Alan Bewell makes a similar point, but with specific reference to the Romantic period. Although there have always been connections "between foreign diseases and foreign places," he identifies Leonhard Ludwig Finke's 1792 two-volume *Versuch einer allgemeinen medicinisch-praktischen Geographie* (Attempt at a general medical-practical geography) as the first modern effort "to understand the geographic distribution of disease *scientifically*."[29] This text heralded a century of similar studies that made and altered national identities through a process of "describing the biomedical boundaries of the modern world."[30] The emphasis on geography and boundaries gives some indication of how disease was often understood in terms of landscape, climate, and location. Bewell posits that "the dominant model of epidemic disease transmission was not contagion, but contamination"; in other words, polluted places rather than infected people communicated disease.[31]

There is still some disagreement among medical historians as to which of these models gained dominance in the Romantic era, but I think it is generally fair to say that ideas about dirt, disease, and decay were in flux. As we saw in chapter 3, both models—contagion through individuals and contamination through environment—circulated simultaneously in this period. In Cruikshank's representations of George's Oriental court at Brighton, Sarah Baartman's monstrously shaped body is very much a product of the South African climate and landscape: the erotic zones of her exaggerated body are as queer as the strange, dark exoticism of her homeland. Yet, she is also the polluted carrier of contagious matter; she is the conduit through which the English court becomes infected. Medical and literary writers may emphasize one model over the other; the main point is that disease, foreign locations, and foreign peoples were closely entwined in the British imagination.

Indeed, the historical trajectory of this imaginative triangle is revealing. Developments in public health in the Victorian period demonstrate how narratives about foreignness had real material consequences for social policy and global medicine. Medical maps, which accentuated boundaries, established national difference, and defined areas as healthy or pathological, greatly influenced and were influenced by the British perceptions of the colonies. In her study of the rise of medical cartography in the 1850s and 1860s, Pamela K. Gilbert reveals how attitudes about the global origins and spread of disease, which were manifest in epidemiological maps, affected legislation and social policy.[32] Taking as her case study the cholera epidemics in India and England, Gilbert shows how maps established ideas of Britain as progressive while India appeared regressive or degenerate. They also created the impression of a great distance between the tropical, disease-producing, and *inherently* diseased colony and an essentially healthy Britain. The belief was that, although there were devastating outbreaks of cholera in low-lying, unsanitary, and poorer urban areas in London, those areas could be cleaned up and reformed. England could make itself invulnerable to foreign contaminants. In contrast, areas in colonial India were cartographically represented as unmanageable, unhygienic, and *naturally* pathological. Cholera spread from its origins in the Ganges Delta (or Bengalla Delta) to metropolitan Britain, where it killed huge numbers of Britons.

Medical mapping reveals the ways that lines are drawn, differences established, and national identities solidified. Such developments in epidemiology and in the spatial imagining of disease shed light on earlier representations of national identity, disease, and the regent's body in the decades before the cholera epidemics. There are rather surprising connections between the mapmaker's attempt to render transparent the otherwise opaque movements of disease and the caricaturist's visual representations of the regent's exotic exchanges with dangerous foreigners. In fact, the research on models of disease provides an important context for understanding the public reaction to a regent who had transplanted the architecture, food, and customs of foreign nations onto English soil. George IV's tastes produced public anxiety in a time when the public was already anxious about the consequences of foreign travel and the imperialist project. Exploration narratives and scientific treatises about Africa, Asia, and other parts of the globe were also narratives about disease and death. English sailors, scientists, and explorers were hammered by malaria, typhus, dysentery, and venereal disease. Many worried that returning Britons and foreign visitors exposed those who stayed at home to these diseases. Cross-cultural exchange would at least change, at worst imperil, the nation's constitution.

PIGGISH KINGS, HOMEGROWN CANNIBALS, AND RADICAL VEGETARIANS

> New Discoveries of the Earth discover new Diseases: for besides the common swarm, there are endemial and local Infirmities proper unto certain Regions, which in the whole Earth make no small number: and if Asia, Africa, and America should bring in their List, Pandoras Box would swell, and there must be a strange Pathology.
> SIR THOMAS BROWNE, Doctor of Physic, *A Letter to a Friend* (1690)

The dangers associated with increased movement about the globe and the epidemiological realities of travel entered ever greater numbers of literary, medical, and political texts in the early nineteenth century. Of course, these concerns existed much earlier, as indicated by Sir Thomas Browne's musings on the subject of epidemics, disease, and death in the passage above. But in the first decades of the nineteenth century, doctors became increasingly preoccupied with the disease profile of populations. They were keen to understand the relationship between race, geography, and vulnerability to illness. By the time the George IV took the throne, the issue of the circulation of foreign pathologies had become pivotal in political, medical, and literary writing. Some Romantic-era authors, including the poet laureate Robert Southey, viewed past centuries rather nostalgically, as a time before Britons were threatened by foreign invasion by disease. There was something more authentically English about medieval society and something more vigorous about the "animal economy" of Renaissance bodies. When the world became crisscrossed with trade routes, over which people and goods seemed to move at alarming speed and scale, Britons became weakened, polluted by their contact with the outside world.

Southey's *Sir Thomas More* (1824) is a series of dialogues in which modern England comes off unfavorably in a comparison with the early sixteenth century. Southey uses the past to criticize the present, and one of his targets is the global trade in goods, which he sees as an importation of "evils" like disease. "Pigs, Spanish dollars, and Norway rats are not the only commodities that have performed the circumnavigation, and are to be found wherever European ships have touched," he writes. "Diseases also find their way from one part of the inhabited globe to another."[33] Impressive strides had been made in medical science by the renowned seventeenth-century physician Thomas Sydenham and the eighteenth-century surgeon John Hunter, yet modern Britons were under an unstoppable threat from imported disease. These foreign contagions were especially frightening because they were unfamiliar and undetectable, which posed a great challenge to medical progress: "the physician works in the dark, and has to deal with what is hidden and mysterious."[34] Fascinatingly, Southey relies on a vision of a natural past similar to that of Cadogan, but targets foreign-born disease more than luxury as the corrupting source. Ancient Britons were healthier, he writes, because they did not face "formidable endemic or contagious maladies" which were "not indigenous."[35] With a wistful nostalgia, he suggests that in Thomas More's time at least one could recognize one's enemy.

The pig is one of Southey's circumnavigating articles of trade, but for Percy Bysshe Shelley the pig symbolizes a whole set of homegrown problems. Shelley's 1820 play *Oedipus Tyrannus; or, Swellfoot the Tyrant* (1820) recalls both Edmund Burke's labeling of the working classes as "the swinish multitude" and the many rejoinders from radicals like Thomas Spence, who cheekily named his political journal *Pig's Meat*. In *Oedipus Tyrannus*, British subjects are farmyard pigs, ruled over by King Swellfoot, an unmistakable rendering of George IV. As his name indicates, Swellfoot suffers from the notorious diseases of high living. His goutish foot parallels his "kingly paunch," which

> Swells like a sail before a favouring breeze,
> And these most sacred nether promontories
> Lie satisfied with layers of fat.[36]

Like the real king, who witnessed the loathing of his subjects in the daily newspapers and heard their resentment shouted at him on the way to the opera house, Swellfoot would like to believe that his cocoon of fat protects him from the world, but it fails as a partition between him and harsh political realities.

Timothy Morton suggests that Shelley's representation of the populace as animals "establishes possibilities of expressing social relationships biologically" while at the same time "politicizing the natural world."[37] This cross-penetration of the biological and the political provides Shelley with the opportunity to make and remake both bodily and sociopolitical identities. This can be seen in the spoof "Advertisement" to the play, where the supposed narrator, an ancient Theban, clearly sets himself and his philosophy at variance with Swellfoot and his tyranny. The Theban "treats the PIGS" with "tenderness"; and even though he is himself only a pig, he is an "*Epicuri de grege porcus* [a pig of the Epicurean flock]."[38] Through his example, the epicurean pig-narrator suggests that the lowly citizen who exercises moderation and discrimination is the real figure of taste, while the excesses and license of the privileged king mark him as outmoded. In the new century, quality came before quantity, discrimination before excessive display. It may sound as if the Theban epicurean pig could be one of the nineteenth-century gastronomes of the last chapter, for he is a man of taste and reason. He belongs firmly in this chapter, however, because as we will see, the tale he tells is one that sets a home-grown populace against a distinctly alien king whose taste for the exotic signals his bigotry against his own subjects.

Ruled as they are by their tasteless and insensible king, the pig-citizens in Shelley's play cannot exercise tasteful moderation and rational judgment. Starving and homeless, they can only search in vain for "hog-wash or grains, or ruta baga." A chorus of swine describes how their emaciated bodies are racked with disease: they have caught "the murrain" (a highly infectious disease resembling anthrax that affects domestic animals), "the mange" (an infectious disease of the skin that results in hair loss), and "the scab and itch."[39] These diseases, which first attack animals and can then be transmitted to humans, indicate how radically dehumanized British subjects have become. The issue of taste and communalism are negated in a world in which humans do not have their basic needs met, let alone have access to the advantages of civilization.

The king's tastes (and the taxation policies that support such tastes) forge a direct correlation between his expanding body and the reduction of the bodies of his subjects. Shelley has been described as a "physiological critic" who, following in the footsteps of his father-in-law and erstwhile mentor William Godwin, articulates an "ideopathology" in his play. Shelley's contention, as Alan Bewell notes, is "that the real causes of the emergence and transmission of disease are to be found not in climate or nature but in the sphere of ideas, in human ignorance."[40] Shelley's observation, made in an 1815 letter to Thomas Jefferson Hogg, that "the human beings which surround us infect us with their opinions" is not metaphorical.[41] There is a destructive cycle at work: tyranny keeps people ignorant; ignorance then breeds disease. Another sequence of events, which will eradicate ignorance, must replace this cycle. Newly acquired knowledge and understanding lead to a desire for political reform; political reform then leads to health reform.

The infector-infected relationship is symbiotic. As the bodies of the pig-populace become leaner, the king's swells to enormous proportions. Swellfoot's body becomes a marker of gross unnaturalness because, to borrow the French philosopher Jean Baudrillard's phrase, "there are no obese animals."⁴² Baudrillard is speaking here of the cultural implications of fat in twentieth-century America, but the idea applies equally to Shelley's critique of George IV. Against the obscenely inflated body of the king, Shelley's animals appear the higher beings because they suffer from "natural" diseases that are not of their own making. In these years, obesity (or to use the nineteenth-century term, corpulence) is a disease of civilization, but increasingly it is an immoral disease produced by a perverse and distorted culture. Fat is increasingly aligned with intemperance, dissipation, and irrationality and by the nineteenth-century, with unnaturalness. The idea that lean is natural is expressed most clearly by the inventor of the stomach pump, Edward Jukes, who promises that "the most corpulent man or woman may with the aid of diet and exercise be reduced to their *natural* size."⁴³ Fat is pathological; lean is normal.

The unnaturally obese King Swellfoot is responsible for turning his subjects into unnatural beings, though of a different kind. While the king's appetites consume all resources, the starving bodies of his subjects undergo grave physiological changes, so that piglets are unable to feed from the milkless bodies of their mothers. "I suck, but no milk will come from the dug," one piglet wails, while the sow advises her litter that "tis in vain to tug" as her body has nothing to give.⁴⁴ Yet another sow goes much further, voicing her desire to cannibalize her children. "I could almost eat my litter," she admits, yet even this is impossible since their bodies are fleshless.⁴⁵ Shelley's representation of the cannibal mother demonstrates how, as one critic notes, extreme hunger "starves compassion, exiling one from any sense of loyalty to a larger community."⁴⁶ Gnawing stomachs, raging fever, and rotting flesh make it impossible to feel higher emotions like sympathy. Not only are familial and communal relations impossible to sustain, but the remarkable exchanges between the would-be cannibal sow and her litter suggest both a more insidious breakdown of social order and a denaturing of the human body.

Shelley's representation of George IV as Swellfoot and his reference to a cannibalizing populace presents a dystopic view in which grotesque eating practices are signs of a monstrous politics. The cannibal was a politically meaningful and incredibly malleable trope in this period; it was also the most alien of figures, signifying precivilized or regressive humanity as well as the most extreme kinds of foreignness. In fact, in this period, as Roxann Wheeler and Peter Kitson show, foreignness and degeneracy fuse in representations of cannibalism.⁴⁷ The cannibal was a fiercely contested and incredibly powerful tool in the public opinion game of the 1790s—for French revolutionaries, British radicals, and loyalists alike. In *Oedipus Tyrannus*, Shelley participates in the constellation of debates that had, since the onset of the French Revolution, used the cannibal to capture the fears that buttressed competing political points of view. In France, orators and authors had employed the image of the cannibal throughout the Revolution's course. In the hopeful early days, republicans characterized the government of the ancien régime—with its phalanx of cannibalizing deputies—as a voracious, monstrous parent that consumed its numerous children.

After the onset of violence, however, this trope was appropriated much more widely. In his work on the visual and literary representations of revolution, Ronald Paulson points out that the figure of the cannibal recalled, with alarming immediacy, the image of "the king killed and supplanted" and indicated the way in which "the generations of the revolution . . . succeeded each other with frightening rapidity."[48] On 13 March 1793, the Girondist leader Pierre Vergniaud invoked the cannibal in his critique of the French National Convention, articulating what would become a catchphrase that encapsulated the dark side of revolution. Like the mythical Saturn, he said, "the revolution devours its own children."[49] Likewise, the contemporary diarist Louis Du Broca recounts how the revolutionary tribunal that sent thousands to the guillotine was comprised of "beasts of prey, fed with human blood!"[50] He describes how during the September massacres of 1792, the "sight of blood continually flowing seemed only to increase the rage of the assassins" so that they forced their victims to join in their feast.[51] Joining a faction of other propagandists, Broca provides his English readers with gory anecdotes of personal tragedy: when one young girl flung herself between the sword and her aged father, "one of the monsters" promised to save his life if she drank a glass of another victim's blood.[52] As the ultimate crime against nature, cannibalism captured for alarmed observers the unbounded violence of republican fervor.

In Britain, the trope of the cannibal followed a fairly similar trajectory. In the early days, reformers used the cannibal to capture the self-consuming quality of the existing structure of public and private life. Thomas Paine famously used the motif of the monstrous cannibal-parent to denote how, under the existing laws of primogeniture, the second- and third-born children of the landed classes were simply "begotten to be devoured."[53] While kings and their politicians devoured the resources of the nation, the wealthy feasted on the entrails of the poor; in the home, despotic fathers and insensible mothers preyed on the bowels of their own young. For conservative observers, it was the Revolution that created cannibals out of average, generally peaceable citizens. As early as 1790, the lone reactionary voice of Edmund Burke agitated vociferously against a revolutionary fervor that whetted the "palates" of those for whom "the sufferings of monarchs make a delicious repast."[54] He accused the revolutionary government of staging spectacles of violence "to stimulate" the people's "cannibal appetites."[55]

By mid-decade, Burke's claims proved prescient and his seemingly lone alarmist voice found a chorus of supporters. There were personal anecdotes: "The French my Friends have been known to drink the warm-Life Blood of those they have murdered," one Suffolk observer wrote to his loyalist association leader in December 1792.[56] There were also pseudonymous antirevolutionary pamphleteers that latched on to Burke's language to spread alarm among working-class readers. In the guise of John Nott, Birmingham buckle maker, Theodore Price compared the godless "French Cannibals (as Mr. Burke justly called 'em for he said they cut out Gentlemens hearts, and squeezed the blood into wine and drank it)" to foreign savages. France's "bloody minded barbarians are worse than the Antipoads that kill'd and chop'd our brave sailor Captain Cook to pieces and mayhap the same cause makes them act the same."[57] In *A Bone to Gnaw for Democrats* (1795) and in *The Bloody Buoy* (1797), the Tory William Cobbett described how republicans had turned France into a "theatre of carnage" with their "menaces and cannibal gesticulations."[58] In these years, he declared, "man was becoming the *food* of man."[59] "Blood was the food of the republican cannibals," echoed the Scottish loyalist Thomas Hardy.[60] In his 1796 *First Letter on a Regicide Peace*, Burke added further fuel to the fire he had started, exclaiming frantically in what had become his signature style that "the practice of *cannibals*" had spread throughout France, so that republicans were now "devouring, as a nutriment of their ferocity, some part of the bodies of those they have murdered." They not only drank "the blood of their victims," he informed readers but also forced "the victims themselves to drink the blood of their kindred slaughtered before their faces."[61]

Recent work on the social and political meanings of cannibalism highlights the cultural significance of this discourse. The figure of the foreign cannibal, Kristen Guest observes, has long been "associated with absolute alterity and used to enforce boundaries between a civilized 'us' and a savage 'them.'"[62] This is clearly the case with the examples above: loyal Britons drew a firm line between themselves and their regressive, anarchic, and foreign neighbors. In *Oedipus Tyrannus*, Shelley's representations of the cannibalizing pigs highlight the sense of alterity between ruler and ruled, yet Shelley's point is that these animal-cannibals are created *within* and *by* the world's most civilized nation. Britain may have avoided revolutionary excess, but its populace submissively and sycophantically bowed to its oppressors. These English pig-subjects may have begun life as the most natural of creatures, but continual poverty and confinement transformed them into almost vestigial creatures. Even in this regressed state, though, they had a political legitimacy that the king had no claim to.

Although the savagery that haunts the ostensibly well-ordered nation originates from within its boundaries, Shelley also Orientalizes that savagery. There is something distinctly foreign about Swellfoot's tastes, practices, and behaviors, and his exoticism is intimately connected to his corruption. When the corpulent king *does* lose his appetite—due to the stress of having to face the fierce public outcry against his persecution of his wife, Queen Caroline—he seeks comfort in luxurious, exotic foods. "I feel the gout flying about my stomach" he moans, and he demands to be served "a glass of Maraschino punch" to calm it.[63] His sidekick Mammon insists that the king can regain his appetite with "a simple kickshaw by your Persian cook."[64] One would not normally characterize a Persian kickshaw as good old down-home English comfort food. This dish not only indicates a king who cannot or will not identify with his people but also suggests something about the "unnaturalness" of the colonial system that brought the dish to his table. Empire is about tyranny, unhealthy competition, and violence. For Britain, it is also about a loss of autonomy and a lack of self-determination.

Shelley outlines this clearly in the extended notes to his long poem *Queen Mab*, also published separately as *A Vindication of Natural Diet*. "How would England," he asks, "depend on the caprices of foreign rulers, if she contained within herself all the necessaries, and despised whatever they possessed of the luxuries of life? How could they starve her into compliance with their views? . . . On a natural system of diet we should require no spices from India; no wines from Portugal, Spain, France, or Madeira; none of those multitudinous articles of luxury, for which every corner of the globe is rifled, and which are the causes of so much individual rivalship, such calamitous and sanguinary national disputes."[65] Shelley's natural, locally produced vegetarian diet creates and supports an equitable politics (more about how his vegetarianism fits in later). The consumption of foreign foodstuffs supports the injustices inherent in empire and makes otherwise autonomous, freedom-loving nations dependent and vulnerable. The taste for luxury and exotic flavors is deeply problematic, since one becomes what one eats. Those who consume produce from a corrupt, enervated, or oppressed nation imbibe corruption and cruelty with each bite, until they unknowingly assume the very qualities they consciously deplore. For this reason, Shelley conceives of empire as, to borrow Alan Bewell's apt phrase, "essentially an eating disorder."[66]

SWEET-TOOTHED MONARCHS AND THE NATURAL SYSTEM OF DIET

Exotic tastes lead to inhumane acts and greedy politics, at home and abroad. Whereas in *Sir Thomas More* Southey worries about how the global circulation of goods brings disease to British shores, in *Oedipus Tyrannus* Shelley portrays a homegrown form of injustice that feeds on, and is fed by, global exploitation and violence. However, for all their differences of opinion, both poets agree about the role of sugar in the chain of human suffering. In one of his sonnets on the slave trade, Southey places the blame for driving the transatlantic slave trade on sweet-toothed Britons who "sip the blood-sweeten'd beverage!"[67] His rhetoric echoes that of a host of anti-saccharite campaigners, including the Quaker William Fox, who characterizes slave traders and plantation owners as "virtually the agents of the consumer": they may hold rum and sugared tea "to our lips, steeped in the blood of our fellow-creatures; but they cannot compel us to accept the loathsome portion."[68]

The public campaign against the consumption of sugar and its relation to privilege and luxury are captured in another well-known James Gillray image, *Anti-saccharrites; or, John Bull and His Family Leaving Off the Use of Sugar* (27 March 1792) (figure 6.5). It is worth noting that this image was published the same year as the two Gillray caricatures of the royal family dining, which featured in the previous chapter. This time George III and Queen Charlotte are accompanied by their six cosseted and largely home-bound daughters. Once again, the king and queen demonstrate their frugality but this time also their allegiance to the anti-saccharite movement, which saw households boycotting sugar in a time when, as Ann Mellor puts it, consumption of sugar "constituted a national addiction."[69] Part of the reason Charlotte finds the taste of sugarless tea "nice" is because, ostensibly, it will save "the poor Blackeemoors" some hard labor; but more to the point, it will save the royal household so "much expence." Although as usual Gillray grossly caricaturizes Charlotte, the monarchy is presented as again generally fulfilling a morally exemplary role. The same miserly qualities are on display here as in Gillray's *Temperance Enjoying a Frugal Meal* (1792), but *Anti-saccharrites* is still a fairly posi-

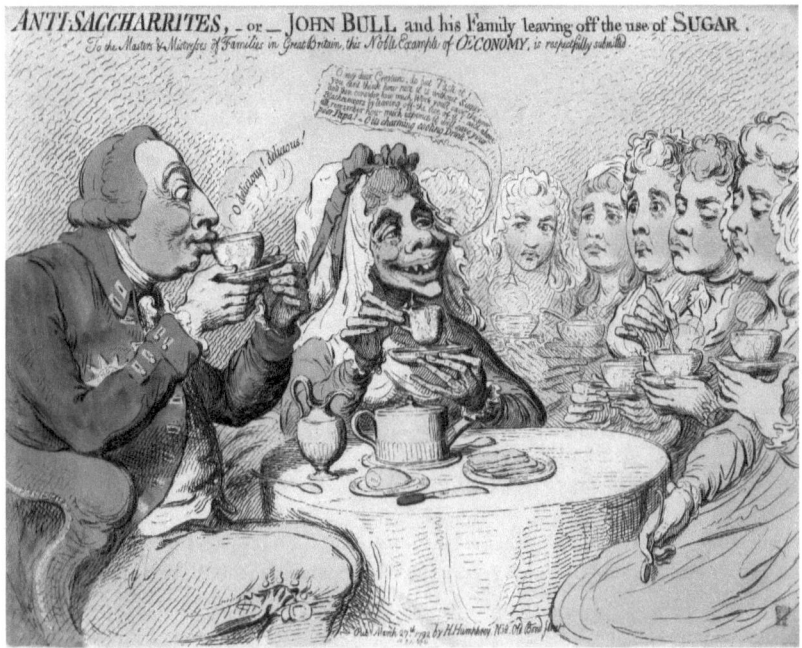

Figure 6.5 James Gillray, *Anti-saccharrites; or, John Bull and His Family Leaving Off the Use of Sugar* (1792 © Trustees of the British Museum, London)

tive image of how the monarchy can set a "Noble Example of Œconomy" for "the Masters & Mistresses of Families in Great Britain."

However, in the very same year, a less affirmative take on this almost exact scene was offered by Isaac Cruikshank. *The Gradual Abolition off* [sic] *the Slave Trade; or, Leaving of* [sic] *Sugar by Degrees* (15 April 1792) (figure 6.6) refashions Gillray's caricature, published a month earlier, but here the anti-saccharite movement in the royal household is rather less successful. At a much more generously stocked table, Princess Elizabeth (second from the left) comments, "I cant leave of a good thing so soon, I am sure of late I have been very moderate, but I must have a bit now & then." The queen and her confidante and Keeper of Robes, Mrs. Schwellenberg (far right) are Cruikshank's real marks. Queen Charlotte weighs out tiny pieces of sugar on a scale typically used for coinage and gold, while Mrs. Schwellenberg grasps a bottle of brandy, expressing her willingness to swap rum for good cognac instead. A sugar by-product, molasses, was distilled into rum and manufactured in New England, forming part of the triangular trade of goods and slaves between Africa, American,

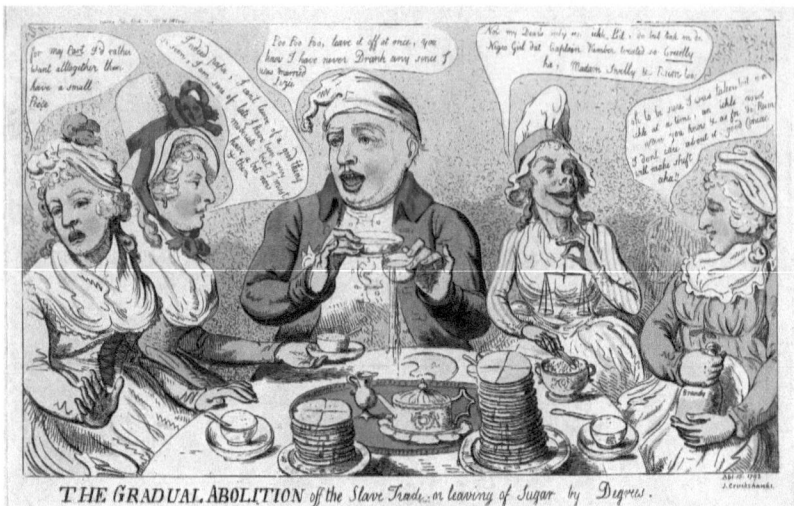

Figure 6.6   Isaac Cruikshank, *The Gradual Abolition off* [sic] *the Slave Trade; or, Leaving of* [sic] *Sugar by Degrees* (1792 © Trustees of the British Museum, London)

and Europe. Cruikshank's portrayal of Charlotte mirrors Gillray's, as if indicating an intention to re-present, in more negative terms, the latter artist's image of the royal table and its tea takers specifically. There is a two-fold message in Cruikshank's image. First, Charlotte's dining choices have less to do with ethics or a concern for human liberty and more to do with her own desire to stockpile proceeds. Second, while she is not the consumer par excellence that her son is, her tastes are still connected to foreign affairs and colonial tyranny. Her foreign tastes might not reach as far as the Orient, but her much-loved Mrs. Schwellenberg is foreign enough. Her presence at table reminds viewers that Britain's monarchy originated in Germany.

In his satirical novel *Melincourt*, Thomas Love Peacock includes a chapter devoted to an anti-saccharite fete. One character, the wildly enthusiastic campaigner Mr. Forester, makes a speech over a dinner of solely local food. Foreign ingredients and condiments, including the currant jelly that would normally accompany the venison, is banished (much to the chagrin of some of the guests). Forester pronounces sugar destructive on many counts, as it is

> oeconomically superfluous . . . [since] in the middling classes of life it is a formidable addition to the expenses of a large family. . . . It is physically pernicious, as its destruction of the teeth, and its effects on

the health of children, much pampered with sweetmeats, sufficiently demonstrate.... It is morally atrocious, from being the primary cause of the most complicated corporeal suffering ... and the most abject mental degradation.... It is politically abominable, for covering with every variety of wretchedness some of the fairest portions of the earth.[70]

On an individual level, says Peacock, sugar is destructive of domestic economy, health, mind, and body, while on a global level it causes enormous human misery. Sugar precludes any possibility of peaceable exchange between nations, for in spite of the symbiotic nature of the relationship between Britain and her colonies, the difference between *us* and *them* is immeasurable: "Slaves cannot breathe in the air of England.... Who is there among you that is not proud of this distinction? ... Not any thing—not an atom of any thing, should enter an Englishman's dwelling, on which the Genius of Liberty had not set his seal."[71] For English people, liberty had identifiable meanings; in Peacock's sense, it made Britain distinct among the globe's nations. Through a long history of political struggle and negotiation, the English constitution had secured universal civil liberties for all inhabitants. Unlike France, which could only pay lip service to liberty, Britons enjoyed real rights and freedoms, which had been refined and balanced with law and moral restraint. The genius of England's liberty was being threatened, however, by the contaminating "atoms" of foreign nations.

To return to Shelley, the issue of taste is never far away from discussions of disease and political corruption in his work, and questions of taste are inseparable from ideas about progress, reform, and perfectibility. In this Shelley was heavily influenced by the perfectibilist tradition, which began with Greek philosophy and continued through to Nicolas de Condorcet, Jean-Jacques Rousseau, and William Godwin. Those who advocated the "perfectibility of man" posited that humans had an infinite ability to improve and, with the use of reason, to adapt to changing environments. Language and cultural expressions of taste were important manifestations of this distinctly human ability to advance. Enlightenment theories of taste were, Denise Gigante observes, "underwritten by a commitment to an ideal of human perfectibility."[72] Since taste was indicative of, and integral to, true human progress, then the reform of one's daily eating habits and routines could extend life, improve human sociability, and increase equality and happiness on an individual and even a global scale. Shelley makes this point in *Queen Mab* and *Vindication of Natural Diet*, where he outlines his vision for the eradication of disease and debility through adoption of a vegetarian and pure water diet.

Shelley's vegetarianism may not seem directly relevant to the question of national identity and to debates surrounding the foreign-local axis, but his advocacy of national self-sufficiency and his natural system of diet are actually inseparable. For Shelley, British produce and eating practices are part of a homegrown politics that celebrates candor, integrity, personal liberty, and a natural equality. Moreover, his philosophy of human perfectibility is bound to ideas about the body, taste, and dietetics. Shelley's republicanism, his civic humanism, and his ideas about masculine virtue are informed by classical ideals but are reformulated for a distinctly English modern nation. His self-presentation (in *Queen Mab* and *Vindication of Natural Diet*) as a purposeful, self-controlled, enlightened, and socially responsible reformer contrasts sharply with the antimonarchist representations of an obese, foreign, and parasitic George IV in other of his writings, particularly his play *Oedipus Tyrannus*.

Influenced by Cheyne's writing on the vegetarian diet and Joseph Ritson's 1802 *Essay on Abstinence from Animal Food, as a Moral Duty*, Shelley's ideas about political and social reform were tied to his advocacy of dietary reform. Part of a circle of vegetarian republicans, which included Richard Phillips (publisher of Ritson and Tom Paine) and the Scottish Jacobin émigré John Oswald, Shelley served up his republicanism with a side of vegetarianism and temperance. Scholars have detailed how, in the 1790s and the early decades of the nineteenth century, a regimented vegetarian diet became a marker of "a revolutionary sobriety" and "a straight, masculine civic humanism" rather than "the effeminate weakness that it signified later."[73] A first edition of Ritson's book on ethical vegetarianism indicates how the claim to masculine, liberal ideals was buttressed by an abstemious diet and disciplined modes of caring for the self. On the flyleaf of one particular copy, an early nineteenth-century annotator referenced the vegetarianism of the dissenter and supporter of the French Revolution Gilbert Wakefield, as well as the eighteenth-century protopsychologist David Hartley. The handwritten comments are as follows:

> Gilbert Wakefield was very abstemious in the article of diet, and in his latter years rarely indulged himself in animal food—Indeed he became from principle, a decided enemy to the use of it altogether. . . .
>
> Dr Hartley considers this subject in the practical part of his great work—. Upon the whole, he concludes that the use of animal food is permitted, yet he freely allows "that taking away the lives of animals,

in order to convert them into food, does great violence to the principles of benevolence and competition."[74]

Ritson's annotator clearly links diet with the formation of individual character and the general cast of society. Since values like compassion and fortitude have a clear dietary basis, then controlling one's intake, and being thoughtful about it, demonstrates social responsibility and a manly sense of personal accountability.

The sympathetic relationship between moderation, masculinity, and sensibility remains a theme in later writing on vegetarianism—even when it was not overtly political. In his 1828 treatise *Sure Methods of Improving Health . . . by Regulating the Diet and Regimen*, Thomas John Graham argues that although animal food is acceptable, overindulgence (particularly with the addition of alcohol) destroys one's health and jeopardizes one's ability to function. For Graham, a vegetable diet does not produce the constitutional disorders that an animal diet does; moreover, it has a wonderful effect on intelligence, creativity, and character. Vegetarianism, Graham argues, has "a beneficial influence on the powers of the mind; and tends to preserve a delicacy of feeling, a liveliness of imagination, and acuteness of judgment, seldom enjoyed by those who live principally on meat."[75] While these are not openly political statements, there are subtle political principles at work here. The positive personal characteristics associated with a controlled diet are the same as those espoused by civic humanists. Careful, controlled eaters demonstrate a responsible care of the self, display masculine moderation, and claim a certain kind of communal responsibility. Corpulent, swollen-footed, boozy-faced individuals are selfish and irrational. If they could not regulate their own bodies, they surely could not regulate the body politic.

In his *Vindication of Natural Diet*, Shelley rereads humanity's trajectory of violence, disease, and want through two seemingly conflicting lenses: myth and medicine. He reinterprets foundational myths, so that the biblical fall and the Promethean allegory are narratives of humanity's grim descent into meat eating. The classical myth becomes a parable of ethical vegetarianism. By giving humans fire, Prometheus enabled humans to cook meat, also allowing them to disguise the bloody reality of the carnivorous diet they had adopted. The vulture that preyed daily on Prometheus's liver was "the vulture of disease," a direct result of eating food (meat) that was unnatural (and thus disease bearing).[76] This diet changed the human constitution: the taste of animal blood made previously peaceful humans bloody minded. Shelley supports his literary exegesis with hard science, drawing on the work of comparative anatomists who argue that humans were originally herbivorous or frugivorous (fruit eating). His contentions are informed both by Ritson, who observed that since "the teeth and intestines of man" resembled "those of frugivorous animals, he should, naturally, be range'd in this class," and by Cuvier (of Hottentot Venus fame), who identified physiological similarities between humans, frugivorous apes, and other vegetation-eating animals.[77]

As may have become obvious, Shelley was among those who expressed a Rousseauvian nostalgia for a pre-urban, premodern world. Along with other radical vegetarians, he envisioned a time and place in which, according to their natural inclinations and physiology, humans were vegetarians. This nostalgia is indicative of what Timothy Morton identifies as "the inconsistent logic of Romantic vegetarianism"; that is, in this thinking there is an attempt both to "rise above one's carnal animality" and also to locate "a way of returning to nature."[78] As we have seen throughout this book, this inconsistent logic is intrinsic to a wide variety of nostalgic, Rousseauvian appeals to nature. Equally, there is the realization, then as now, that humanity cannot return to noble savagery even if it wanted to, or if such a thing ever existed. The idea that modern health practices and moral codes can be decided by "nature" (or what we think we know of it) is a deeply flawed one. Nature is not separable from culture; nor, I think, would we want it to be. Shelley found ways, however, of reconciling this nature-culture/past-present dilemma, in all its many contradictions. His inconsistent logic is resolved by trading nostalgia for evolution and by redefining "nature" to suit the present. For British vegetarian republicans, who were "revolutionary from the assembly room to the dinner plate, nature is an unfinished project that hails humanity from the future."[79] Nineteenth-century Britons may have left off ancestral practices, but they could not simply return to that past. Moderns had to learn from the trajectory of history in order to ameliorate current and future problems. In other words, vegetarianism was a fusing of culture and nature, in a way that reconciled past and present—but always looked firmly to the future and to local, homegrown food.

Indeed, Shelley brought his revised myths and contemporary medical knowledge to bear on recent political events. If Parisian revolutionaries had drunk only pure water and feasted on vegetables, they would not have supported Robespierre, nor would they have been capable of callously standing by while their fellow citizens were brutally butchered.[80] Shelley discovered that, as Morton puts it, "the scientific, diachronic view of early humankind could be mapped on to historical, social and synchronic views of the working classes and colonial subjects."[81] In other words, the long trajectory of human history, profoundly connected as it is with the history of eating, elucidates moments of struggle and suffering, including the terrifying events in Paris in 1792 or the working-class discontent and Luddism of England in 1812. For Shelley, the long record of human consumption paralleled an equally long chronicle of human decline, punctuated by violent events. The legacy of tyranny and war could be traced back to the beginnings of human selfishness. In a state of nature, humans were not, as Hobbes had posited, so awfully self-interested that their short lives were brutal affairs; rather, they were benevolent, peaceful vegetarians who, because they had no taste for blood, did not tyrannize one another.

To further understand "the unfinished project" that hails Shelley from the future, I want to return briefly to George IV as Swellfoot of the exotic tastes and to the British citizen as cannibalizing pig. Read through Shelley's vegetarian ethics, the cannibal pig is a native Briton who no longer has the option to eat healthy, indigenous food. Britons' subjected bodies have adopted the type of debased and uncivilized lust for flesh usually associated with South Sea Islanders and other foreigners. The native Briton has become a symbol of racial degeneracy—but this degeneracy is set in motion by an Orientalized king. As such, the citizen's body registers the tyranny inherent in a monarchical system of government, even a modern constitutional monarchy. The king's corpulent body is also a register, but of the retreat of authority. He has no self-command; in fact, his appetite is only slaked when continuous pressure is applied by his disgruntled pigs. He is unable to exercise the bodily self-control and ethical conscience of a vegetarian Shelley or to demonstrate the good taste and refined sensibility of a gastronome.

In this chapter, we have seen how *excess, foreign,* and *contagious* were bridging terms that linked otherwise seemingly unrelated, or at least only very loosely related, fields of inquiry. These links between medicine, morality, politics, and geography operated on wider cultural attitudes more consistently and with greater effect than in previous eras. Practices surrounding the body and care of the self were associated with ideas about national identity, race, and place and they began to figure more prominently in the realm of politics. Importantly, as the case of George IV demonstrates, the bodies, tastes, habits, and practices of public figures were used to forge these connections. In this politically charged age of revolution, propagandists adopted medical terms to tar their enemies and to bring about the redistribution of political power. To be goutish, to display immoderation at table, to overindulge in exotic foodstuffs, to surround oneself with filthy foreign goods was also to threaten national identity, to be socially irresponsible, and to jeopardize political stability.

Coda

Medicine, Politics, and the Production of the Modern Body

This book has been about the relationship between medicine and politics. It has also been about the multifarious and perplexing connections between the public and publicity and discipline and governmentality.

Before I draw the six chapters together, I want to pick up where the last two chapters left off, with an aging, fat, gout-ridden king. For the end of his story, and the narratives about excess and disease that dogged him until his death, reveal much about the accumulation, circulation, and functioning of medical discourses about self-control, taste, and healthfulness. George IV occupied a crucial position at a time when both medicine and politics became more closely and densely connected to that by now familiar constellation of concerns: personal probity, attachment to family, responsibility to community, and a willingness to play a productive role in nation building. The good citizen, that is, *each* good citizen, was required to demonstrate political accountability, a willingness to regulate his or her health, and a dutiful devotion to home, hearth, and nation. Just who was articulating those requirements remains a question. Where did this disciplinary message originate? Who was enforcing it? The final years of the king's life provide at least partial answers.

From about 1824 until his death in 1830, the hugely unpopular George IV closed up the gates to St. James's Palace and barricaded himself at Windsor. He had the extensive grounds fenced and thickly planted to thwart the prying eyes of the public. He decreed that servants who looked at him would be discharged from their duties and that any visitors to the grounds should never "turn their eyes to the window, lest the king should be passing under it."[1] He slathered his aging and fleshy face with powder and paint in an effort to protect himself from his political detractors and from the censorious gaze of the public. The Duchess of Gloucester described the king as "enormous, like a feather bed," and his correspondence and the eyewitness reports of doctors and friends make it clear how painfully aware he was of his profound unpopularity.[2] As contemporary satirical poems, caricatures, political pamphlets, and newspaper columns attest, his gouty, swollen body provided his critics with innumerable opportunities to deride him for his debauched life and his political incapacity.

Public disapproval of the king's body and his habits resulted at least in part from newly overlapping attitudes about excess, fat, and irresponsibility. George must have been somewhat bewildered by the incredible hostility directed at him and, more specifically, his body. The relationship between the king and the public, as it played out in the newspapers, and as he recorded it in his correspondence, raises crucial issues about who constituted the public and how it had access to the monarchy. Obviously, we can never know *exactly* who the public is. However, through the work of Jürgen Habermas, Craig Calhoun, John Brewer, John Barrell, and other scholars we know that print culture was widening in the eighteenth and nineteenth centuries, readership was increasing, the middle classes were expanding, and meanings were being negotiated and opinions disseminated in a plethora of social spaces.[3] As collective knowledge was constituted, so the public was formed.

That journalists could report their disapprobation of the royal family's behavior underscores how this system worked and how close was the public's physical proximity to the royals. As Linda Colley has shown, the sense of closeness between the court and the people was a peculiarly English phenomenon of late eighteenth- and nineteenth-century society. Unlike the isolated French monarchs who were insulated in their "beehive court" at Versailles, the British royal circle was not a self-contained entity; rather, George III's court *was* the theater and the opera house and the seashore at Weymouth.[4] This aspect of English spatial politics proved a boon for some members of the royal family and disastrous for others. Well aware that London crowds could demonstrate either incredible generosity or astounding hostility, newspapers exploited this proximity by urging readers to make their views known, whether in the street or at the theater. By the time the Prince of Wales was made regent, newspapers were tracking his every move and informing "decent" readers of his whereabouts so that they could publicly demonstrate their discontent through verbal insults or by hurling refuse at his carriage.[5] Any number of newspapers, on any given day, reported on a variety of public arenas for the expression of discontent:

the opera, the park, the crowd-lined streets the regent traveled through on the way to his coronation.

As audiences widened and scandal became an integral part of political debate and a means of expressing social anxieties, the business of gossip became much more regulative and of greater consequence. George IV's astonished and fearful responses to personal attacks in the press illustrate the newly regulative role of newspapers. Undoubtedly one of the greatest targets of scandal's censorious eye for forty years of his life, he reportedly took in 546 copies of eight different daily newspapers at Carlton House, where he was said to have "read every newspaper quite through."[6] His correspondence records his sense of being "exposed" and catalogs his very real fears that scurrilous reportage could lead to his personal downfall and to the downfall of the entire British monarchy. On one occasion, for example, he shared with his mother his fear that scandalous publications were tearing "to pieces every private character . . . my own among the rest . . . in open defiance of all law and decency."[7] His letters are full of these types of comments. For many years, he paid editors to refrain from publicizing his exorbitant expenditures, from poking fun at his physique, and from informing the public about his scandalous affairs. At one time, he arranged, through his most trusted member of staff, to buy the *Morning Post* outright in order to prevent it from writing nasty things about him.[8] In 1812, the radical editors of the *Examiner*, Leigh and John Hunt, published Charles Lamb's poem "The Triumph of the Whale." The following passage gives a sense of its tenor:

> Name or title what has he?
> Is he Regent of the Sea?
> From this difficulty free us,
> Buffon, Banks or sage Linnaeus.
> With his wondrous attributes
> Say what appellation suits.
> By his bulk, and by his size,
> By his oily qualities,
> This (or else my eyesight fails),
> This should be the PRINCE OF WHALES.[9]

In this poem we see a wonderfully tongue-in-cheek turn to science—and to the famous taxonomists the Comte de Buffon, Sir Joseph Banks, and Carl Linnaeus—in order to classify the monstrous figure of the king. Such scientific classification paralleled parliamentary efforts, urged on by the public, to reclassify and redefine the role of monarch. At any rate, George was well aware of how representations like this one spoke to and for a body of readers that was growing in size and significance, as well as dissatisfaction. The year after this poem appeared, the Hunt brothers were found guilty of seditious libel for publishing a similarly cutting satire. Unquestionably, this prosecution, like others, was motivated by the king himself.

Lamb's poem, like the satirical images and texts discussed in the last two chapters, may have been directed at the corpulent king, but they were also part of wider attitudinal changes about what fat represented—as well as other "pathological" symptoms. We know that the medical manuals and treatises of the period targeted the same public that was, in turn, targeting the bodies of public figures. A quick sampling of the language of these manuals indicates their role in a newly temperate, restrained era in which individuals were pressured to demonstrate their personal probity, domestic values, and civic responsibility through, among other things, their bodily habits and rituals. By the mid-nineteenth century, those who could not or did not regulate themselves at the table—those whose fat, goutish bodies indicated a lack of conformity—could hardly be trusted to exercise command over themselves in other spheres. One treatise is particularly instructive: Twenty years after the death of George IV, the physician Thomas King Chambers complained tellingly about an earlier generation of physicians who did not treat fatness with seriousness. In *Corpulence; or, Excess of Fat in the Human Body* (1850), he blasted doctors who had treated the issue of weight with "amusement." Humor had no place in medical case studies, since obesity was a "pathological state" that required serious consideration.[10] Equally critical was the issue of treatment: fighting fat involved constant management and total dedication to a strict regimen that brought the patient's desires and excessive behavior under control. The obese patient "must be taught to view himself as his worst enemy," Chambers cautioned, and must endeavor to hold an "hourly watch over the instinctive desires."[11]

This is precisely the type of disciplinary, panoptic language that Foucault addresses in *Discipline and Punish*. The instruction to see one's desires, appetites, and indeed oneself as an enemy indicates how punitive and governmental the language surrounding obesity and intemperance had become. Moderating one's intake was a sign of credibility and social accountability. As a case study, then, the public response to the body and private habits of George IV *and* the wider circulating discourses about eating and corpulence reveals changing definitions of health and disease, normality and pathology. But crucially, these definitions were not so much administered as dispersed. Material conditions, medical discoveries, and political events produce real findings and give rise to knowledge, but the resulting knowledge-discourse interface operates like moving tentacles in all directions.

• • •

To sum up, in this project I have attempted to intervene in the vast and important area of research often called the history of the body. As I hope I have demonstrated, medical developments in physiology, anatomy, and epidemiology have never been isolated. Evolving theories about sexuality and reproduction, cleanliness and contamination, diet and drink, foreignness and epidemics, migrated from medical circles into wider culture and, in particular, into the arena of politics. As we have seen, a whole realm of political writers and artists employed a vocabulary rich in anatomical terms: my goal has been to reveal the effects of this migrating vocabulary, on all types of bodies, wherever they are found along the political spectrum.

The case studies in this book should be seen as symptomatic of a grasping after certainty in an age of uncertainty. Marie Antoinette's body was appropriated and metaphorically anatomized in support of a discriminatory politics against public women. Mary Wollstonecraft's death from puerperal fever demonstrated woman's biological unsuitability for politics. William Godwin's allegedly emotionless machine-like approach to her death revealed an affinity between his utilitarian political philosophy and the cold objectivity of medical anatomists. Thomas Paine's supposedly unhygienic, brandy-soaked body and his refusal to have children indicated his constitutional infidelity. The antirevolutionary use of medicopolitical discourse targeted the bodies, habits, and sexual practices of political radicals. George IV's bodily symptoms were refashioned as signs of his political apathy and incapacity. In a period of political exigency, pathologizing the bodies of political figures was a way to make visible, or to form into a narrative, the political dangers such figures were seen to embody. The public anatomizing of their diseases, practices, and rituals was part of a cultural and political emphasis on transparency, and it anticipated what would be an even greater emphasis on the body's ability to "speak the truth of nature" in the Victorian period.[12]

These case studies reveal the modern tradition of trying to read the body to understand such intangible and unknowable phenomena as desire, intention, character, and intelligence. This tradition includes the Enlightenment physiognomist Johann Caspar Lavater's search for character in facial structures; the Victorian phrenologists Johann Spurzheim and Franz Joseph Gall's search for the same in the bumps on the skull; Jean-Martin Charcot's attempts to document hysteria by meticulously photographing the faces of suffering women; and Cesare Lombroso's efforts to identify criminality by cataloging the craniums of prisoners. In her book about pathology in Victorian culture, Erin O'Connor traces a similar tradition, which also includes the French naturalist Georges Cuvier's attempt to "dissect the bestial truth of black female sexuality in the distinctive labia and buttocks of the female Hottentot."[13] And so it seems we return again to George IV's body, which as we have seen, was caricaturized as the Hottentot Venus and made to speak volumes about the two figures' mutual foreignness and excessive sexuality. The pathologizing of political figures, like scientific attempts to read the body, is buttressed by the belief that identity is "thoroughly embodied" and that human character and desire might be "so elaborately materialized that one's moral, mental, and emotional fibers could be read in the telling characters of flesh and bone."[14] This is an accurate assessment, but as I hope I have shown, physicians did not stop at reading the body—they also wanted the body to look, to behave, to *be* a certain way.

Kathleen Brown is right to say, taking a cue from Norbert Elias's *Civilizing Process*, that "political and economic institutions leave their imprint on our bodies."[15] We are profoundly shaped, materially and psychically, by our environments, including all the cultural mechanisms in operation within them. Our bodies, then—and knowledge about them—influence our political institutions. The wide variety of medical topics addressed here, including sexual dysfunction, reproduction, anatomy, hygiene, disease, and dietetics, connect to an equally wide variety of cultural phenomena that in earlier eras would be seen as outside the purview of medicine, including family, morality, politics, and social structures. Health concerns are never removed from moral imperatives, nor are they disconnected from cultural or aesthetic matters like taste, sensibility, and refinement. Language demonstrates this: we commonly use phrases like "health of the nation" or "health of the constitution"; we talk about having "healthy communities" and having "healthy work environments"; more to the point, we refer to healthy or dysfunctional family lives and healthy or toxic marriages. In other words, ideas about health and pathology are part of defining the normative standards by which our "conduct is conducted." Medicine provides norms by which we self-orientate, self-regulate, and self-govern. For these reasons, it is fair to say that medicopolitical discourse in the late eighteenth and nineteenth centuries was most often conservative, although as with most things, this was not universally the case. Medicine fed and was fed by an emergent middle-class ideology that promoted restraint and regulation, at times alongside an emphasis on progress and liberty.

This is borne out by the very high occurrence of medicalized normative categories (and bridging terms) in the medical and political literature of the period, including *natural, clean, rational, civilized,* and *moral*—and their opposites *unnatural, unsanitary, unreasonable, foreign,* and *immoral.* Ultimately, this is a project about categories and beliefs that seem natural, normal, and innate. It is about the rise of modern definitions of the normal and the abnormal; the natural and the unnatural; the healthy and the pathological. It is about what practices, rituals, bodies, and individual characteristics we assign to those categories. My goal has been to trace the ways these categories come into being, how they become defined, and how they become established as "truth." Finally, this book is about the regulative effects these categories have had, and continue to have, on individual and wider identities.

Notes

INTRODUCTION

1. William Hunter, *Correspondence of William Hunter*, ed. C. Helen Brock (London: Pickering & Chatto, 2008), 1:19. Unless otherwise indicated, quotations preserve historical spellings.

2. Helkiah Crooke, *Microcosmographia: The Body of Man* (London: William Iaggard, 1615), 13.

3. Ian Hacking, *The Taming of Chance* (Cambridge: Cambridge University Press, 1990), 65.

4. Jean-Jacques Rousseau, *Émile; or, Education* (1762), trans. Barbara Foxley (London: J. M. Dent and Sons, 1993), 23; see 20–23.

5. Edmund Burke, *Reflections on the Revolution in France and on the Proceedings in Certain Societies in London Relative to that Event* (London: J. Dodsley, 1790), 49.

6. Ibid., 90.

7. Ibid., 128.

8. Timothy Morton, *Shelley and the Revolution in Taste: The Body and the Natural World* (Cambridge: Cambridge University Press, 1994), 40.

9. Burke, *Reflections on the Revolution*, 107.

10. Ibid., 106.

11. Charles Pigott, *The Jockey Club; or, A Sketch of the Manners of the Age*, 7th ed. (London: H. D. Symonds, 1792) 1:119–120.

12. John Brewer, "This, That and the Other: Public, Social and Private in the Seventeenth and Eighteenth Centuries," in *Shifting the Boundaries: Transformation of the Languages of Public and Private in the Eighteenth Century*, ed. Dario Castiglione and Lesley Sharpe (Exeter, UK: Exeter University Press, 1995), 9.

13. See John Barrell, *The Spirit of Despotism: Invasions of Privacy in the 1790s* (Oxford: Oxford University Press, 2006).

14. Michael McKeon, *The Secret History of Domesticity: Public, Private*

and the Division of Knowledge (Baltimore: Johns Hopkins University Press, 2005), 106.

15. For more on the relationship between public and private in 1790s Britain, see John Barrell's *Spirit of Despotism* and his *Imagining the King's Death: Figurative Treason, Fantasies of Regicide, 1793–1796* (Oxford: Oxford University Press, 2000). On the way that scandal and moral discourse played a part in political culture, see Anna Clark, *Scandal: The Sexual Politics of the British Constitution* (Princeton: Princeton University Press, 2004); Corinna Wagner, "Press Scandal and the Struggle for Cultural Authority in the 1790s," *Nineteenth-Century Studies* 22 (2008): 1–14; and Corinna Wagner, "Domestic Invasions: John Thelwall and the Exploitation of Privacy," in *John Thelwall: Radical Romantic and Acquitted Felon*, ed. Steve Poole (London: Pickering & Chatto, 2009), 95–106.

16. J. Brewer, "This, That and the Other," 18.

17. "The Two Cultures" is the title of an influential 1959 Rede Lecture by British novelist and scientist C. P. Snow, subsequently published as *The Two Cultures and the Scientific Revolution* (Cambridge: Cambridge University Press, 1959). Throughout his career, Roy Porter drew numerous points of connection between the history of medicine and social history more generally; see especially *Bodies Politic: Disease, Death and the Doctors in Britain, 1650–1900* (Ithaca: Cornell, 2001) and *Flesh in the Age of Reason* (London: Penguin/Allen Lane, 2003). George Rousseau demonstrates how the study of the human nervous system gave rise to the culture of sensibility and the production of sentimental literature; see especially *Nervous Acts: Essays on Literature, Culture and Sensibility* (Houndmills, UK: Palgrave, 2004). See also Ludmilla Jordanova, *Sexual Visions: Images of Gender in Science and Medicine between the Eighteenth and Twentieth Centuries* (Hemel Hempstead, UK: Harvester/Wheatsheaf; Madison: University of Wisconsin, 1989). In *Sexual Visions*, Jordanova traces the ways biology and gender intersected to create key ideological constructs such as "nature" and "culture" in the eighteenth century. In *Body Criticism: Imaging the Unseen in Enlightenment Art and Medicine* (Cambridge, MA: MIT Press, 1991), Barbara Maria Stafford focuses on the important relationship between visual culture and medicine, as do Jordanova and Porter, the latter of whom urges scholars to consider visual representations of medicine and medics "within the wider cultural pool" (in *Bodies Politic*, 12). For literary scholars who have drawn important connections between science, medicine, and literature, see Alan Richardson, *British Romanticism and the Science of the Mind* (Cambridge: Cambridge University Press, 2001); Sharon Ruston, *Shelley and Vitality* (Houndmills, UK: Palgrave, 2005); and James Robert Allard, *Romanticism, Medicine, and the Poet's Body* (Aldershot, UK: Ashgate, 2007). In a provocative study, Paul Youngquist has shown how the anatomical identification of difference—of monstrosity—is intimately caught up with such modern phenomena as "liberalism, free-market-economics, British nationalism, and professionalized medicine"; see

Monstrosities: Bodies and British Romanticism (Minneapolis: University of Minnesota Press, 2003), xv.

18. G. Rousseau, *Nervous Acts*, 6.

19. Nikolas Rose, "Medicine, History and the Present," in *Reassessing Foucault: Power, Medicine and the Body*, ed. Colin Jones and Roy Porter (1994; reprint, London: Routledge, 1998), 49.

20. This point has been made convincingly by Roger Cooter and Mary Fissell in *The Cambridge History of Science: Eighteenth-Century Science*, ed. Roy Porter (Cambridge: Cambridge University Press, 2004), 4:146.

21. Mary E. Fissell, *Vernacular Bodies: The Politics of Reproduction in Early Modern England* (Oxford: Oxford University Press, 2006), 9.

22. For more on the use of narrative, see Mark Bevir, "Rethinking Governmentality: Towards Genealogies of Governance," *European Journal of Social Theory* 13, no. 4 (2010): 434.

23. Jordanova, *Sexual Visions*, 27.

24. Michel Foucault, *Discipline and Punish: The Birth of the Prison*, trans. Alan Sheridan (New York: Vintage, 1995).

25. Bevir, "Rethinking Governmentality," 431.

CHAPTER 1

1. Lynn Hunt, "The Many Bodies of Marie-Antoinette: Political Pornography and the Problem of the Feminine in the French Revolution," in *Marie Antoinette: Writings on the Body of the Queen*, ed. Dena Goodman (London: Routledge, 2003), 117. See also Robert Darnton, "The High Enlightenment and the Low-Life of Literature," in *The Literary Underground of the Old Regime* (Cambridge, MA: Harvard University Press, 1982), 1–40.

2. See Goodman, *Marie Antoinette*; Lynn Hunt, *The Family Romance of the French Revolution* (Berkeley: University of California Press, 1992); Lynn Hunt, ed., *The Invention of Pornography: Obscenity and the Origins of Modernity, 1500–1800* (New York: Zone Books, 1993); Sarah Maza, *Private Lives and Pubic Affairs: The Causes Célèbres of Prerevolutionary France* (Berkeley: University of California Press, 1993); and Chantal Thomas, *The Wicked Queen: The Origins of the Myth of Marie-Antoinette* (New York: Zone Books, 1999).

3. Adriana Craciun, *Fatal Women of Romanticism* (Cambridge: Cambridge University Press, 2003), 10.

4. Iain McCalman, "The Making of a Libertine Queen: Jeanne de La Motte and Marie-Antoinette," in *Libertine Enlightenment: Sex, Liberty and License in the Eighteenth Century*, ed. Peter Cryle and Lisa O'Connell (Houndmills, UK: Palgrave, 2004), 113.

5. Thomas Laqueur, "Orgasm, Generation, and the Politics of Reproductive Biology," in *The Making of the Modern Body: Sexuality and Society in the Nineteenth Century*, ed. Thomas Laqueur and Catherine Gallagher (Berkeley: University of California Press, 1987), 2.

6. James Parsons, *A Mechanical and Critical Enquiry into the Nature of Hermaphrodites* (London: London: J. Walthoe, 1741), 31–33.

7. Thomas Laqueur, *Making Sex: Body and Gender from the Greeks to Freud* (Cambridge, MA: Harvard University Press, 1990), 207.

8. Youngquist, *Monstrosities*, 132.

9. J.-J. Rousseau, *Émile*, 386.

10. Ibid., 385.

11. Ibid.

12. Ibid.

13. *La godmiché* [The royal dildo] (n.p., 1789), in Thomas, *Wicked Queen*, 201.

14. *L'autrichienne en goguettes; ou, L'orgie royale* [The Austrian woman on the rampage; or, The royal orgy] (n.p., 1789), in Thomas, *Wicked Queen*, 205–206; *Bord . . . R . . .* [The royal bordello] (n.p., [1789?]), in ibid., 225.

15. *The Royal Dildo*, in Thomas, *Wicked Queen*, 201.

16. George Rousseau has identified a "paradigmatic shift from a uterine to a nervous model of hysteria," while Mark Micale has argued for a shift back to the uterine model (a "re-eroticization" of hysteria). In contrast, Mary Peace has argued convincingly that the disease had never been de-eroticized. See George Rousseau, "'A Strange Pathology'" in *Hysteria beyond Freud*, ed. Sander Gilman et al. (Berkeley: University of California Press, 1993), 91–221; Mark Micale, *Approaching Hysteria: Disease and Its Interpretations* (Princeton, NJ: Princeton University Press, 1995); and Mary Peace, "The Economy of Nymphomania: Luxury, Virtue, Sentiment and Desire in Mid-Eighteenth Century Medical Discourse," in *At the Borders of the Human: Beasts, Bodies and Natural Philosophy in the Early Modern Period*, ed. Erica Fudge, Ruth Gilbert, and Susan Wiseman (Houndmills, UK: Palgrave, 2002), 248–250.

17. M. D. T. de Bienville, *Nymphomania; or, A Dissertation Concerning the Furor Uterinus*, trans. Edward Sloane Wilmot (London: J. Bew, 1775), xiv.

18. Ibid., 31, 36.

19. Ibid., 31, 36.

20. Lynn Hunt, *Politics, Culture and Class in the French Revolution* (1984; reprint, Berkeley: University of California Press, 2004), 44.

21. L. Hunt, "Many Bodies," 121.

22. Michel Foucault, *Power/Knowledge*, ed. Colin Gordon (1972; reprint, New York: Pantheon, 1980), 153.

23. Michel Foucault, "The Birth of Social Medicine," in *The Essential Foucault*, ed. Paul Rabinow and Nikolas Rose (New York: New Press, 2003), 320.

24. *The Austrian Woman*, in Thomas, *Wicked Queen*, 209.

25. Bienville, *Nymphomania*, 257.

26. *Les amours de Charlot et Toinette* [The love life of Charlie and Toinette] (n.p., 1779), in Thomas, *Wicked Queen*, 186.

27. Barrell, "The Last Interview," in *Imagining the King's Death*, 49–86. See also David Bindman, *The Shadow of the Guillotine: Britain and the French Revolution* (London: British Museum Publications, 1989).

28. Barrell, *Imagining the King's Death*, 62.
29. *Tomahawk*, 26 January 1795.
30. *Tomahawk*, 26 January 1795 (emphasis added).
31. Joseph Priestley, *Letters to the Right Honourable Edmund Burke, Occasioned by His Reflections on the Revolution in France* (Dublin: J. Sheppard et al., 1791), 16; John Thelwall, "Report on the State of Popular Opinion, and the Causes of the Rapid Diffusion of Democratic Principles, Part the Second," *The Tribune* 2, no. 25 (1795): 221.
32. Thomas Christie, *Letters on the Revolution of France* (1791), in *Political Writings of the 1790s*, ed. Gregory Claeys (London: Pickering & Chatto, 1995), 2:246.
33. Stafford, *Body Criticism*, 2.
34. Bienville, *Nymphomania*, vii.
35. *The Ladies Dispensatory; or, Every Woman Her Own Physician: Treating of the Nature, Causes, and Various Symptoms, of All the Diseases, Infirmities* (London: James Hodges, 1739) 107, 109.
36. John Aiken, *Principles of Midwifery; or, Puerperal Medicine*, 3rd ed. (London: J. Murray, 1786), 136.
37. On women's sexuality and religion, see Carroll Smith-Rosenberg, *Disorderly Conduct: Visions of Gender in Victorian America* (New York: Knopf, 1985). On the role of changing economic climate and nymphomania, see Anne Digby "Women's Biological Straitjacket," in *Sexuality and Subordination: Interdisciplinary Studies of Gender in the Nineteenth Century*, ed. Susan Mendus and Jane Rendall (London: Routledge, 1989), 192–220.
38. Carol Groneman, "Nymphomania: The Historical Construction of Female Sexuality," in *Deviant Bodies: Critical Perspectives on Difference in Science and Popular Culture*, ed. Jennifer Terry and Jacqueline Urla (Bloomington: Indiana University Press, 1995), 226.
39. Elizabeth Colwill, "Pass as a Woman, Act Like a Man: Marie Antoinette as Tribade in the Pornography of the French Revolution," in Goodman, *Marie Antoinette*, 144.
40. Ibid., 144.
41. *La journée amoureuse* (n.p., n.d.), 18, also reprinted in Colwill, "Pass as a Woman," 150. See also Ann Jones and Peter Stallybrass, "Fetishizing Gender: Constructing the Hermaphrodite in Renaissance Europe," in *Body Guards: The Cultural Politics of Gender Ambiguity*, ed. Julia Epstein and Kristina Straub (New York: Routledge, 1991), 90.
42. Mary Sheriff, "Woman? Hermaphrodite? History Painter? On the Self-Imaging of Elizabeth Vigée-Lebrun," *The Eighteenth Century* 35 (1994): 3–27, see especially p. 7; Colwill, "Pass as a Woman," 152.
43. Helen Deutsch and Felicity Nussbaum, introduction to *Defects: Engendering the Modern Body* (Ann Arbor: University of Michigan Press, 2000), 7, 8. See also Andrew Curran and Patrick Graille, "The Faces of Eighteenth-Century Monstrosity," *Eighteenth-Century Life* 21, no. 2 (1997): 1–15.

44. Georges Canguilhem, *The Normal and the Pathological*, trans. Carolyn R. Fawcett (1978; reprint, New York: Zone Books, 2007), 239.

45. Craciun, *Fatal Women of Romanticism*, 128.

46. John Hunter married Home's sister, Anne, in 1771; Home was Hunter's pupil before becoming his teaching, research, and surgical assistant. Although their relationship was often troubled and there is evidence that Home traded on Hunter's reputation, Home persuaded the British government to buy Hunter's anatomical museum and to house it at the Royal College of Surgeons. In 1817 Home was named master of the Royal College of Surgeons, where he endowed the Hunterian Oration and gave courses in comparative anatomy.

47. Everard Home, "An Account of the Dissection of an Hermaphrodite Dog: To Which Are Prefixed, Some Observations on Hermaphrodites in General," *Philosophical Transactions of the Royal Society of London* 89 (1799): 159.

48. Ibid., 242.
49. Ibid., 165.
50. Ibid., 162.
51. Ibid., 162–163.
52. Ibid., 242.
53. Ibid., 164.
54. Ibid., 165.

55. Richard Sha, "Scientific Forms of Sexual Knowledge in Romanticism," *Romanticism on the Net* 23 (August 2001), 9, www.erudit.org/revue/ron/v/n23/005993ar.html.

56. Parsons, *Mechanical and Critical Enquiry*, 10–11.

57. Qtd. in Sha, "Scientific Forms of Sexual Knowledge," 46.

58. Lucy Bland, "Trial by Sexology? Maud Allan, Salome, and the 'Cult of the Clitoris' Case," in *Sexology in Culture: Labelling Bodies and Desires*, ed. Lucy Bland and Laura Doan (Chicago: University of Chicago Press, 1998), 184.

59. *Fureurs uterines de Marie-Antoinette, femme de Louis XVI* (n.p., n.d.), 8, in Thomas, *Wicked Queen*, 120.

60. The attitude would be expressed some years later by Napoleon's disdain for nunneries, which as he said, "assail the very roots of population" and weaken the nation; he would only allow nuns "to make perpetual vows at fifty years of age; for then their task is fulfilled." Qtd. in June Burton, *Napoleon and the Woman Question: Discourses of the Other Sex in French Education, Medicine and Medical Law, 1799–1815* (Lubbock: Texas Tech University Press, 2007), 4. Also see chap. 1 of that book for similar comments.

61. Gérard Walter, ed., *Actes du tribunal révolutionnaire* (Paris: Mercure de France, 1968), 96, qtd. in Thomas, *Wicked Queen*, 146. See also *Authentic Trial at Large of Marie Antoinette, Late Queen of France, before the Revolutionary Tribunal at Paris*, (London: Chapman & Co, 1793).

62. *Le Moniteur Universal*, 20 October 1793, qtd. in L. Hunt, "Many Bodies," 123.
63. Ibid.
64. John Adolphus, *Biographical Memoirs of the French Revolution* (London: T. Cadell, Jun. & W. Davies, 1799), 1:150.
65. Ibid., 1:149–150.
66. Helen Maria Williams, *Letters Containing a Sketch of the Politics of France, 1793–94* (London: G. G. & J. Robinson, 1795), 2:54.
67. "Ode to Jacobinism," *Anti-Jacobin or Weekly Examiner* 20 (26 March 1798), 157.
68. William Hamilton, *Letters on the Principles of the French Democracy and Their Application and Influence on the Constitution and Happiness of Britain and Ireland* (Dublin: G. Bonham, 1792), 29.
69. Edmund Burke, *First Letter on a Regicide Peace, from Two Letters . . . on the Proposals for Peace with the Regicide Directory of France* (1796), in *The Impact of the French Revolution*, ed. Iain Hampsher-Monk (Cambridge: Cambridge University Press, 2005), 307.
70. William Cobbett, *The Bloody Buoy, Thrown Out as a Warning to the Political Pilots of America; or, a Faithful Relation of a Multitude of Acts of Horrid Barbarity, such as the Eye Never Witnessed, the Tongue Never Expressed, or the Imagination Conceived, until the Commencement of the French Revolution*, 3rd ed. (1796; reprint, Philadelphia: N.p., 1823), 34–35.
71. Ibid., 35.
72. See Johann Caspar Lavater, "Girl with Birthmarks," in *Essays on Physiognomy: For the Promotion of the Knowledge and the Love of Mankind*, trans. Thomas Holcroft, 18th ed. (London: Ward, Lock and Co., 1789), 376–379; 433–434.
73. Jane Sharp, *The Midwives Book; or, The Whole Art of Midwifery* (London: Simon Miller, 1671), 186–187, 118.
74. Nicholas de Venette, *The Mysteries of Conjugal Love Reveal'd*, 8th ed. (London: N.p., 1707), 388–389.
75. Ibid., 390.
76. Ibid., 392, 407.
77. Lavater, "Girl with Birthmarks," 433–434.
78. Elizabeth Nihell, *A Treatise on the Art of Midwifery* (London: A. Morley, 1760), 61, 236.
79. Lisa Foreman Cody, *Birthing the Nation: Sex, Science and the Conception of Eighteenth-Century Britons* (Oxford: Oxford University Press, 2006), 147.
80. John Cook, *The New Theory of Generation, According to the Best and Latest Discoveries in Anatomy* (London: J. Buckland, 1762), 254–255.
81. John Leake, *A Lecture Introductory to the Theory and Practice of Midwifery* (London: R. Baldwin, 1782), 25–26.
82. Ibid., 26.

83. Rosi Braidotti, *Nomadic Subjects: Embodiment and Sexual Difference in Contemporary Feminist Theory* (New York: Columbia University Press, 1994), 80.

84. Margrit Shildrick, *Embodying the Monster: Encounters with the Vulnerable Self* (London: Sage, 2002), 29 (emphasis added).

85. John Marten, *Onania; or, The Heinous Sin of Self-Pollution, and All Its Frightful Consequences*, 19th ed. (London: C. Corbett, 1759), 13–14, 31.

86. J.G. Zimmermann, "Warnung an Aeltern, Erzieher und Kinderfreunde wegen der Selbstbefleckung, zumal bey ganz jungen Mädchen," *Neues Magazin für Ärzte* 1 (1779): 51.

87. Michael Stolberg, "An Unmanly Vice: Self-Pollution, Anxiety, and the Body in the Eighteenth Century," *Social History of Medicine*, 13, no. 1 (2000): 1–22.

88. See Peter Gay, *The Bourgeois Experience: Victoria to Freud*, vol. 1, *Education of the Senses* (New York: Norton, 1984).

89. Thomas W. Laqueur, *Solitary Sex: A Cultural History of Masturbation* (New York: Zone Books, 2003), 21.

90. *Lettres de cachet* were infamous legal orders, bearing the king's signature, that entitled family members and friends to imprison one another. They became a significant point of debate in the months leading up to the Revolution, as they signified the link between familial and state tyranny. A father's *lettre de cachet* against a rebellious son, for instance, was the definitive symbol of the entwined nature of political tyranny and familial degradation under the old regime. These legal orders demonstrated how, under the authority of corrupt laws and the sanction of a distant father-king who cared little for his subjects, family members were entitled, even encouraged, to persecute their own dependents.

91. A.F.M. Willich, *Lectures on Diet and Regimen*, 2nd ed. (London: Longman & Rees, 1799), 548.

92. Ibid., 547.

93. See, for example, Robert Darby, "A Post-Modernist Theory of Wanking: Solitary Sex," *Journal of Social History* 38, no. 1 (2004): 205–210.

94. Michel Foucault, *History of Sexuality*, trans. Robert Hurley (New York: Vintage, 1990), 1:281. Although Foucault's argument that personal health issues and moral codes cannot be disengaged from the state of the nation applies to France, his conclusions are also relevant to England.

95. Marten, *Onania*, 83 (emphasis added).

96. Helen Maria Williams, *Letters Written in France, in the Summer 1790, to a Friend in England* (London: T. Cadell, 1790). This vital promise underwrote the National Assembly's introduction of *tribunaux de famille*, which were councils that disentangled family difficulties. As Thomas Christie, the radical editor of the *Analytical Review*, explained for his British audience, "When a parent, or tutor, has weighty grounds of dissatisfaction with the conduct of a child or pupil, whom he can no longer restrain," or when disagreements arise between "grandfather and grandchild, brothers and sisters, uncles and nephews," they appeared before a council of relatives for judgment.

These tribunals, Christie explained, were an expression of the assembly's desire "to democratize family life" by "removing its despotic and aristocratic characteristics, while leaving it in place as the bedrock of society." The new state was keen to rebuild families, and families were intent on rebuilding the state as a family. Christie, *Letters on the Revolution*, vol. 2.

97. Anna Letitia Barbauld, *Civic Sermons, Number II* (London: J. Johnson, 1792), 6.

98. Christie, *Letters on the Revolution*, 120.

99. Ibid., 217–218.

100. Qtd. in Mary Sheriff, "The Portrait of the Queen," in Goodman, *Marie Antoinette*, 47.

101. Christie, *Letters on the Revolution*, 120 (emphasis added).

102. Ibid., 217.

103. Ibid., 237.

104. Ibid., 220.

105. The three parts of *The Jockey Club* were published separately in Britain in many editions, but they were published together in one volume in New York. For ease of referencing and to avoid confusion, I use this collated American edition unless otherwise noted. Charles Pigott, *The Jockey Club* (American reprint; New York: Thomas Greenleaf, 1793), 167.

106. Ibid., 165.

107. Ibid., 167.

108. Ibid., 166.

CHAPTER 2

1. These manuals were, in some ways, part of a much longer history of suspicion about the corrupt milk of wet nurses, stretching back to the classical period. The famous botanist and physician Carl Linnaeus, for example, reiterated Erasmus's claim that the filthy, corrupted milk of immoral and disease-ridden wet nurses had given rise to Nero's alcoholism and Caligula's cruelty. See Londa Schiebinger, *Nature's Body: Sexual Politics and the Making of Modern Science* (London: HarperCollins, 1993), 68.

2. Mary Wortley Montagu, *Letters of the Right Honourable Lady M——y W——y M——e* (London: Thomas Martin, 1790), 180–181.

3. Schiebinger, *Nature's Body*, 4.

4. See Ruth Perry, "Colonizing the Breast: Sexuality and Maternity in Eighteenth-Century England," *Journal of the History of Sexuality* 2, no. 2 (1991): 204–234; Julie Kipp, *Romanticism, Maternity, and the Body Politic* (Cambridge: Cambridge University Press, 2007); Laura Brace, "Rousseau, Maternity and the Politics of Emptiness," *Polity* 39 (2007): 361–383; and Rebecca Kukla, *Mass Hysteria: Medicine, Culture, and Mother's Bodies* (Lanham, MD: Rowman & Littlefield, 2005).

5. George D. Sussman, *Selling Mothers' Milk: The Wet-Nursing Business in France, 1715–1914* (Urbana: University of Illinois Press, 1982), 110.

6. J.-J. Rousseau, *Émile*, 15.
7. Elizabeth Wingrove, *Rousseau's Republican Romance* (Princeton. NJ: Princeton University Press, 2000), 159.
8. J.-J. Rousseau, *Émile*, 15.
9. Jean-Jacques Rousseau, *Considerations on the Government of Poland* (1772), trans. Willmoer Kendall (Indianapolis: Hackett, 1985), 19.
10. Mary Wollstonecraft, *A Vindication of the Rights of Woman* (London: J. Johnson, 1792), 334.
11. Kukla, *Mass Hysteria*, 42, 41, 49 (emphasis added).
12. William Cadogan, *An Essay upon Nursing and the Management of Children*, 9th ed. (London: R. Florsfield, 1772), 14–15.
13. Ibid., 45.
14. Ibid., 20.
15. Ibid., 21.
16. Aiken, *Principles of Midwifery*, 3rd ed., 67. In the first edition, in 1785, this statement was only a footnote; it became embedded in the text by the third edition.
17. William Moss, *An Essay on the Management, Nursing and Diseases of Children*, 2nd ed. (Egham, UK: C. Boult, 1794), 138.
18. Ibid., 466.
19. Ibid., 462–463.
20. Cadogan, *Essay upon Nursing*, 33.
21. Hugh Smith, *Letters to Married Women* (London: G. Kearsley, 1767), 76.
22. Cadogan, *Essay upon Nursing*, 34.
23. Kukla, *Mass Hysteria*, 48–49.
24. Perry, "Colonizing the Breast," 231.
25. Kukla, *Mass Hysteria*, 29.
26. Ibid., 48–49.
27. Colwill, "Pass as a Woman," 142.
28. Dorothy McLaren, "Marital Fertility and Lactation, 1570–1720," in *Women in English Society*, ed. Mary Prior (London: Methuen, 1985), 45; see also 27.
29. *Rambler's Magazine*, 1783, 318.
30. Charles Pigott, *The Female Jockey Club*, 3rd ed. (London: D.I. Eaton, 1794), 16–17.
31. Thomas Hardy, *The Patriot, Addressed to the People, on the Present State of Affairs in Britain and in France*, 2nd ed. (Edinburgh: J. Dickson, 1793), 49.
32. William Cobbett, "The Republican Judge," in *Porcupine's Works* (London: Cobbett, 1801), 12:316.
33. Member of Parliament, and of His Majesty's Privy Council, *An Exposure of the Domestic and Foreign Attempts to Destroy the British Constitution* (London: J. Stockdale, 1792), 9.
34. W.C. Proby, *Modern Philosophy and Barbarism: or, A Comparison*

between the Theory of Godwin and the Practice of Lycurgus (London: R. H. Westley, [1798]), 5.

35. An alternative account has it that he remarked, "I see you suckled your children yourself." Either way, the message is the same. *The Court Journal: Court Circular and Fashionable Gazette* (London: H. Colburn, 1835), 7:37. And see Madame Campan, *Private Journal of Madame Campan, Comprising Original Anecdotes of the French Court*, ed. M. Maigne (Philadelphia: A. Small, 1825), 61.

36. Lynn Salkin Sbiroli, "Generation and Regeneration: Reflections on the Biological and Ideological Role of Women in France (1786–96)," in *Literature and Medicine during the Eighteenth Century*, ed. Marie Mulvey Roberts and Roy Porter (London, 1993), 266.

37. Louis Du Broca, *Interesting Anecdotes of the Heroic Conduct of Women, previous to, and during the French Revolution* (Baltimore: Fryer & Clark, 1804), 32.

38. Broca, *Interesting Anecdotes*, 158.

39. *Biographical Anecdotes of the Founders of the French Republic* (London: R. Phillips, 1797), 246.

40. Ibid., 247.

41. Henry James Pye, *The Democrat: Interspersed with Anecdotes of Well Known Characters* (London: William Lane, 1795), 2:30.

42. *Bon Ton*, September 1792, 241.

43. Isaac D'Israeli, *Flim Flams! Or the Life and Errors of My Uncle and the Amours of My Aunt* (London: John Murray, 1805), 1:b1, b5.

44. Jean-Jacques Rousseau, *Politics and the Arts: Letter to M. d'Alembert on the Theatre* (1758), trans. Alan Bloom (Ithaca, NY: Cornell University Press, 1968) 100–101.

45. *Bon Ton*, September 1792, 241.

46. Marilyn Yalom, *A History of the Breast* (New York: Alfred A. Knopf, 1997), 3.

47. *The Royal Dildo*, in Thomas, *Wicked Queen*, 193–194.

48. *Les enfans de Sodome à l'Assemblée Nationale* (1790), in Lynn Hunt, "Pornography and the French Revolution," in L. Hunt, *Invention of Pornography*, 309.

49. Ewa Lajer-Burcharth, "The Aesthetics of Male Crisis: The Terror in the Republican Imaginary and in Jean-Louis David's Work from Prison," in *Femininity and Masculinity in Eighteenth-Century Art and Culture*, ed. Gillian Perry and Michael Rossington (Manchester: Manchester University Press, 1994), 222.

50. Count Thomas O'Neil, *Narrative of the Incarceration of Count O'Neil, and the Massacre of His Family in France, etc.* (London: Charles Squire, 1814), 22.

51. Ibid., 75.

52. Ibid., 48.

53. Ibid., 52.

54. Anna Clark, *Struggle for the Breeches: Gender and the Making of the British Working Class* (Berkeley: University of California Press, 1995), 154.

55. There is much debate on the issue of changing perceptions of homosexuality in this century. See Stephen Garton, *Histories of Sexuality: Antiquity to Sexual Revolution* (New York: Routledge, 2004); George Rousseau, "The Pursuit of Homosexuality in the Eighteenth Century: 'Utterly Confused Category' and/or Rich Repository?" in *'Tis Nature's Fault: Unauthorized Sexuality During the Enlightenment*, ed. Robert Perks Maccubbin (Cambridge: Cambridge University Press, 1987) 132–168; Laurence Senelick, "Mollies or Men of Mode? Sodomy and the Eighteenth-Century London Stage," *Journal of the History of Sexuality* 1 (1990): 33–67; Randolph Trumbach, "Sodomitical Subcultures, Sodomitical Roles, and the Gender Revolution of the Eighteenth Century: The Recent Historiography," in Maccubbin, *'Tis Nature's Fault*, 109–121; Randolph Trumbach, "Erotic Fantasy and Male Libertinism in Enlightenment England," in L. Hunt, *Invention of Pornography*, 253–282; Martin Duberman, Martha Vicinus, and George Chauncey, eds., *Hidden from History: Reclaiming the Gay and Lesbian Past* (London: Penguin, 1991); and Tim Hitchcock, *English Sexualities, 1700–1800* (Houndmills, UK: Palgrave, 1997).

56. Herman Boerhaave, *Boerhaave's Academical Lectures on the Lues Venerea*, trans. Jonathan Watham (London: J. Rivington, 1763), 23.

57. Nikolai Detlef Falck, *A Treatise on the Venereal Disease* (London: For the author, 1772), 108.

58. Qtd. in Clark, *Struggle for the Breeches*, 154.

59. Cobbett, *Bloody Buoy*, 187.

60. Michèle Cohen argues that in the eighteenth century Britons became suspicious of the French traditions of *politesse* and the *honnête homme*. These terms refer to the practice, in place since the seventeenth century, in which men refined their social skills by conversing with—and attempting to impress—women in salons. See Michèle Cohen, *Fashioning Masculinity: National Identity and Language in the Eighteenth Century* (London: Routledge) 1996.

61. "Sex Museum Displays Hillary Rodham Clinton Bust," *USA Today*, 11 August 2006, www.usatoday.com/news/offbeat/2006-08-11-clinton-bust_x.htm.

62. Pierre Saint-Amand, "Terrorizing Marie Antoinette," *Critical Inquiry* 20 (Spring 1994): 391.

63. Ibid., 382.

CHAPTER 3

1. *Admirable Satire on the Death, Dissection, Funeral Procession, and Epitaph, of Mr. Pitt* (London: C. Smith, 1795), 5.

2. *Morning Post*, 7 July 1791.

3. *Courier*, 22 January 1795.

4. *Courier*, 28 November 1794, 29 December 1794.

5. *Courier*, 15 December 1794.

6. *Admirable Satire*, 13.

7. The *True Briton*, on 5 January 1797, unflaggingly assured readers "of the approaching nuptials" of Pitt and Eden; a week later, on 11 January 1791, the *Morning Post* stated compellingly that "Mr. PITT should unite with EDEN," as he would then "not be far from Paradise."

8. *Admirable Satire*, 12.

9. In one *Morning Post* squib, from 8 February 1793, the Tory ministry is made to declare how proud it is to be "chaste and good" and "frigid."

10. This phrase is borrowed from A Friend to Social Order, *Thoughts on Marriage and Criminal Conversation, with some hints of appropriate means to check the progress of the latter; comprising remarks on the life, opinions, and example of the late Mrs. Wollstonecraft Godwin: Respectfully addressed and inscribed to the Right Honourable Lord Kenyon, Lord Chief Justice of the Court of King's Bench* (London: F. C. Rivington, et al., 1799), 54.

11. Tim Fulford, *Romanticism and Masculinity: Gender, Politics and Poetics in the Writing of Burke, Coleridge, Cobbett, Wordsworth, DeQuincey and Hazlitt*, (Houndmills, UK: Macmillan, 1999), 20.

12. *Anti-Jacobin Review* 1 (1798): 94–102. More than one periodical chose the word *concubinage* to characterize Wollstonecraft's personal relations: see *The Scientific Magazine and Free-Mason's Repository* 10 (1798): 403–404.

13. *Anti-Jacobin Review* (August 1805) in William Godwin, introduction to *Fleetwood: or, The New Man of Feeling* (1805), ed. Gary Handwerk and A. A. Markley (Peterborough, ON: Broadview, 2001), 530. Also see *European Magazine* (also known as *The London Review and Literary Journal*) 33 (1798): 246–251.

14. William Godwin, *Enquiry Concerning Political Justice* (1793), 3rd ed. (London: G. G. and J. Robinson, 1798) 2:508.

15. Matthew Grenby, *The Anti-Jacobin Novel: British Conservatism and the French Revolution* (Cambridge: Cambridge University Press, 2001), 66.

16. Ibid., 75.

17. Godwin, *Political Justice*, 2:510.

18. Coleridge attacked Godwin and the principles of *Political Justice* in his 1795 Bristol lectures and in *The Watchman* of 1796.

19. William Godwin, *Considerations on Lord Grenville's and Mr. Pitt's Bills* (London: J. Johnson, 1795), 2.

20. Although Godwin's precise motives for turning on Thelwall are open to debate, it seems certain that, as John Barrell surmises, Thelwall must have felt betrayed by what seemed to be an attempt to define his "philosophical disquisitions" as somehow "beyond the reach of law." Barrell, *Imagining the King's Death*, 587. It is significant that Thelwall had previously referred to Godwin as his "philosophical father": Godwin's condemnation of the political immoderation of the popular radical movement reads like a heartless rejection of a son who had sought his father's approval. The exact intellectual relationship between the two radicals remains rather opaque. See Peter Marshall,

William Godwin (New Haven, CT: Yale University Press, 1984), 140. Acting the part of the forsaken son, Thelwall interpreted Godwin's characterization of his politics as an intrinsically personal public attack and so felt justified in attacking on equally personal grounds, in an equally public medium.

21. John Thelwall, preface to *The Tribune, a Periodical Publication, Consisting Chiefly of the Political Lectures of J. Thelwall*, no. 2 (London: Symonds et al., 1796), xiv–xv.

22. *Morning Chronicle*, 21 April 1795.

23. Thelwall, *Tribune*, 2:xv (second emphasis added).

24. Ibid.

25. William Godwin, *Memoirs of the Author of "A Vindication of the Rights of Woman"* (London: J. Johnson and G. G. and J. Robinson, 1798), 176. Unless otherwise noted, citations to the *Memoirs* are from this edition.

26. Ibid., 183.

27. Ibid., 184.

28. Ibid., 181–182.

29. Ibid., 188.

30. *European Magazine* 33 (1798): 246–245.

31. Charles Lucas, *The Infernal Quixote: A Tale of the Day* (1801), ed. M. O. Grenby (reprint, Peterborough, ON: Broadview, 2004), 84; *British Critic* 12 (1798): 228–233, in *William Godwin Reviewed*, ed. Kenneth W. Graham (New York: AMS Press, 2001), 144. See also *Monthly Mirror* 5 (1798): 153–157.

32. William Godwin, qtd. in William D. Brewer, *The Mental Anatomies of William Godwin and Mary Shelley* (Madison, NJ: Fairleigh-Dickinson University Press, 2001), 15.

33. Tilottama Rajan, "Framing the Corpus: Godwin's 'Editing' of Wollstonecraft in 1798," *Studies in Romanticism* 39 (Winter 2000): 531.

34. Mitzi Myers, "Godwin's Memoirs of Wollstonecraft: The Shaping of the Self and Subject," *Studies in Romanticism* 20 (Fall 1981): 312, 303.

35. Angela Monsam, "Biography as Autopsy in William Godwin's *Memoirs of the Author of 'A Vindication of the Rights of Woman'*" *Eighteenth-Century Fiction* 21, no. 1 (2008): 110–111.

36. Ibid., 124.

37. Ibid.

38. Sha, "Scientific Forms of Sexual Knowledge," 2.

39. Martin Kemp, "'The Mark of Truth': Looking and Learning in some Anatomical Illustrations from the Renaissance and Eighteenth Century," in *Medicine and the Five Senses*, ed. W. F. Bynum and Roy Porter (Cambridge: Cambridge University Press, 1993), 113.

40. Ibid., 105.

41. Ibid., 117.

42. As a novice medical illustrator, Rymsdyk produced plates for William Smellie, *Sett* [sic] *of Anatomical Tables with Explanations, and an Abridge-*

ment of the Practice of Midwifery (London: N.p., 1754). This could be counted as an earlier example of the flesh-and-blood school of illustration.

43. Jan van Rymsdyk and Andrew van Rymsdyk, *Museum Britannicum*, 2nd ed. (London: J. Moore, 1791), vi.

44. Youngquist, *Monstrosities*, 135.

45. Ibid.

46. Courtney Wennerstrom, "Cosmopolitan Bodies and Dissected Sexualities: Anatomical Mis-stories in Ann Radcliffe's *Mysteries of Udolpho*," *European Romantic Review* 16, no. 2 (2005): 197.

47. William Hunter, *The Anatomy of the Human Gravid Uterus* (Birmingham: John Baskerville, 1774), n.p.

48. Both of these tales can be found in Corinna Wagner, ed., *Gothic Evolutions: Poetry, Tales, Context, Theory* (Peterborough, ON: Broadview, 2013).

49. Anne Millard, qtd. in Ruth Richardson, *Death, Dissection and the Destitute*, 2nd ed. (Chicago: University of Chicago Press, 2000), 95.

50. Youngquist, *Monstrosities*, 135.

51. Wennerstrom, "Cosmopolitan Bodies," 197.

52. For more on this debate, see the introduction and chapter 1 of Ruston, *Shelley and Vitality*.

53. Burke, *Reflections on the Revolution*, 115 (emphasis added).

54. Ibid., 115.

55. Thomas Carlyle, "Signs of the Times" (1829), in *Thomas Carlyle: Selected Writings*, ed. Alan Shelston (Harmondsworth, UK: Penguin, 1971), 69.

56. Thomas Carlyle, *Sartor Resartus* (Boston: James Munroe, 1840), 120.

57. Carlyle had just read Godwin's *History of the Commonwealth of England*, 4 vols. (London, 1824–28). He also commented that Godwin was "long-winded" and "dull as ditchwater." Thomas Carlyle to John Forster, 12 April 1839, *Collected Letters*, 11:72, doi:10.1215/lt-18390412-TC-JF-01.

58. Godwin, *Political Justice*, viii.

59. *Anti-Jacobin Review* 1 (1798): 94–102, in K. W. Graham, *Godwin Reviewed*, 139.

60. *The Scientific Magazine and Free-Mason's Repository* 10 (1798): 403–404, in K. W. Graham, *Godwin Reviewed*, 155 (emphasis added).

61. Robert Southey, letter dated 1 July 1804, qtd. in the introduction to William Godwin, Memoirs of the Author of "A Vindication of the Rights of Woman," ed. Pamela Clemit and Gina Luria Walker (Peterborough, ON: Broadview, 2001), 11.

62. *Monthly Mirror* 5 (1798): 153–157, in K. W. Graham, *Godwin Reviewed*, 149.

63. James Neu, *A Tear Is an Intellectual Thing: The Meanings of Emotion* (Oxford: Oxford University Press, 2000), 102.

64. John Brown, *The Elements of Medicine* (London: J. Johnson, 1795), 1:15.

65. Anne Mallory, "Burke, Boredom, and the Theater of Counterrevolution," *PMLA* 118, no. 2 (2003): 228, 226.

66. John Arbuthnot, *Law Is a Bottomless Pit; or, The History of John Bull* (1712; reprint, Glasgow: Robert Urie, 1766), 19.

67. Samuel Romilly, *Thoughts on the Probable Influence of the French Revolution on Great-Britain* (Dublin: P. Byrne, 1790), 4.

68. Godwin, *Political Justice*, 1:127. Charles Lamb was the first to term Godwin's dilemma the "famous fire cause," and it stuck. Godwin made changes in later editions, for instance, substituting the mother with the father. For a detailed analysis of this dilemma its different versions, see Robert Lamb, "The Foundations of Godwinian Impartiality," *Utilitas* 18, no. 2 (2006): 134–153.

69. Godwin, *Political Justice*, 1:128.

70. Proby, *Modern Philosophy and Barbarism*, 39.

71. Ibid., 16.

72. Lucas, *Infernal Quixote*, 178, 181.

73. Thomas Green, *An Examination of the Leading Principle of the New System of Morals, as That Principle Is Stated and Applied in Mr. Godwin's Enquiry Concerning Political Justice* (London: T.N. Longman, 1798), 46–47. Godwin is fictionalized as a whole range of unfeeling zealots: for instance, as "Myope" in Elizabeth Hamilton's *Memoirs of Modern Philosophers* (1800), a character whose "enthusiasm" is "the produce of an inflammable imagination . . . blinded by the glare of its own bewildering light." Elizabeth Hamilton, *Memoirs of Modern Philosophers* (1800), ed. Claire Grogan (Peterborough, ON: Broadview, 2000), 145.

74. See section on Amazonian republican women in chapter 2. See also D'Israeli, *Flim Flams!*, 1:b1, b5.

75. Ibid., 1:b6, 3:165.

76. Ibid., 3:152.

77. Ibid., 3:172.

78. Ibid., 3:173–174.

79. Marquis de Sade, *La nouvelle Justine* (1797), qtd. in Simone de Beauvoir, "Must We Burn Sade?" trans. Annette Michelson, in Marquis de Sade, *"The 120 Days of Sodom" and Other Writings*, trans. Austryn Wainhouse and Richard Seaver (New York: Grove Press, 1966), 39.

80. Marquis de Sade, *Justine* (1791), in *"Justine," "Philosophy in the Bedroom" and Other Writings*, trans. Austryn Wainhouse and Richard Seaver (New York: Grove Press, 1990), 551. For an insightful discussion of this, see Wennerstrom, "Cosmopolitan Bodies," 201–203.

81. Sade, *Justine*, 552.

82. Qtd. in Iwan Bloch, *Marquis de Sade: His Life and Works* (Amsterdam: Fredonia, 2002), 86; for more on the Rose Keller affair, see 156–162.

83. Qtd. in ibid., 159.

84. Madame du Deffand to Horace Walpole 1768, in David Coward's introduction to Marquis de Sade, *"The Misfortunes of Virtue" and Other Early Tales* (Oxford: Oxford University Press, 1999), xix.

85. Beauvoir, "Must We Burn Sade?," 58.

86. Wollstonecraft, *Vindication*, 279.
87. Ibid., 2, 5, 135.
88. Mary Wollstonecraft, *Maria; or, The Wrongs of Woman*, in *Posthumous Works of the Author of "A Vindication of the Rights of Woman,"* ed. William Godwin (London: J. Johnson, 1798), 2:136.
89. Qtd. in Ashley Tauchert, *Mary Wollstonecraft and the Accent of the Feminine* (Houndmills, UK: Palgrave, 2002), 57.
90. Ibid., 57.
91. Qtd. in ibid., 53.
92. Qtd. in ibid., 53.
93. Ibid., 13.
94. Richard Polwhele, *The Unsex'd Females: A Poem, Addressed to the Author of "The Pursuits of Literature"* (1798) (New York: William Cobbett, 1800), 39.
95. This "moral," Thompson notes, "has been repeated ever since." E. P. Thompson, *The Romantics: England in a Revolutionary Age* (Woodbridge, Suffolk, UK: Merlin, 1997), 72. Similarly, Vivien Jones observes that "this particularly gendered death seems to defy so cruelly some of the most fundamental tenets of Wollstonecraft's own feminism." Vivien Jones, "The Death of Mary Wollstonecraft," *British Journal for Eighteenth-Century Studies* 20, no. 2 (1997): 187.
96. C. G. Salzmann, *Elements of Morality, for the Use of Children*, trans. Mary Wollstonecraft (London: J. Johnson, 1790), 1:i, ii, iv.
97. Ibid., 1:xii–xiii.
98. Ibid., xviii (emphasis added).
99. *British Critic* 12 (1798): 228–233 (emphasis added). This critic mistakenly attributes the authorship of the work to Wollstonecraft. Compare this with the Platonist Thomas Taylor's comments in his *Vindication of the Rights of Brutes* (London: Edward Jeffery, 1792). He criticizes Wollstonecraft for using a bold tone to disguise unsophisticated and outlandish arguments and mocks her for wanting to remove the social, political, and even the biological boundaries that separated male and female, adult and child. Referring to the Salzmann text, Taylor declares that even a simpleton would have thought to inform children "how the genital parts . . . are to be employed in a natural way." Yet the woman-philosopher had presented this solution as an "original" new idea, disguised with bold, inflated rhetoric. Wollstonecraft's proposition was, Taylor mocked, "a most striking proof of . . . the truth of her grand theory, *the equality of the female nature with the male*" (82).
100. Wollstonecraft, *Vindication*, 278.
101. Polwhele, *Unsex'd*, 15.
102. Ibid., 26.
103. Laqueur, *Solitary Sex*, 204.
104. Foucault, *History of Sexuality*, 1:104. For more on masturbation and the tarring of Marie Antoinette, see the previous chapter.

105. G. J. Barker-Benfield, *Culture of Sensibility: Sex and Society in Eighteenth-Century Britain* (Chicago: Chicago University Press, 1996).

106. Ann Jessie Van Sant, *Eighteenth-Century Sensibility and the Novel: The Senses in Social Context* (Cambridge: Cambridge University Press, 1993), 15.

107. Polwhele, *Unsex'd*, 26–27.

108. Samantha George, *Botany, Sexuality and Women's Writing, 1760–1830: From Modest Shoot to Forward Plant* (Manchester, UK: Manchester University Press, 2007).

109. Darwin's *The Botanic Garden* (London: Joseph Johnson, 1791) is a set of two long poems, *The Loves of the Plants* and *The Economy of Vegetation*. The more titillating *Loves of the Plants* was published anonymously by Joseph Johnson in 1789.

110. Wollstonecraft, *Vindication*, 278.

111. Godwin, *Memoirs*, 111–112.

112. Ibid., 112.

113. Ibid., 31.

114. Barker-Benfield, *Culture*, 35–36.

115. Ibid.

116. George Cheyne, *The English Malady; or, A Treatise of Nervous Diseases of all Kinds, as Spleen, Vapours, Lowness of Spirits, Hypochondriacal, and Hysterical Distempers*, (London: G. Strahan in Cornhill, 1733), 52.

117. William Cullen, *First Lines of the Practice of Physic*, 3rd ed. (Edinburgh: William Creech, 1783), 3:1–3.

118. Neil Vickers disagrees with Alan Richardson's reading of Romantic medicine and literature as distinctly materialist and thus hostile to "mind-brain dualism." Rather Vickers argues that "most doctors of the 1790s accepted that the brain was the seat of the mind, though expressed in the form of physical events in the brain (and some thought, in other parts of the body as well), were distinct from, and often more powerful than, the mechanical actions of the organic body." Neil Vickers, *Coleridge and the Doctors* (Oxford: Oxford University Press, 2004), 6–7. See also A. Richardson, *British Romanticism*.

119. Cullen, *First Lines*, 3:384.

120. A. F. M. Willich, *Lectures on Diet and Regimen*, 2nd ed. London: Longman & Rees, 1799), 540.

121. Ibid., 547.

122. Ibid., 554.

123. Ibid., 554–555.

124. Bernard Mandeville, *A Treatise of the Hypochondriack and Hysterick Diseases* (1730; Delmar, NY: Scholars' Facsimiles and Reprints, 1976), 269–270.

125. G. Rousseau, *Nervous Acts*, 54.

126. Janet Todd, *Mary Wollstonecraft: A Revolutionary Life* (London: Weidenfeld and Nicholson, 2000), 357.

127. See, for instance, the *British Critic* 9 (March 1797).
128. A Friend to Social Order, *Thoughts on Marriage*, vi.
129. *British Critic* 12 (1798): 228–233, in K. W. Graham, *Godwin Reviewed*, 143.
130. *Anti-Jacobin Review* 21 (August 1805): 337–358, qtd. in Godwin, *Fleetwood*, 530.
131. Ibid. The *European Magazine* also congratulated the two women who, "to the honour of the sex," showed that new philosophy could not "obliterate all sense of decorum." See *European Magazine* 33 (1798): 246–251, in K. W. Graham, *Godwin Reviewed*, 147.
132. *The Scientific Magazine and Free-Mason's Repository* 10 (1798): 403–404, in K. W. Graham, *Godwin Reviewed*, 155.
133. *European Magazine* 33 (1798): 246–251, in K. W. Graham, *Godwin Reviewed*, 146.
134. *Critical Review* (1798): 414–417, in K. W. Graham, *Godwin Reviewed*, 144.

CHAPTER 4

1. Pigott, *Jockey Club*, American reprint, lxviii.
2. Ibid., v.
3. Jonathan Mee, "Libertines and Radicals in the 1790s: The Strange Case of Charles Pigott I," in Cryle and O'Connell, *Libertine Enlightenment*, 186.
4. Qtd. in Jonathan Mee, "The Political Showman at Home: Reflections on Popular Radicalism and Print Culture in the 1790s," in *Radicalism and Revolution in Britain, 1775–1848: Essays in Honour of Malcom I. Thomis*, ed. Michael T. Davis (Houndmills, UK: Palgrave, 2000), 42.
5. Reeves Papers, 11 December 1792, British Library, London (hereafter BL), MS 16, 922, vol. 4, f. 97.
6. Reeves Papers, 12 November 1792, BL, MS 16, 919, vol. 1, f. 1.
7. Reeves Papers, [December] 1792, BL, MS 16, 923, f. 198.
8. Member of the Jockey Club, *An Answer to Three Scurrilous Pamphlets, Entitled "The Jockey Club,"* 2nd ed. (London: J. S. Jordan, [1792]), 12.
9. Ibid., 11–12.
10. Ibid., 14.
11. Ibid., 10.
12. Ibid., 10–11.
13. Laurence Sterne, *Tristram Shandy*, ed. Ian Campbell Ross (1760–67; reprint, Oxford: Oxford University Press, 1998), 127.
14. Roy Porter and George Rousseau, *Gout: The Patrician Malady* (New Haven, CT: Yale University Press, 1998), 1.
15. Thomas Paine, *Common Sense* (Philadelphia: W. and T. Bradford, 1776), 5.
16. *A Bird in the Hand Is Worth Two in the Bush; or, A Dialogue between*

John Frankly and George Careful ([London], 1792), in Claeys, *Political Writings of the 1790s*, 7:287–288.

17. George Chalmers [Francis Oldys], *The Life of Thomas Pain, the Author of the "Rights of Man": With a Defence of His Writings* (1791), 5th ed. (reprint, London: Stockdale, 1793). George Chalmers, alias "Francis Oldys," was a government propagandist who, although he had never met Paine, claimed an intimate familiarity with his subject's private life. I am using the fifth edition here, with the added preface. In all of the many editions and printings of his "defence," Chalmers insisted on using the original spelling of "Pain" instead of what he called the "fictitious" appellation "Paine," for he believed the added "e" was an example of how the lowly revolutionary had inappropriately "exercised a freedom, which only great men enjoy for honourable ends" (2).

18. Mercure Daniel Conway, *Life of Thomas Paine*, 3rd ed. (New York: Putnam & Sons, 1893), 1:xxiii.

19. Sir Brooke Boothby, *Observations on the Appeal from the New to the Old Whigs, and on Mr. Paine's Rights of Man* (London: John Stockdale, 1792), 273.

20. *New Year's Gift for Mr. Thomas Paine, in Return for His "Rights of Man": Humbly Presented by the Citizens of Caledonia* (Edinburgh: N.p., 1792), 6.

21. Mary Douglas, *Purity and Danger: An Analysis of Concepts of Pollution and Taboo* (London: Routledge, 2002), 4.

22. Ibid.

23. John Wood, *A Full Exposition of the Clintonian Faction and the Society of the Columbian Illuminati with an Account of the Writer of the Narrative, and the Characters of His Certificate Men* (Newark: For the author, 1802), 11.

24. John Adams to Benjamin Waterhouse, 29 October 1805, qtd. in Craig Nelson, *Thomas Paine: Enlightenment, Revolution, and the Birth of Modern Nations* (New York: Viking, 2006), 89.

25. Isaac Hunt, *Rights of Englishmen: An Antidote to the Poison Now Vending by the Transatlantic Republican Thomas Paine* (London: J. Bew, 1791), 8.

26. James Cheetham, *The Life of Thomas Paine* (New York: Southwick & Pelsue, 1809), 267–268.

27. Dani Cavallaro and Alexandra Warwick, *Fashioning the Frame* (Oxford: Berg, 2001), xvii.

28. Shildrick, *Embodying the Monster*, 68.

29. Kathleen Brown, *Foul Bodies: Cleanliness in Early America* (New Haven, CT: Yale University Press, 2009), 117.

30. Cheetham, *Life of Thomas Paine*, 271.

31. Edward Mangin, *George the Third: A Novel* (London: James Carpenter, 1807), 2:95–96.

32. Cheetham, *Life of Thomas Paine*, 279.

33. Ibid., 250, 282.

34. Ibid., 287–288.

35. Ibid., 288.

36. Ibid.

37. J.-J. Rousseau, *Émile*, 26.
38. Virginia Smith, *Clean: A History of Personal Hygiene and Purity* (Oxford: Oxford University Press, 2007), 247.
39. John Armstrong, *The Art of Preserving Health: A Poem* (London: A. Millar, 1744), 5–6.
40. John Alderson, *Essay on the Nature and Origin of the Contagion of Fevers* (Hull, UK: G. Prince, 1788), 1.
41. Ibid., 34.
42. Ibid., 35.
43. Armstrong, *Art of Preserving Health*, 5.
44. Raymond Williams, *The Country and the City* (London: Chatto & Windus, 1973), 43.
45. Charles Rosenberg, *Explaining Epidemics and Other Studies in the History of Medicine* (Cambridge: Cambridge University Press, 1992), 293–304.
46. Ibid., 295.
47. Alderson, *Contagion of Fevers*, 18.
48. Willich, *Diet and Regimen*, 220–221 (emphasis added).
49. Bernhard Christoph Faust, *Catechism of Health: For the Use of Schools, and for Domestic Instruction*, trans. J. H. Basse (London: C. Dilly, 1794), 52.
50. Porter and Rousseau, *Gout*, 1.
51. William Clayton, *Lecture on Dirt Delivered to the Harrow Young Men's Society* (London: Wertheim and Macintosh, 1852), 4.
52. Ibid., 22
53. Ibid., 6.
54. Ibid., 4.
55. Willich, *Diet and Regimen*, 236.
56. Ibid., 235.
57. Alderson, *Contagion of Fevers*, 36.
58. See Barrell, *Spirit of Despotism*, 63–70.
59. Clayton *Lecture on Dirt*, 2.
60. I. Hunt, *Rights of Englishmen*, 8.
61. Eve Kosofsky Sedgwick, "The Character in the Veil: Imagery of the Surface in the Gothic Novel," *PMLA* 96, no. 2 (1981): 255.
62. Ibid., 255.
63. Erving Goffman, *Stigma: Notes on the Management of Spoiled Identity* (London: Penguin, 1990); Gerhard Falk, *Stigma: How We Treat Outsiders* (Amherst, MA: Prometheus Books, 2001).
64. Goffman, *Stigma*, 15
65. Grant Thorburn, *The Life and Writings of Grant Thorburn* (New York: Edward Walker, 1852), 102.
66. Charles Harrington Elliot, *The Republican Refuted; in a Series of Biographical, Critical and Political Strictures on Thomas Paine's "Rights of Man"* (London: W. Richardson, 1791), 37.
67. Daniel 4:33.
68. Carver, qtd. in Cheetham, *Life of Thomas Paine*, 30, and in John S.

Harford, *The Account of the Life, Death, and Principles of Thomas Paine*, (Bristol: J. M. Gutch, 1819), 52. Both biographers transcribed these personal details from William Carver's letter to Paine (a letter he apparently never sent).

69. Willich, *Lectures on Diet*, 223.

70. Chalmers, *Life of Thomas Pain*, 7.

71. Martin Lluelyn, *An Elegie on the Death of the Most Illustrious Prince, Henry Duke of Gloucester*, 2nd ed. (Oxford: H. Hall, 1660), 5; Henry Jones, *Innoculation; or, Beauty's Triumph, a Poem in Two Cantos* (Bath, UK: C. Pope, 1768), 7.

72. Henry Bold, *Poems, Lyrique, Macaronique, Heroique* (London: Henry Brome, 1664), qtd. in David Shuttleton, *Small Pox and the Literary Imagination, 1660–1820* (Cambridge: Cambridge University Press, 2007), 40.

73. Shuttleton, *Small Pox*, 81.

74. Ibid., 75.

75. Chalmers, *Life of Thomas Pain*, 67.

76. Ibid.

77. Julia Kristeva, *Powers of Horror: An Essay in Abjection*, trans. Leon S. Roudiez (New York: Columbia University Press, 1982), 73.

78. Faust, *Catechism*, 76.

79. Ibid., 78.

80. Ibid., 76–77.

81. See for instance Harford, *Life, Death, and Principles*, 21. The story is that the feverishly ill Paine's cell door was left open to allow for a breeze; as a result, the executioner's mark was made on the inside rather than the exterior of the door, so that when it was then closed, the executioners missed seeing the mark.

82. Cheetham, *Life of Thomas Paine*, 188.

83. Ibid., 99.

84. Harford, *Life, Death, and Principles*, 4–5.

85. Cheetham, *Life of Thomas Paine*, 274.

86. Harford, *Life, Death, and Principles*, 142.

87. Chalmers, *Life of Thomas Pain*, 7.

88. Ibid., 12–13.

89. Ibid., 17.

90. Ibid., 19.

91. Ibid.

92. Ibid., 30. See also Durey, *Transatlantic Radicals*, 32–33, 36, 152, 271–273.

93. Cheetham, *Life of Thomas Paine*, 33.

94. See Foucault, *History of Sexuality*, vol. 1.

95. Chalmers, *Life of Thomas Pain*, 23.

96. Elliot, *Republican Refuted*, 3 (first emphasis added). The loyalist writer Hannah More masterfully appropriated and redefined radical key words. For instance, in her popular tract *Village Politics*, 2nd ed. (London: F. & C. Rivington, 1792), the character Jack Anvil asks his *Rights of Man*–reading

friend Tom Hood why he looks so miserable. To Tom's reply that he wants a new constitution, Jack scoffs: "Indeed, I thought thou hadst been a desperate healthy fellow. Send for the doctor then" (4).

97. *Life and Character of Mr. Thomas Paine, Put in Metre, and Inscribed to the Society against Levellers and Republicans* ([London: N.p., 1793?]), one broadside sheet.

98. Elliot, *Republican Refuted*, 4–5.

99. Ibid., 5.

100. Lawrence Stone, *The Family, Sex and Marriage in England, 1500–1800* (London: Weidenfeld & Nicholson, 1977), 219; Ruth Perry, *Novel Relations: The Transformation of Kinship in English Literature and Culture, 1748–1818* (Cambridge: Cambridge University Press, 2004), 197.

101. See, for instance, Wagner, "Press Scandal," 1–14.; Wagner, "Domestic Invasions" ; Cohen, *Fashioning Masculinity*; and Leonore Davidoff and Catharine Hall, *Family Fortunes: Men and Women of the English Middle Class, 1780–1850*, 2nd ed. (London: Routledge, 2002).

102. Elliot, *Republican Refuted*, 6.

103. Cobbett, *Bloody Buoy*, 145.

104. Ibid., 144.

105. Cheetham, *Life of Thomas Paine*, 267.

106. Dr. Manley, qtd. in ibid., 302–303.

107. Ibid., 279.

108. Bevir, "Rethinking Governmentality," 423. Foucault describes these ideas in "The Subject and Power," trans. Leslie Sawyer, *Critical Inquiry* 8, no. 4 (Summer 1982): 777–795. Sawyer's translation does not include the direct quote "the conduct of conduct," but it is there in the original French article, where Foucault writes, "L'exercice du pouvoir consiste à 'conduire des conduites' et à aménager la probabilité. Le pouvoir, au fond, est moins de l'ordre de l'affrontement entre deux adversaires, ou de l'engagement de l'un à l'égard de l'autre, que de l'ordre du 'gouvernement.'" Michel Foucault, "Why Study Power: The Question of the Subject," in *Dits et écrits IV* (Paris: Gallimard, 1994), 237.

109. Norbert Elias, *The Civilizing Process: Sociogenetic and Psychogenetic Investigations*, trans. Edmund Jephcott, revised ed., ed. Eric Dunning et al. (Oxford: Blackwell, 2000), 365.

110. Ibid.

111. I. Hunt, *Rights of Englishmen*, 8.

112. William Cobbett, *The Life of Thomas Paine* (London: J. Wright, 1797), 22. There were several versions of these pamphlets, reprinted from an original review Cobbett wrote for *The Political Censor; or, Review of the Most Interesting Occurrences* (Philadelphia), September 1796, 1–49.

113. Conway, *Life of Thomas Paine*, xvi.

114. Interestingly, Roosevelt partially retracted this statement in a letter, claiming that his comments were based on observations made by Governor Morris, who was minister in France during the Terror. Morris had visited

Paine, whom he found "in bed, where he had stayed for some days without getting out, to perform the offices of nature." "If this is not 'filthy,'" Roosevelt writes, "I don't know what is," in a letter in private holding, sold at auction, Swann Auction Galleries, New York. See Paul Fraser Collectibles, www.paulfrasercollectibles.com/section.asp?catid=73&docid=2879.

115. Howard Fast, *Citizen Tom Paine* (New York: Grove Press, 1943), 79.

116. Ibid., 239.

117. These descriptions of Paine appear in all of the following: Philip S. Foner, introduction to *Thomas Paine: The Age of Reason* (New York: Citadel Press, 1974), 40, xliii; Gregory Claeys, *Thomas Paine: Social and Political Thought* (Boston: Unwin Hyman, 1989), 192; and Michael Foot and Thomas Kramnick, *The Thomas Paine Reader* (Harmondsworth, UK: Penguin, 2004), 17.

CHAPTER 5

1. Porter and Rousseau, *Gout,* 55. The sections about gout in this chapter owe much to this thorough and intelligent study of gout and the cultural issues surrounding the disease. Of particular importance are the conclusions Porter and Rousseau draw about the political aspects of the debate on the causes of gout.

2. Thomas Sydenham, *The Whole Works of that Excellent Practical Physician, Dr. Thomas Sydenham,* trans. John Pechey, 6th ed. (London: R. Wellington, 1715), 342.

3. Dorothy George has the artist as John Cawse, but Andrew Norton has suggested that Cawse was not known to have produced prints after 1801 and that this image is in the style of William Heath around this time (see the British Museum online commentary for this image, www.britishmuseum.org/research/search_the_collection_database/search_object_details.aspx?objectid=1480828&partid=1&searchText=Louis+XVIII+heath&fromADBC=ad&toADBC=ad&numpages=10&images=on&orig=%2fresearch%2fsearch_the_collection_database.aspx&currentPage=1.

4. Porter and Rousseau, *Gout,* 87.

5. Alan Bewell, *Romanticism and Colonial Disease* (Baltimore: Johns Hopkins University Press, 1999), 133.

6. To Dorothea Gibbon, letter 288, 7 January 1775, qtd. in Porter and Rousseau, *Gout,* 89.

7. To Dorothea Gibbon, letter 568, 29 March 1783, qtd. in Porter and Rousseau, *Gout,* 90.

8. Richard Kentish, *Advice to Gouty Persons* (1789), 2nd ed. (London: J. Murray & J. Johnson et al., 1791), 17.

9. William Cadogan, *A Dissertation on the Gout, and All Chronic Diseases, Jointly Considered as Proceeding from the Same Causes; What Those Causes Are; and a Rational and Natural Method of Cure Proposed,* 5th ed. (London: J. Dodsley, 1771), 97.

10. William Stevenson, *A Successful Method of Treating the Gout by Blistering* (Bath, UK: R. Cruttwell, 1779), 58–59.

11. Stevenson's biblical references recall Paine's biblical analogies to British hereditary traditions in *Common Sense,* published three years earlier, in 1776. Paine refers to the biblical story of the military general Gideon, who was offered a kingship for his military prowess. In the wake of his victory on the battlefield, the Jewish people expressed their gratitude, "saying, Rule thou over us, thou and thy son and thy son's son." But Paine claims that the wise Gideon refused the offer of a hereditary kingdom because he had come to recognize that monarchy was "a degradation" and that hereditary succession, which bestowed perpetual preference on one family, was "an insult." See Paine, *Common Sense,* 20, 23. For more on developing attitudes, see Jay Fliegelman, *Prodigals and Pilgrims: The American Revolution Against Patriarchal Authority, 1750–1800* (Cambridge: Cambridge University Press, 1985), 1.

12. Thomas Paine, *Rights of Man* (London: J. S. Jordan, 1791).

13. Porter and Rousseau, *Gout,* 124.

14. Thomas Beddoes, *Hygeia: Essays Moral and Medical* (1802; reprint, London: Thoemmes Continuum, 2004), 2:138.

15. Ibid., 2:98.

16. Ibid.

17. George Cheyne, *An Essay on the True Nature and Due Method of Treating the Gout,* 4th ed. (London: G. Strahan, 1722), 132.

18. William Buchan, *Domestic Medicine,* 2nd ed. (London: Strahan & Cadell, 1772), 103.

19. Robert Campbell, *The London Tradesman* (London: T. Gardner, 1747), 38.

20. One of the Faculty, *The Restorer of Health and Physician of Nature* (London: E. Hodson, 1792), 21.

21. Thomas Jeans, *A Treatise on the Gout* (Southampton, UK: T. Baker, 1792).

22. Stevenson, *Successful Method,* xviii.

23. See also Gillray's *Toasting Muffins, vide Royal Breakfast* (1791) and its companion piece, *Frying Sprats, vide, Royal Supper* (1791), in the British Museum's online collection, www.britishmuseum.org.

24. Marilyn Morris, *British Monarchy and the French Revolution* (New Haven, CT: Yale University Press, 1998), 175. Although it might have been an exaggeration to call George III's rise in popularity in the 1780s and 1790s as an apotheosis, Morris rightly points out that he was often preferred to Prime Minister William Pitt, who was "accused after 1788 of usurping the crown" (161; see also 163).

25. Richard Godfrey, *James Gillray: The Art of Caricature* (London: Tate, 2001), 174. Godfrey's comment refers to Gillray's *Affability* (1795), where George III appears as the homespun Farmer George, a fine example of the teasing attitude often adopted toward the king by satirists.

26. Charles Pigott, *A Political Dictionary, Explaining the True Meanings of*

Words, illustrated and exemplified in the lives, morals, character and conduct of the following most illustrious persons, and among many others (London: D. I. Eaton, 1795), 83.

27. Christopher Hibbert, *George III: A Personal History* (London: Viking, 1998), 170.

28. Ibid., 171.

29. Unquestionably, this marriage emphasized the fundamental personal and political differences between father and son. Many supporters of George III argued that this marriage was an act of filial recalcitrance that both physically and emotionally wounded a loving father. One court observer recounted how George III "was so hurt" at "the bare suspicion . . . that his son should have acted contrary to the laws of succession," and it "so preyed upon his mind," that as "with other family disturbances, it produced a violent paroxysm of a disorder which was near proving fatal to his life." *The Deathbed Confessions of the Late Countess of Guernsey, to Lady Anne H*******, 16th ed. (Glasgow: J. Carmichael et al., 1821), 7.

30. John Horne Tooke, *A Letter to a Friend on the Reported Marriage of His Royal Highness the Prince of Wales* (London: J. Johnson, 1787), 22, 6.

31. Ibid., 19.

32. Ibid., 21–22.

33. Pigott, *Female Jockey Club*, 8.

34. Ibid., 2.

35. Ibid., 5.

36. Ibid., 3.

37. Ibid., 8.

38. Ibid., 7–8.

39. Ibid., 10.

40. Stevenson, *Successful Method*, 117.

41. William Augustus Miles, *A Letter to the Prince of Wales, on a Second Application to Parliament, to Discharge Debts Wantonly Contracted since May 1787*, 10th ed. (London: J. Owen, 1795), xxii, xv.

42. A 1713 newspaper advertisement provides a fascinating example of how, earlier in the century, disease fell under the banner of "broken constitutions." "The Practical Scheme" to cure "Secret Injuries" was targeted at those who suffered from "Broken Constitutions; By Fast Living; Former Ill Cures; Salivations, and Mercury." Qtd. in Porter and Rousseau, *Gout*, 129. Besides promising "A New System of the GOUT," this scheme contained "A Rational Account of the Cause, Nature, Seat and Cure of Gleets [gonorrhea] and Other Such WEAKNESSES, etc." that accompanied those who, among other things, had experienced "Over-Strainings" and "Self-Abuse." Part of the practical scheme also included a full explication of "the Horrid Nature, and Most Miserable Consequences of Self-Abuse in Particular, the Ruin and Bane of the More Flourishing part of Mankind, Punished in the Person of Onan" (129).

43. Denise Gigante, *Taste: A Literary History* (New Haven, CT: Yale University Press, 2005), 177–179.

44. Immanuel Kant, *Anthropology from a Pragmatic Point of View* (1798; reprint, Cambridge: Cambridge University Press, 2006), 139.
45. Ibid., 180.
46. Ibid., 181.
47. Peter Melville, "'A Friendship of Taste': The Aesthetics of Eating Well in Kant's *Anthropology from a Pragmatic Point of View*," in *Cultures of Taste/ Theories of Appetite: Eating Romanticism*, ed. Timothy Morton (Houndmills, UK: Palgrave, 2004), 205.
48. Kant, *Anthropology*, 139–140.
49. William Wadd, *Comments on Corpulency* (London: John Ebers, 1829), 53.
50. Kant, *Anthropology*, 133.
51. Melville, "'Friendship of Taste,'" 213.
52. Miles, *Letter to the Prince of Wales*, xv.
53. Kant, *Anthropology*, 148.
54. Ibid.
55. Ibid., 147.
56. Ibid.
57. Stephen Mennell, "Eating in the Public Sphere in the Nineteenth and Twentieth Centuries," in *Eating Out in Europe: Picnics, Gourmet Dining and Snacks Since the Late Eighteenth Century*, ed. Marc Jacobs and Peter Scholliers (Oxford: Berg, 2003), 247.
58. Denise Gigante, ed., *Gusto: Essential Writings in Nineteenth-Century Gastronomy* (New York: Routledge, 2005), xxx.
59. Jean-Anthelme Brillat-Savarin, *Physiologie du Goût: A Handbook of Gastronomy; New and Complete Translation* (1826; reprint, New York: J. W. Boulton, 1884), reprinted in Gigante, *Gusto*, 154.
60. Gigante, *Gusto*, xxxii.
61. Alexandre Balthazar Laurent Grimod de la Reynière, *The Gourmand's Almanac*, in Gigante, *Gusto*, 18.
62. Stephen Mennell, *All Manners of Food: Eating and Taste in Britain and France from the Middle Ages to the Present* (Chicago: Illini Books, 1996), 32.
63. Ibid., 33.
64. Ibid., 34.
65. Dick Humelbergius Secundus [Gabriel Hummelberger], *Apacian Morsels; or, Tales of the Table, Kitchen, and Larder, with Reflections on the Dietic Productions of Early Writers* (1829), 2nd ed. (London: Whittaker, Treacer & Co., 1834), 58–59.
66. Gigante, *Gusto*, xix.
67. Ange Denis Macquin, *Tabella Cibaria: The Bill of Fare* (London: Sherwood, Neeley and Jones, 1820), 15.
68. Brillat-Savarin, *Brillat-Savarin's "Physiologie du Goût,"* in Gigante, *Gusto*, 161, 145.
69. Lancelot Sturgeon, *Essays, Moral, Philosophical, and Stomachical,*

on the Important Science of Good-Living (1822), 2nd ed. (London: G. & W. B. Whittaker, 1823), 3–4.

70. William Kitchiner, *The Cook's Oracle: Containing Receipts for Plain Cookery* (1822; reprint, Boston: Munroe & Francis, 1831), 11. Kitchiner's book was first published in 1817 in London as *Apicius Redevivus; or, The Cook's Oracle: Actual Experiments Instituted in the Kitchen of a Physician*.

71. Ibid., 12.
72. Ibid., 14.
73. C. J. Lawrence, "William Buchan: Medicine Laid Open," *Medical History* 19, no. 1 (January 1975): 25.
74. Buchan, *Domestic Medicine*, xix.
75. Cheyne, *English Malady*, 56.
76. Foucault, *History of Sexuality*, 2:100.
77. Ibid., 101.
78. William Nisbet, *A Practical Treatise on Diet* (London: R. Phillips, 1801), 3, 2.
79. Ibid., 14.
80. Ibid., 3.
81. Hunter, *The Works of John Hunter*, ed. James F. Palmer (London: Longman et. al., 1835) 1:247–248.
82. Ibid., 1:247.
83. William Kitchiner, *The Art of Invigorating and Prolonging Life, by Food, Clothes, Air, Exercise, Wine, Sleep, &c. and Peptic Precepts, pointing out Agreeable and Effectual Methods to Prevent and Relieve Indigestion . . . to which is added the Pleasure of Making a Will* (London: Hurst, Robinson & Co., 1822), 167.
84. Kitchiner, *Cook's Oracle*, 265.
85. Ibid., 263.
86. Ibid., 166.
87. Ibid.
88. Secundus [Hummelberger], *Apacian Morsels*, 88.
89. Ibid., 177.

CHAPTER 6

1. Edmund Burke, *Thoughts on the Cause of the Present Discontents* (London: J. Dodsley, 1770), 29.
2. Helen S. Conant, "Kitchen and Dining Room," *Harper's New Monthly Magazine* 54 (1876–77): 425, in Gigante, *Gusto*, xlii–xliii.
3. Onno Oerlemans, *Romanticism and the Materiality of Nature* (Toronto: Toronto University Press, 2004), 102; Beatrice Fink, "You Are Not Necessarily What You Eat," in *The Eighteenth-Century Body: Art, History, Literature, Medicine*, ed. Angelica Goodden (Bern: Peter Lang, 2002), 108.
4. See Fink, "You Are Not Necessarily What You Eat," 108. And for a slightly different translation, see Brillat-Savarin, *Brillat-Savarin's "Physiologie du Goût,"* in Gigante, *Gusto*, 144.

5. George Cheyne, *The Natural Method of Cureing Diseases of the Body, and the Disorders of the Mind Depending on the Body* (London: George Strahan, 1742), 82.

6. Ibid., 85.

7. Bewell, *Romanticism and Colonial Disease*, 136–139.

8. Qtd. in ibid., 135.

9. Robert Huish, *Memoirs of George IV: Descriptions of His Private and Public Life* (London: Kelley, 1830), 83.

10. Junius, *Last Letter of Junius, Addressed to the Prince Regent* (Sheffield, UK: J. T. Saxton, 1812), 32.

11. Ibid., 32.

12. Huish, *Memoirs of George IV*, 507.

13. Princess Lieven to Metternich, 27 October 1820, qtd. in Christopher Hibbert, *George IV* (London: Penguin, 1988), 521.

14. The Comtesse de Boigne was referring to a slightly earlier incarnation of the Pavilion in 1817, in her *Memoirs of the Comtesse de Boigne*, ed. Charles Nicollaud (London: Heinemann, 1907), 2:248.

15. *Brighton Herald*, 27 January 1821, qtd. in John Evans, *An Excursion to Brighton, with an Account of the Royal Pavilion* (Chiswick, UK: C. Whittingham, 1821), 41.

16. Lady Bessborough to Granville Leveson Gower on her visit to the Pavilion in 1805, in Lord Granville Leveson Gower, *Lord Granville Leveson Gower . . . Private Correspondence, 1781–1821*, ed. Castalia Countess Grenville (London: Murray, 1916), 2:120.

17. See Mary Douglas, *Purity and Danger: An Analysis of Concepts of Pollution and Taboo* (London: Routledge, 2002); Claude Lévi-Strauss, *The Raw and the Cooked* (1964), trans. John and Doreen Weightman (London: Penguin, 1986); Roland Barthes, *Mythologies* (1972), trans. Annette Lavers (London: Vintage, 2000); Pierre Bourdieu, *Distinction: A Social Critique of the Judgement of Taste* (1984) (Abingdon, UK: Routledge, 2010); John Ruskin, "The Nature of Gothic," in *The Stones of Venice*, vol. 2 (New York: John Wiley, 1860); A. W. N. Pugin, *Contrasts*, 2nd ed. (London: Charles Dolman, 1841); and Henri Lefebvre, *The Production of Space*, trans. Donald Nicholson-Smith (Oxford: Blackwell, 1991).

18. William Hone, *The Joss and His Folly* (London: William Hone, 1820), 2, 1. As is typical, the registers of foreignness were mixed: for other observers, George ruled over a Taj Mahal–inspired British seraglio. See Huish, *Memoirs or George IV*, 525.

19. Qtd. in Sander L. Gilman, *Fat Boys* (Lincoln: University of Nebraska Press, 2004), 160.

20. For more on the Hottentot Venus, see Yvette Abrahams, "Images of Sara Bartman: Sexuality, Race and Gender in Early Nineteenth Century Britain," in *Nation, Empire, and Colony: Historicizing Race and Gender*, ed. Ruth Roach Pierson and Nupur Chaudhuri (Indianapolis: Indiana University Press, 1998), 220–236; Anne Fausto-Sterling, "Gender, Race and Nation:

The Comparative Anatomy of 'Hottentot' Women in Europe, 1815–1817," in *Feminism and the Body*, ed. Londa Schiebinger (Oxford: Oxford University Press, 2000), 203–233; Zine Magubane, "Which Bodies Matter? Feminism, Postructuralism, Race, and the Curious Theoretical Odyssey of the 'Hottentot Venus,'" *Gender and Society* 15, no. 6 (2001): 816–834; Sander S. Gilman, "Black Bodies, White Bodies: Toward an Iconography of Female Sexuality in Late Nineteenth Century Art, Medicine, and Literature," *Critical Inquiry* 12 (Autumn 1985): 204–242; and Schiebinger, *Nature's Body*, 160–172.

21. See Schiebinger, *Nature's Body*, 164.
22. Ibid., 168.
23. Fausto-Sterling, "Gender, Race and Nation," 203–233.
24. Cadogan, *Dissertation on the Gout*, 55.
25. Ibid., 64 (emphasis added).
26. William Blake, *Visions of the Daughters of Albion* (1792), in *The Complete Poetry and Prose of William Blake*, ed. David V. Erdman (New York: Doubleday, 1988), 46, lines 20–22.
27. Cadogan, *Dissertation on the Gout*, 64.
28. Susan Sontag, *Illness as Metaphor and AIDS and Its Metaphors* (London: Penguin, 2002), 134.
29. Bewell, *Romanticism and Colonial Disease*, 29.
30. Ibid., 17.
31. Ibid., 30.
32. Pamela K. Gilbert, "Mapping Colonial Disease: Victorian Medical Cartography in British India," in *Framing and Imagining Disease in Cultural History*, ed. George Rousseau et al. (Houndmills, UK: Palgrave, 2003), 111.
33. Robert Southey, *Sir Thomas More; or, Colloquies on the Progress and Prospects of Society* (London: John Murray, 1824), 1:57–58.
34. Ibid., 1:57.
35. Ibid., 1:58.
36. Percy Bysshe Shelley, *Oedipus Tyrannus; or, Swellfoot the Tyrant* (London: J. Johnston, 1820), Act 1, Scene 1, p. 7, lines 3–6.
37. Timothy Morton, "Porcine Poetics: Shelley's *Swellfoot the Tyrant*" in *The Unfamiliar Shelley*, ed. Timothy Webb and Alan Mendel Weinberg (Farnham, UK: Ashgate, 2009), 283.
38. Shelley, *Oedipus*, Act 1, Scene 1, p. 10, lines 47, 44.
39. Ibid., line 44.
40. Bewell, *Romanticism and Colonial Disease*, 207.
41. Percy Bysshe Shelley, *The Letters of Percy Bysshe Shelley*, ed. F. L. Jones (Oxford: Clarendon, 1964), 1:430. Also qtd. in Bewell, *Romanticism and Colonial Disease*, 207.
42. Jean Baudrillard, "The Obese," in *Fatal Strategies*, trans. Jim Fleming (London: Pluto Press, 1999), 30.
43. Edward Jukes, *On Indigestion and Costiveness: A Series of Hints to Both Sexes*, 2nd ed. (London: John Churchill, 1833) 293, qtd. in Gilman, *Fat Boys*, 64 (emphasis added).
44. Shelley, *Oedipus*, Act 1, Scene 1, lines 51, 49.

45. Ibid., line 50.
46. Samuel Gladden, "Shelley's Agenda Writ Large: Reconsidering *Oedipus Tyrannus; or, Swellfoot the Tyrant,*" *Romantic Circles Praxis Series*, paragraph 3, www.rc.umd.edu/praxis/interventionist/gladden/gladden.html.
47. Roxann Wheeler, *The Complexion of Race: Categories of Difference in Eighteenth-Century British Culture* (Philadelphia: University of Pennsylvania Press, 2004); Peter J. Kitson, "Sustaining the Romantic and Racial Self: Eating People in the 'South Seas,'" in Morton, *Cultures of Taste*, 79.
48. Ronald Paulson, *Representations of Revolution, 1789–1820* (New Haven, CT: Yale University Press, 1983), 24.
49. Qtd. in ibid., 24.
50. Broca, *Interesting Anecdotes of the Heroic Conduct of Women, Previous To, and During the French Revolution* (Baltimore: Fryer & Clark, 1804), 136.
51. Ibid., 68.
52. Ibid.
53. Thomas Paine, *"Rights of Man," "Common Sense" and Other Political Writings*, ed. Mark Philp (Oxford: Oxford University Press, 1998), 133.
54. Burke, *Reflections on the Revolution in France*, 107.
55. Ibid., 210
56. "G.X." Reeves Papers, Bungary, Suffolk, 20 December 1792, BL, MS 16, 919, vol. 1, f. 193.
57. [Theodore Price], *Life and Adventures of Job Nott, Buckle Maker of Birmingham* (Birmingham: E. Piercy, 1793), 5, 6.
58. William Cobbett, *A Bone to Gnaw for the Democrats; or, Observations on a Pamphlet Entitled "The Political Progress of Britain"* (1795), in *William Cobbett: Selected Writings*, ed. Leonora Nattrass (London: Pickering & Chatto, 1998), 1:136.
59. Cobbett, *Bloody Buoy*, 36.
60. Hardy, *Patriot*, 45.
61. Burke, *First Letter on a Regicide Peace*, 308.
62. Kristen Guest, introduction to *Eating their Words: Cannibalism and the Boundaries of Cultural Identity* (Albany: State University of New York Press, 2001), 2.
63. Shelley, *Oedipus*, 39, Act 2, Scene 2, p. 39, lines 31–32.
64. Ibid., line 23.
65. Percy Bysshe Shelley, *A Vindication of Natural Diet* (1813; reprint, London: F. Pitman, 1884), 20–21.
66. Bewell, *Romanticism and Colonial Disease*, 208.
67. Robert Southey, "Poems Concerning the Slave Trade: Sonnet III," in *Poetical Works of Robert Southey* (New York: D. Appleton, 1839), 110.
68. William Fox, *An Address to the People of Great Britain, on the Propriety of Abstaining from West Indian Sugar and Rum*, 25th ed. (London: M. Gurney, 1792), 2.
69. Ann Mellor, "Sex, Violence, and Slavery: Blake and Wollstonecraft," *Huntington Library Quarterly* 58, nos. 3–4 (1995): 347.

70. Thomas Love Peacock, *Melincourt* (London: T. Hookham, 1817), 2:189–190.
71. Ibid., 190.
72. Gigante, *Taste*, 174.
73. Morton, *Shelley and the Revolution in Taste*, 52. Morton refers to Orrin Wang's "Romantic Sobriety," *Modern Language Quarterly* 60, no. 4 (1999): 469–493.
74. Joseph Ritson, *An Essay on Abstinence from Animal Food, as a Moral Duty* (London: Richard Phillips, 1802), flyleaf. This edition is held by the University of Glasgow.
75. Thomas John Graham, *Sure Methods of Improving Health . . . by Regulating the Diet and Regimen* (London: Simpkin & Marshall, 1827), 8.
76. Shelley, *Vindication*, 10.
77. Georges Cuvier's ideas about vegetarianism and the study of comparative anatomy were taken up by vegetarians throughout the nineteenth century. For just one example, see William A. Alcott, *Vegetable Diet: As Sanctioned by Medical Men, and by Experience in All Ages* (Boston: Marsh, Capen and Lyon, 1838), 88–90.
78. Timothy Morton, "Joseph Ritson, Percy Shelley and the Making of Romantic Vegetarianism," *Romanticism* 12, no. 1 (2006): 59.
79. Ibid.
80. Shelley, *Vindication*, 16.
81. Morton, "Joseph Ritson," 59.

CODA

1. Qtd. in Hibbert, *George IV*, 708.
2. Qtd. in E. A. Smith, *George IV* (New Haven, CT: Yale University Press, 1999): 270.
3. See Craig Calhoun, "The Public Sphere in the Field of Power Social Science," *History* 34, no. 3 (Fall 2010): 301–335; Craig Calhoun, ed., *Habermas and the Public Sphere* (Cambridge, MA: MIT Press, 1993); Jürgen Habermas, *The Structural Transformation of the Public Sphere: An Inquiry into a Category of Bourgeois Society* (Cambridge, MA: MIT Press, 1991); Barrell, *Spirit of Despotism*; and J. Brewer, "This, That and the Other," in Castiglione and Sharpe, *Shifting the Boundaries*, 1–21.
4. Linda Colley, *Britons: Forging the Nation, 1707–1837* (New Haven, CT: Yale University Press, 1992), 199. For more on the issue of proximity, see also Steve Poole, *The Politics of Regicide in England, 1760–1850: Troublesome Subjects* (Manchester: Manchester University Press, 2000).
5. The type of physical, proximate moral corrective, meted out in the newspapers in particular and directed at the very highest levels of society, demonstrates not only how far reaching and pervasive scandal had become but also how average people were recruited to act on their moral values. As just one example of hundreds, when the Prince of Wales was having an affair with the married Lady Jersey, the papers relentlessly pursued her and her

lover like modern-day paparazzi. On any given day, reportage like the following *Times* story would appear: On 6 June 1796, readers were told how the prince had slipped out of Carlton House incognito, so that his own servant had no idea where he was going. On the same evening, it was reported, "Lady Jersey left her house in Pall Mall, INCOG. She has retired, though NOT UNOBSERVED to the house of her daughter, Lady Ann Lambton, in Berkley-Square."

6. Qtd. in Hibbert, *George IV,* 759.

7. A. Aspinall, ed., *Correspondence of George IV* (London: Cassel, 1963), 2:285.

8. See Hibbert, *George IV,* 95–108.

9. Charles Lamb, "The Triumph of the Whale," in *The Works of Charles Lamb,* ed. Charles Noon Talfourd (New York: Harper & Brothers, 1838), 1:160.

10. Thomas King Chambers, *Corpulence; or, Excess of Fat in the Body* (London: Longman et al., 1850), 2, 5.

11. Ibid., 137.

12. Erin O'Connor, *Raw Material: Producing Pathology in Victorian Culture* (Durham, NC: Duke University Press, 2000), 14.

13. Ibid., 14.

14. Ibid.

15. K. Brown, *Foul Bodies,* 3.

Bibliography

NEWSPAPERS AND PERIODICALS

Anti-Jacobin, or Weekly Examiner
Anti-Jacobin Review
Bon Ton
British Critic
Courier
Critical Review
European Magazine
Le Moniteur Universal
Monthly Mirror
Morning Chronicle
Morning Post
Rambler's Magazine
The Scientific Magazine and Free-Mason's Repository
Tomahawk
True Briton
USA Today

MANUSCRIPTS

Reeves Papers. 2 November 1792. British Library, London (hereafter BL), MS 16, 919, vol. 1, f. 1.
———. [December] 1792. BL, MS 16, 923, vol. 5, f. 198.
———. 11 December 1792. BL, MS 16, 922, vol. 4, f. 97.
———. "G. X.," Bungary, Suffolk, 20 December 1792. BL, MS 16, 919, vol. 1, f. 193.
Thomas Carlyle to John Forster, 12 April 1839. *Collected Letters*, 11:72. doi:10.1215/lt-18390412-TC-JF-01.

PRIMARY SOURCES

Admirable Satire on the Death, Dissection, Funeral Procession, and Epitaph, of Mr. Pitt. London: C. Smith, 1795.
Adolphus, John. *Biographical Memoirs of the French Revolution.* 2 vols. London: T. Cadell, Jun. & W. Davies, 1799.
Aiken, John. *Principles of Midwifery; or, Puerperal Medicine.* 3rd ed. London: J. Murray, 1786.
Alcott, William A. *Vegetable Diet: As Sanctioned by Medical Men, and by Experience in All Ages.* Boston: Marsh, Capen and Lyon, 1838.
Alderson, John. *Essay on the Nature and Origin of the Contagion of Fevers.* Hull, UK: G. Prince, 1788.
Arbuthnot, John. *Law Is a Bottomless Pit; or, The History of John Bull.* 1712. Reprint, Glasgow: Robert Urie, 1766.
Armstrong, John. *The Art of Preserving Health: A Poem.* London: A. Millar, 1744.
Aspinall, A., ed. *Correspondence of George IV.* 8 vols. London: Cassel, 1963.
Astruc, John. *A Treatise on All the Diseases Incident to Women.* London: M. Cooper, 1743.
Authentic Trial at Large of Marie Antoinette, Late Queen of France, before the Revolutionary Tribunal at Paris. London: Chapman & Co., 1793.
Barbauld, Anna Letitia. *Civic Sermons, Number II.* London: J. Johnson, 1792.
Beddoes, Thomas. *Hygeia: Essays Moral and Medical.* 3 vols. 1802. Reprint, London: Thoemmes Continuum, 2004.
Bienville, M. D. T. de. *Nymphomania; or, A Dissertation Concerning the Furor Uterinus.* Trans. Edward Sloane Wilmot. London: J. Bew, 1775.
Biographical Anecdotes of the Founders of the French Republic. London: R. Phillips, 1797.
A Bird in the Hand Is Worth Two in the Bush; or, A Dialogue between John Frankly and George Careful. 1792. In *Political Writings of the 1790s,* ed. Gregory Claeys, 7:287–290. London: Pickering & Chatto, 1995.
Blake, William. *Visions of the Daughters of Albion* (1792). In *The Complete Poetry and Prose of William Blake,* ed. David V. Erdman, 45–50. New York: Doubleday, 1988.
Boerhaave, Herman. *Boerhaave's Academical Lectures on the Lues Venerea.* Trans. Jonathan Watham. London: J. Rivington, 1763.
Bold, Henry. *Poems, Lyrique, Macaronique, Heroique.* London: Henry Brome, 1664.
Boothby, Sir Brooke. *Observations on the Appeal from the New to the Old Whigs, and on Mr. Paine's "Rights of Man."* London: John Stockdale, 1792.
Brillat-Savarin, Jean-Anthelme. *Brillat-Savarin's "Physiologie du Goût": A Handbook of Gastronomy.* 1884. In *Gusto: Essential Writings in Nineteenth-Century Gastronomy,* ed. Denise Gigante, 141–174. New York: Routledge, 2005.
Broca, Louis Du. *Interesting Anecdotes of the Heroic Conduct of Women, previous to, and during the French Revolution.* Baltimore: Fryer & Clark, 1804.

Brown, John. *The Elements of Medicine.* 2 vols. London: J. Johnson, 1795.
Brown, Sir Thomas. *A Letter to a Friend.* London: Charles Brome, 1690.
Buchan, William. *Domestic Medicine.* 2nd ed. London: Strahan & Cadell, 1772.
Burke, Edmund. *First Letter on a Regicide Peace, from Two Letters . . . on the Proposals for Peace with the Regicide Directory of France.* 1796. In *The Impact of the French Revolution,* ed. Iain Hampsher-Monk, 302–315. Cambridge: Cambridge University Press, 2005.
———. *Reflections on the Revolution in France and on the Proceedings in Certain Societies in London Relative to that Event.* London: J. Dodsley, 1790.
———. *Thoughts on the Cause of the Present Discontents.* London: J. Dodsley, 1770.
Cadogan, William. *A Dissertation on the Gout, and All Chronic Diseases, Jointly Considered as Proceeding from the Same Causes; What Those Causes Are; and a Rational and Natural Method of Cure Proposed.* 5th ed. London: J. Dodsley, 1771.
———. *An Essay upon Nursing and the Management of Children.* 9th ed. London: R. Florsfield, 1772.
Campan, Madame. *Private Journal of Madame Campan, Comprising Original Anecdotes of the French Court.* Ed. M. Maigne. Philadelphia: A. Small, 1825.
Campbell, Robert. *The London Tradesman.* London: T. Gardner, 1747.
Carlyle, Thomas. *Sartor Resartus.* Boston: James Munroe, 1840.
———. "Signs of the Times." 1829. In *Thomas Carlyle: Selected Writings,* ed. Alan Shelston, 61–85. Harmondsworth, UK: Penguin, 1971.
Chalmers, George [Francis Oldys]. *The Life of Thomas Pain, the Author of the "Rights of Man": With a Defence of His Writings.* 1791. 5th ed. London: Stockdale, 1793.
Chambers, Thomas King. *Corpulence; or, Excess of Fat in the Body.* London: Longman et al., 1850.
Cheetham, James. *The Life of Thomas Paine.* New York: Southwick & Pelsue, 1809.
Cheyne, George. *The English Malady; or, A Treatise of Nervous Diseases of all Kinds, as Spleen, Vapours, Lowness of Spirits, Hypochondriacal, and Hysterical Distempers.* London: G. Strahan in Cornhill, 1733.
———. *An Essay of Health and Long Life.* London: G. Strahan and J. Leake, 1724.
———. *An Essay on the True Nature and Due Method of Treating the Gout.* 4th ed. London: G. Strahan, 1722.
———. *The Natural Method of Cureing Diseases of the Body, and the Disorders of the Mind Depending on the Body.* Part 1. London: George Strahan, 1742.
Christie, Thomas. *Letters on the Revolution of France.* 1791. In *Political Writings of the 1790s,* ed. Gregory Claeys, 2:154–269. London: Pickering & Chatto, 1995.
Clayton, William. *Lecture on Dirt Delivered to the Harrow Young Men's Society.* London: Wertheim and Macintosh, 1852.

Cobbett, William. *The Bloody Buoy, Thrown Out as a Warning to the Political Pilots of America; or, A Faithful Relation of a Multitude of Acts of Horrid Barbarity, such as the Eye Never Witnessed, the Tongue Never Expressed, or the Imagination Conceived, until the Commencement of the French Revolution.* 3rd ed. 1796. Reprint, Philadelphia: N.p., 1823.

———. *A Bone to Gnaw for the Democrats; or, Observations on a Pamphlet Entitled "The Political Progress of Britain."* 1795. In *William Cobbett: Selected Writings,* ed. Leonora Nattrass, 1:109–153. London: Pickering & Chatto, 1998.

———. *The Life of Thomas Paine.* London: J. Wright, 1797.

———. "The Republican Judge." In *Porcupine's Works,* 12:315–330. London: Cobbett, 1801.

The Comtesse de Boigne. *Memoirs of the Comtesse de Boigne.* Vol. 2 (1815–19). Ed. Charles Nicollaud. London: Heinemann, 1907.

Conway, Mercure Daniel. *Life of Thomas Paine.* 3rd ed. New York: Putnam & Sons, 1893.

Cook, John. *The New Theory of Generation, According to the Best and Latest Discoveries in Anatomy.* London: J. Buckland, 1762.

The Court Journal: Court Circular and Fashionable Gazette. Vol. 7. London: H. Colburn, 1835.

Crooke, Helkiah, *Microcosmographia: The Body of Man.* London: William Iaggard, 1615.

Cullen, William. *First Lines of the Practice of Physic.* 3 vols. 3rd ed. Edinburgh: William Creech, 1783.

The Deathbed Confessions of the Late Countess of Guernsey, to a Lady Anne H******. 16th ed. Glasgow: J. Carmichael et al., 1821.

D'Israeli, Isaac. *Flim Flams! Or the Life and Errors of My Uncle and the Amours of My Aunt.* 3 vols. London: John Murray, 1805.

Elliot, Charles Harrington. *The Republican Refuted; in a Series of Biographical, Critical and Political Strictures on Thomas Paine's "Rights of Man."* London: W. Richardson, 1791.

Evans, John. *An Excursion to Brighton, with an Account of the Royal Pavilion.* Chiswick, UK: C. Whittingham, 1821.

Falck, Nikolai Detlef. *A Treatise on the Venereal Disease.* London: For the author, 1772.

Faust, Bernhard Christoph. *Catechism of Health: For the Use of Schools, and for Domestic Instruction.* Trans. J. H. Basse. London: C. Dilly, 1794.

Fox, William. *An Address to the People of Great Britain, on the Propriety of Abstaining from West Indian Sugar and Rum.* 25th ed. London: M. Gurney, 1792.

A Friend to Social Order. *Thoughts on Marriage and Criminal Conversation, with some hints of appropriate means to check the progress of the latter; comprising remarks on the life, opinions, and example of the late Mrs. Wollstonecraft Godwin: Respectfully addressed and inscribed to the Right Hon-*

orable Lord Kenyon, Lord Chief Justice of the Court of King's Bench. London: F.C. Rivington et al., 1799.
Fureurs Uterines de Marie-Antoinette, Femme de Louis XVI. N.p., n.d.
Godwin, William. *Considerations on Lord Grenville's and Mr. Pitt's Bills.* London: J. Johnson, 1795.
——. *Enquiry Concerning Political Justice.* 1793. 2 vols. 3rd ed. London: G.G. and J. Robinson, 1798.
——. *Fleetwood: or, The New Man of Feeling.* 1805. Ed. Gary Handwerk and A.A. Markley. Peterborough, ON: Broadview, 2001.
——. *Memoirs of the Author of "A Vindication of the Rights of Woman."* London: J. Johnson and G.G. and J. Robinson, 1798.
——. *Memoirs of the Author of "A Vindication of the Rights of Woman."* 1798. Ed. Pamela Clemit and Gina Luria Walker. Peterborough, ON: Broadview, 2001.
Gower, Lord Granville Leveson. *Lord Granville Leveson Gower ... Private Correspondence, 1781–1821.* Ed. Castalia Countess Grenville. London: Murray, 1916.
Graham, Thomas John. *Sure Methods of Improving Health ... by Regulating the Diet and Regimen.* London: Simpkin & Marshall, 1827.
Green, Thomas. *An Examination of the Leading Principle of the New System of Morals, as That Principle Is Stated and Applied in Mr. Godwin's "Enquiry Concerning Political Justice."* London: T.N. Longman, 1798.
Grimod de la Reynière, Alexandre Balthazar Laurent. *The Gourmand's Almanac.* In *Gusto: Essential Writings in Nineteenth-Century Gastronomy*, ed. Denise Gigante, 1–55. New York: Routledge, 2005.
Hamilton, Elizabeth. *Memoirs of Modern Philosophers.* 1800. Ed. Claire Grogan. Peterborough, ON: Broadview, 2000.
Hamilton, William. *Letters on the Principles of the French Democracy and Their Application and Influence on the Constitution and Happiness of Britain and Ireland.* Dublin: G. Bonham, 1792.
Hardy, Thomas. *The Patriot, Addressed to the People, on the Present State of Affairs in Britain and in France.* 2nd ed. Edinburgh: J. Dickson, 1793.
Harford, John S. *The Account of the Life, Death, and Principles of Thomas Paine.* Bristol: J.M. Gutch, 1819.
Hays, Mary. *Memoirs of Emma Courtney.* London: G.G. & J Robinson, 1796.
Home, Everard. "An Account of the Dissection of an Hermaphrodite Dog: To Which Are Prefixed, Some Observations on Hermaphrodites in General." *Philosophical Transactions of the Royal Society of London* 89 (1799): 157–178.
Hone, William. *The Joss and His Folly.* London: William Hone, 1820.
Huish, Robert. *Memoirs of George IV: Descriptions of His Private and Public Life.* London: Kelley, 1830.
Hunt, Isaac. *Rights of Englishmen: An Antidote to the Poison Now Vending by the Transatlantic Republican Thomas Paine.* London: J. Bew, 1791.

Hunter, John. *The Works of John Hunter.* Ed. James F. Palmer. 4 vols. London: Longman et. al., 1835.
Hunter, William. *The Anatomy of the Human Gravid Uterus.* Birmingham: John Baskerville, 1774.
———. *Correspondence of William Hunter.* Ed. C. Helen Brock. 2 vols. London: Pickering & Chatto, 2008.
Jeans, Thomas. *A Treatise on the Gout.* Southampton, UK: T. Baker, 1792.
Jones, Henry. *Innoculation; or, Beauty's Triumph, a Poem in Two Cantos.* Bath, UK: C. Pope, 1768.
Junius. *Last Letter of Junius, Addressed to the Prince Regent.* Sheffield, UK: J. T. Saxton, 1812.
Kant, Immanuel. *Anthropology from a Pragmatic Point of View.* 1798. Reprint, Cambridge: Cambridge University Press, 2006.
———. *Critique of Judgment.* 1790. Oxford: Oxford University Press, 2008.
Kentish, Richard. *Advice to Gouty Persons.* 2nd ed. London: J. Murray & J. Johnson et al., 1791.
Kitchiner, William. *The Art of Invigorating and Prolonging Life, by Food, Clothes, Air, Exercise, Wine, Sleep, &c. and Peptic Precepts, pointing out Agreeable and Effectual Methods to Prevent and Relieve Indigestion . . . to which is added the Pleasure of Making a Will.* London: Hurst, Robinson & Co., 1822.
———. *The Cook's Oracle: Containing Receipts for Plain Cookery.* 1822. Reprint, Boston: Munroe & Francis, 1831.
The Ladies Dispensatory; or, Every Woman Her Own Physician: Treating of the Nature, Causes, and Various Symptoms, of all the Diseases, Infirmities. London: James Hodges, 1739.
La journée amoureuse. N.p., n.d.
Lamb, Charles. "The Triumph of the Whale." In *The Works of Charles Lamb,* ed. Charles Noon Talfourd, 1:159–160. New York: Harper & Brothers, 1838.
Lavater, Johann Caspar. *Essays on Physiognomy: For the Promotion of the Knowledge and the Love of Mankind.* Trans. Thomas Holcroft. 18th ed. London: Ward, Lock and Co., 1789.
Leake, John. *A Lecture Introductory to the Theory and Practice of Midwifery.* London: R. Baldwin, 1782.
Life and Character of Mr. Thomas Paine, Put in Metre, and Inscribed to the Society against Levellers and Republicans. [London: N.p., 1793?]
Lluelyn, Martin. *An Elegie on the Death of the Most Illustrious Prince, Henry Duke of Gloucester.* 2nd ed. Oxford: H. Hall, 1660.
Lucas, Charles. *The Infernal Quixote: A Tale of the Day.* 1801. Ed. M. O. Grenby. Reprint, Peterborough, ON: Broadview, 2004.
Macquin, Ange Denis. *Tabella Cibaria: The Bill of Fare.* London: Sherwood, Neeley and Jones, 1820.
Mandeville, Bernard. *A Treatise of the Hypochondriack and Hysterick Diseases.* 1730. Reprint, Delmar, NY: Scholars' Facsimiles and Reprints, 1976.

Mangin, Edward. *George the Third: A Novel*. 3 vols. London: James Carpenter, 1807.
Marten, John. *Onania; or, The Heinous Sin of Self-Pollution, and All Its Frightful Consequences*. 19th ed. London: C. Corbett, 1759.
Member of Parliament, and of His Majesty's Privy Council. *An Exposure of the Domestic and Foreign Attempts to Destroy the British Constitution*. London: J. Stockdale, 1792.
Member of the Jockey Club. *An Answer to Three Scurrilous Pamphlets, Entitled "The Jockey Club."* 2nd ed. London: J. S. Jordan, [1792].
Miles, William Augustus. *A Letter to the Prince of Wales, on a Second Application to Parliament, to Discharge Debts Wantonly Contracted since May 1787*. 10th ed. London: J. Owen, 1795.
Montagu, Mary Wortley. *Letters of the Right Honourable Lady M——y W——y M——e*. London: Thomas Martin, 1790.
More, Hannah. *Village Politics*. 2nd ed. London: F. & C. Rivington, 1792.
Moss, William. *An Essay on the Management, Nursing and Diseases of Children*. 2nd ed. Egham, UK: C. Boult, 1794.
New Year's Gift for Mr. Thomas Paine, in Return for His "Rights of Man": Humbly Presented by the Citizens of Caledonia. Edinburgh: N.p., 1792.
Nihell, Elizabeth. *A Treatise on the Art of Midwifery*. London: A. Morley, 1760.
Nisbet, William. *A Practical Treatise on Diet*. London: R. Phillips, 1801.
Nott, John. *An Appeal to the Residents of Birmingham: Designed as an Answer to Job Nott, Buckle-Maker* [Birmingham]: N.p., 1792.
The Nurse's Guide; or, The Right Method of Bringing Up Young Children: To Which Is Added, an Essay on Preserving Health, and Prolonging Life; With a Treatise of the Gout. London: John Brotherton and Lawton Gilliver, 1729.
"Ode to Jacobinism." *Anti-Jacobin or Weekly Examiner* 20 (26 March 1798), 157.
O'Neill, Count Thomas. *Narrative of the Incarceration of Count O'Neil, and the Massacre of his Family in France, etc*. London: Charles Squire, 1814.
One of the Faculty. *The Restorer of Health and Physician of Nature*. London: E. Hodson, 1792.
Paine, Thomas. *Common Sense*. Philadelphia: W. and T. Bradford, 1776.
———. *Rights of Man*. London: J. S. Jordan, 1791.
———. *"Rights of Man," "Common Sense" and Other Political Writings*. Ed. Mark Philp. Oxford: Oxford University Press, 1998.
Parsons, James. *A Mechanical and Critical Enquiry into the Nature of Hermaphrodites*. London: J. Walthoe, 1741.
Peacock, Thomas Love. *Melincourt*. Vol. 2 of 3 vols. London: T. Hookham, 1817.
Pigott, Charles. *The Female Jockey Club*. 3rd ed. Part 1 of 3 parts. London: D. I. Eaton, 1794.
———. *The Jockey Club, in Three Parts*. American reprint. New York: Thomas Greenleaf, 1793.
———. *The Jockey Club; or, A Sketch of the Manners of the Age*. 7th ed. London: H. D. Symonds, 1792.

———. *A Political Dictionary, Explaining the True Meanings of Words, illustrated and exemplified in the lives, morals, character and conduct of the following most illustrious persons, and among many others.* London: D.I. Eaton, 1795.

Polwhele, Richard. *The Unsex'd Females: A Poem, Addressed to the Author of "The Pursuits of Literature."* 1798. New York: William Cobbett, 1800.

[Price, Theodore]. *Life and Adventures of Job Nott, Buckle Maker of Birmingham.* Birmingham: E. Piercy, 1793.

Priestley, Joseph. *Letters to the Right Honourable Edmund Burke, Occasioned by His Reflections on the Revolution in France.* Dublin: J. Sheppard et al., 1791.

Proby, W.C. *Modern Philosophy and Barbarism; or, A Comparison between the Theory of Godwin and the Practice of Lycurgus.* London: R.H. Westley, [1798].

Pugin, A.W.N. *Contrasts.* 2nd ed. London: Charles Dolman, 1841.

Pye, Henry James. *The Democrat: Interspersed with Anecdotes of Well Known Characters.* 2 vols. London: William Lane, 1795.

Ritson, Joseph. *An Essay on Abstinence from Animal Food, as a Moral Duty.* London: Richard Phillips, 1802.

Romilly, Samuel. *Thoughts on the Probable Influence of the French Revolution on Great-Britain.* Dublin: P. Byrne, 1790.

Rousseau, Jean-Jacques. *Considerations on the Government of Poland.* 1772. Trans. Willmoer Kendall. Indianapolis: Hackett, 1985.

———. *Émile; or, Education.* 1762. Trans. Barbara Foxley. London: J.M. Dent and Sons, 1993.

———. *Politics and the Arts: Letter to M. d'Alembert on the Theatre.* 1758. Trans. Alan Bloom. Ithaca, NY: Cornell University Press, 1968.

Ruskin, John. "The Nature of Gothic." In *The Stones of Venice*, vol. 2. New York: John Wiley, 1860.

Rymsdyk, Jan van, and Andrew van Rymsdyk. *Museum Britannicum.* 2nd ed. London: J. Moore, 1791.

Sade, Marquis de. *Justine.* 1791. In *"Justine," "Philosophy in the Bedroom" and Other Writings*, trans. Austryn Wainhouse and Richard Seaver, 447–743. New York: Grove Press, 1990.

———. *"The Misfortunes of Virtue" and Other Early Tales.* Trans. David Coward. Oxford: Oxford University Press, 1999.

Salzmann, C.G. *Elements of Morality, for the Use of Children.* Trans. Mary Wollstonecraft. 2 vols. London: J. Johnson, 1790.

Secundus, Dick Humelbergius [Gabriel Hummelberger]. *Apacian Morsels; or, Tales of the Table, Kitchen, and Larder, with Reflections on the Dietic Productions of Early Writers.* 1829. 2nd ed., London: Whittaker, Treacer & Co., 1834.

Sharp, Jane. *The Midwives Book: or, The Whole Art of Midwifery.* London: Simon Miller, 1671.

Shelley, Mary. "Appendix B: The Third Edition (1831); Substantive Changes."

In *Frankenstein*, ed. Marilyn Butler (Oxford: Oxford University Press, 2008).
Shelley, Percy Bysshe. *The Letters of Percy Bysshe Shelley*. Ed. F. L. Jones. 2 vols. Oxford: Clarendon, 1964.
———. *Oedipus Tyrannus; or, Swellfoot the Tyrant*. London: J. Johnston, 1820.
———. *A Vindication of Natural Diet*. 1813. Reprint, London: F. Pitman, 1884.
Shipman, Thomas. "Beauty's Enemy." In *Carolina: or, Loyal Poems*, 78–79. London: Samuel Heyrick and William Crook, 1683.
Smellie, William. *Sett* [sic] *of Anatomical Tables with Explanations, and an Abridgement of the Practice of Midwifery*. London: N.p., 1754.
Smith, Hugh. *Letters to Married Women*. London: G. Kearsley, 1767.
Southey, Robert. "Poems Concerning the Slave Trade: Sonnet III." In *Poetical Works of Robert Southey*, 110. New York: D. Appleton, 1839.
———. *Sir Thomas More; or, Colloquies on the Progress and Prospects of Society*. 2 vols. London: John Murray, 1824.
Stephens, Alexander. *Public Characters of 1807*. London: J. Adlard, 1807.
Sterne, Laurence. *Tristram Shandy*. 1760–67. Reprint, Oxford: Oxford University Press, 1998.
Stevenson, William. *A Successful Method of Treating the Gout by Blistering*. Bath, UK: R. Cruttwell, 1779.
Sturgeon, Lancelot. *Essays, Moral, Philosophical, and Stomachical, on the Important Science of Good-Living*. 1822. 2nd ed. London: G. & W. B. Whittaker, 1823.
Sydenham, Thomas. *The Whole Works of that Excellent Practical Physician, Dr. Thomas Sydenham*. Trans. John Pechey. 6th ed. London: R. Wellington, 1715.
Taylor, Thomas. *Vindication of the Rights of Brutes*. London: Edward Jeffery, 1792.
Thelwall, John. Preface to *The Tribune, a Periodical Publication, Consisting Chiefly of the Political Lectures of J. Thelwall*. No. 2. London: Symonds et al., 1796.
———. "Report on the State of Popular Opinion, and the Causes of the Rapid Diffusion of Democratic Principles, Part the Second." *The Tribune* 2, no. 25 (1795).
Thorburn, Grant. *The Life and Writings of Grant Thorburn*. New York: Edward Walker, 1852.
Tooke, John Horne. *A Letter to a Friend on the Reported Marriage of His Royal Highness the Prince of Wales*. London: J. Johnson, 1787.
Venette, Nicholas de. *The Mysteries of Conjugal Love Reveal'd*. 8th ed. London: N.p., 1707.
Wadd, William. *Comments on Corpulency*. London: John Ebers, 1829.
Wathen, Jonathan. *Boerhaave's Academical Lectures on the lues venerea. In which are accurately described, the history, origin, progress, causes, symptoms, and cure of that disease*. Translated from the Latin, with notes. London: J. Rivington, 1763.

Williams, Helen Maria. *Letters Containing a Sketch of the Politics of France, 1793–94.* 2 vols. London: G. G. & J. Robinson, 1795.
———. *Letters Written in France, in the Summer 1790, to a Friend in England.* London: T. Cadell, 1790.
Willich, A. F. M. *Lectures on Diet and Regimen.* 2nd ed. London: Longman & Rees, 1799.
Wollstonecraft, Mary. *A Vindication of the Rights of Woman.* London: J. Johnson, 1792.
———. *Maria; or, The Wrongs of Woman.* In *Posthumous Works of the Author of "A Vindication of the Rights of Woman."* Vol. 2. Ed. William Godwin. London: J. Johnson, 1798.
Wood, John. *A Full Exposition of the Clintonian Faction and the Society of the Columbian Illuminati with an Account of the Writer of the Narrative, and the Characters of His Certificate Men.* Newark: For the author, 1802.
Zimmermann, J. G. "Warnung an Aeltern, Erzieher und Kinderfreunde wegen der Selbstbefleckung, zumal bey ganz jungen Mädchen." *Neues Magazin für Ärzte* 1 (1779): 43–51.

SECONDARY SOURCES

Abrahams, Yvette. "Images of Sara Bartman: Sexuality, Race and Gender in Early Nineteenth Century Britain." In *Nation, Empire, and Colony: Historicizing Race and Gender*, ed. Ruth Roach Pierson and Nupur Chaudhuri, 220–236. Indianapolis: Indiana University Press, 1998.
Allard, James Robert. *Romanticism, Medicine, and the Poet's Body.* Aldershot, UK: Ashgate, 2007.
Barker-Benfield, G. J. *Culture of Sensibility: Sex and Society in Eighteenth-Century Britain.* Chicago: Chicago University Press, 1996.
Barrell, John. *Imagining the King's Death: Figurative Treason, Fantasies of Regicide, 1793–1796.* Oxford: Oxford University Press, 2000.
———. *The Spirit of Despotism: Invasions of Privacy in the 1790s.* Oxford: Oxford University Press, 2006.
Barthes, Roland. *Mythologies.* 1972. Trans. Annette Lavers. London: Vintage, 2000.
Baudrillard, Jean. *Fatal Strategies.* Trans. Jim Fleming. London: Pluto Press, 1999.
Beauvoir, Simone de. "Must We Burn Sade?" Trans. Annette Michelson. In Marquis de Sade, *"The 120 Days of Sodom" and Other Writings*, trans. Austryn Wainhouse and Richard Seaver, 3–64. New York: Grove Press, 1966.
Bevir, Mark. "Rethinking Governmentality: Towards Genealogies of Governance." *European Journal of Social Theory* 13, no. 4 (2010): 423–441.
Bewell, Alan. *Romanticism and Colonial Disease.* Baltimore: Johns Hopkins University Press, 1999.
Bindman, David. *The Shadow of the Guillotine: Britain and the French Revolution.* London: British Museum Publications, 1989.

Bland, Lucy. "Trial by Sexology? Maud Allan, Salome, and the 'Cult of the Clitoris' Case." In *Sexology in Culture: Labelling Bodies and Desires*, ed. Lucy Bland and Laura Doan, 183–193. Chicago: Chicago University Press, 1998.
Bloch, Iwan. *Marquis de Sade: His Life and Works*. Amsterdam: Fredonia, 2002.
Bourdieu, Pierre. *Distinction: A Social Critique of the Judgement of Taste*. 1984. Abingdon, UK: Routledge, 2010.
Brace, Laura. "Rousseau, Maternity and the Politics of Emptiness." *Polity* 39 (2007): 361–383.
Braidotti, Rosi. *Nomadic Subjects: Embodiment and Sexual Difference in Contemporary Feminist Theory*. New York: Columbia University Press, 1994.
Brewer, John. "This, That and the Other: Public, Social and Private in the Seventeenth and Eighteenth Centuries." In *Shifting the Boundaries: Transformation of the Languages of Public and Private in the Eighteenth Century*, ed. Dario Castiglione and Lesley Sharpe, 1–21. Exeter, UK: Exeter University Press, 1995.
Brewer, William. *The Mental Anatomies of William Godwin and Mary Shelley*. Madison, NJ: Fairleigh-Dickinson University Press, 2001.
Brown, Kathleen M. *Foul Bodies: Cleanliness in Early America*. New Haven, CT: Yale University Press, 2009.
Burton, June. *Napoleon and the Woman Question: Discourses of the Other Sex in French Education, Medicine and Medical Law, 1799–1815*. Lubbock: Texas Tech University Press, 2007.
Calhoun, Craig, ed. *Habermas and the Public Sphere*. Cambridge, MA: MIT Press, 1993.
———. "The Public Sphere in the Field of Power Social Science." *History* 34, no. 3 (Fall 2010): 301–335.
Canguilhem, Georges. *The Normal and the* Pathological. Trans. Carolyn R. Fawcett. 1978. Reprint, New York: Zone Books, 2007.
Cavallaro, Dani, and Alexandra Warwick. *Fashioning the Frame*. Oxford: Berg, 2001.
Claeys, Gregory. *Thomas Paine: Social and Political Thought*. Boston: Unwin Hyman, 1989.
Clark, Anna. *Scandal: The Sexual Politics of the British Constitution*. Princeton, NJ: Princeton University Press, 2004.
———. *Struggle for the Breeches: Gender and the Making of the British Working Class*. Berkeley: University of California Press, 1995.
Cody, Lisa Foreman. *Birthing the Nation: Sex, Science and the Conception of Eighteenth-Century Britons*. Oxford: Oxford University Press, 2006.
Cohen, Michèle. *Fashioning Masculinity: National Identity and Language in the Eighteenth Century*. London: Routledge, 1996.
Colley, Linda. *Britons: Forging the Nation, 1707–1837*. New Haven, CT: Yale University Press, 1992.
Colwill, Elizabeth. "Pass as a Woman, Act Like a Man: Marie Antoinette as

Tribade in the Pornography of the French Revolution." In *Marie Antoinette: Writings on the Body of the Queen*, ed. Dena Goodman, 139–169. New York: Routledge, 2003.

Cooter, Roger, and Mary Fissell. *The Cambridge History of Science: Eighteenth-Century Science*. Vol. 4 of 7 vols. Ed. Roy Porter. Cambridge: Cambridge University Press, 2004.

Craciun, Adriana. *Fatal Women of Romanticism*. Cambridge: Cambridge University Press, 2003.

Curran, Andrew, and Patrick Graille. "The Faces of Eighteenth-Century Monstrosity." *Eighteenth-Century Life* 21, no. 2 (1997): 1–15.

Darby, Robert. "A Post-Modernist Theory of Wanking: Solitary Sex." *Journal of Social History* 38, no. 1 (2004): 205–210.

Darnton, Robert. "The High Enlightenment and the Low-Life of Literature." In *The Literary Underground of the Old Regime*, 1–40. Cambridge, MA: Harvard University Press, 1982.

Davidoff, Leonore, and Catharine Hall. *Family Fortunes: Men and Women of the English Middle Class, 1780–1850*. 2nd ed. London: Routledge, 2002.

Davidson, Arnold. *The Emergence of Sexuality: Historical Epistemology and the Formation of Concepts*. Cambridge, MA: Harvard University Press, 2004.

Deleuze, Giles. *Foucault*. Minneapolis: University of Minnesota Press, 1988.

Deutsch, Helen, and Felicity Nussbaum. Introduction to *Defects: Engendering the Modern Body*, 1–28. Ann Arbor: University of Michigan Press, 2000.

Digby, Anne. "Women's Biological Straitjacket." In *Sexuality and Subordination: Interdisciplinary Studies of Gender in the Nineteenth Century*, ed. Susan Mendus and Jane Rendall, 192–220. London: Routledge, 1989.

Douglas, Mary. *Purity and Danger: An Analysis of Concepts of Pollution and Taboo*. London: Routledge, 2002.

Duberman, Martin, Martha Vicinus, and George Chauncey, eds. *Hidden from History: Reclaiming the Gay and Lesbian Past*. London: Penguin, 1991.

Durey, Michael. *Transatlantic Radicals and the Early American Republic*. Wichita: University of Kansas Press, 1997.

Elias, Norbert. *The Civilizing Process: Sociogenetic and Psychogenetic Investigations*. Trans. Edmund Jephcott. Revised ed. Ed. Eric Dunning et al. Oxford: Blackwell, 2000.

Falk, Gerhard. *Stigma: How We Treat Outsiders*. Amherst, MA: Prometheus Books, 2001.

Fast, Howard. *Citizen Tom Paine*. New York: Grove Press, 1943.

Fausto-Sterling, Anne. "Gender, Race and Nation: The Comparative Anatomy of 'Hottentot' Women in Europe, 1815–1817." In *Feminism and the Body*, ed. Londa Schiebinger, 203–233. Oxford: Oxford University Press, 2000.

Fink, Beatrice. "You Are Not Necessarily What You Eat." In *The Eighteenth-Century Body: Art, History, Literature, Medicine*, ed. Angelica Goodden, 107–114. Bern: Peter Lang, 2002.

Fissell, Mary E. *Vernacular Bodies: The Politics of Reproduction in Early Modern England*. Oxford: Oxford University Press, 2006.

Fliegelman, Jay. *Prodigals and Pilgrims: The American Revolution Against Patriarchal Authority, 1750–1800.* Cambridge: Cambridge University Press, 1985.
Foner, Philip S., ed. Introduction to *Thomas Paine: The Age of Reason,* 7–42. New York: Citadel Press, 1974.
Foot, Michael, and Thomas Kramnick. *The Thomas Paine Reader.* Harmondsworth, UK: Penguin, 2004.
Foucault, Michel, "The Birth of Social Medicine." In *The Essential Foucault,* ed. Paul Rabinow and Nikolas Rose, 319–337. New York: New Press, 2003.
———. *Discipline and Punish: The Birth of the Prison.* Trans. Alan Sheridan. New York: Vintage, 1995.
———. *Flesh in the Age of Reason.* London: Penguin/Allen Lane, 2003.
———. *The History of Sexuality.* Vol. 1, *Introduction.* Trans. Robert Hurley. New York: Vintage, 1990.
———. *The History of Sexuality.* Vol. 2, *The Use of Pleasure.* Trans. Robert Hurley. New York: Vintage, 1990.
———. *The History of Sexuality.* Vol. 3., *The Care of the Self.* Trans. Robert Hurley. New York: Vintage, 1990.
———. *Power/Knowledge.* Ed. Colin Gordon. 1972. Reprint, New York: Pantheon, 1980.
———. "The Subject and Power." Trans. Leslie Sawyer. *Critical Inquiry* 8, no. 4 (Summer 1982): 777–795.
———. "Why Study Power: The Question of the Subject." In *Dits et écrits IV.* Paris: Gallimard, 1994.
Fulford, Tim. *Romanticism and Masculinity: Gender, Politics and Poetics in the Writing of Burke, Coleridge, Cobbett, Wordsworth, DeQuincey and Hazlitt.* Houndmills, UK: Macmillan, 1999.
Garton, Stephen. *Histories of Sexuality: Antiquity to Sexual Revolution.* New York: Routledge, 2004.
Gay, Peter. *The Bourgeois Experience: Victoria to Freud.* Vol. 1, *Education of the Senses.* New York: Norton, 1984.
George, Samantha. *Botany, Sexuality and Women's Writing, 1760–1830: From Modest Shoot to Forward Plant.* Manchester: Manchester University Press, 2007.
Gigante, Denise, ed. *Gusto: Essential Writings in Nineteenth-Century Gastronomy.* New York: Routledge, 2005.
———. *Taste: A Literary History.* New Haven, CT: Yale University Press, 2005.
Gilbert, Pamela K. "Mapping Colonial Disease: Victorian Medical Cartography in British India." In *Framing and Imagining Disease in Cultural History,* ed. George Rousseau et al., 111–128. Houndmills, UK: Palgrave, 2003.
Gilman, Sander L. "Black Bodies, White Bodies: Toward an Iconography of Female Sexuality in Late Nineteenth Century Art, Medicine, and Literature." *Critical Inquiry* 12 (Autumn 1985): 204–242.
———. *Fat Boys.* Lincoln: University of Nebraska Press, 2004.
Gladden, Samuel. "Shelley's Agenda Writ Large: Reconsidering *Oedipus*

Tyrannus; or, Swellfoot the Tyrant." *Romantic Circles Praxis Series.* www.rc.umd.edu/praxis/interventionist/gladden/gladden.html.

Godfrey, Richard. *James Gillray: The Art of Caricature.* London: Tate, 2001.

Goffman, Erving. *Stigma: Notes on the Management of Spoiled Identity.* London: Penguin, 1990.

Goodman, Dena, ed. *Marie Antoinette: Writings on the Body of the Queen.* London: Routledge, 2003.

Graham, Kenneth W., ed. *William Godwin Reviewed.* New York: AMS Press, 2001.

Grenby, Matthew. *The Anti-Jacobin Novel: British Conservatism and the French Revolution.* Cambridge: Cambridge University Press, 2001.

Groneman, Carol. "Nymphomania: The Historical Construction of Female Sexuality." In *Deviant Bodies: Critical Perspectives on Difference in Science and Popular Culture,* ed. Jennifer Terry and Jacqueline Urla, 219–249. Bloomington: Indiana University Press, 1995.

Guest, Kristen. Introduction to *Eating their Words: Cannibalism and the Boundaries of Cultural Identity,* 1–9. Albany: State University of New York Press, 2001.

Habermas, Jürgen. *The Structural Transformation of the Public Sphere: An Inquiry into a Category of Bourgeois Society.* Cambridge, MA: MIT Press, 1991.

Hacking, Ian. *The Taming of Chance.* Cambridge: Cambridge University Press, 1990.

Halberstam, Judith. *Skin Shows: Gothic Horror and the Technology of Monsters.* Durham, NC: Duke University Press, 1995.

Hibbert, Christopher. *George III: A Personal History.* London: Viking, 1998.

———. *George IV.* London: Penguin, 1988.

Hitchcock, Tim. *English Sexualities, 1700–1800.* Houndmills, UK: Palgrave, 1997.

Hunt, Lynn. *The Family Romance of the French Revolution.* Berkeley: University of California Press, 1992.

———, ed. *The Invention of Pornography: Obscenity and the Origins of Modernity, 1500–1800.* New York: Zone Books, 1993.

———. "The Many Bodies of Marie-Antoinette: Political Pornography and the Problem of the Feminine in the French Revolution." In *Marie Antoinette: Writings on the Body of the Queen,* ed. Dena Goodman, 117–138. London: Routledge, 2003.

———. *Politics, Culture and Class in the French Revolution.* 1984. Reprint, Berkeley: University of California Press, 2004.

Jones, Ann, and Peter Stallybrass. "Fetishizing Gender: Constructing the Hermaphrodite in Renaissance Europe." In *Body Guards: The Cultural Politics of Gender Ambiguity,* ed. Julia Epstein and Kristina Straub, 80–111. New York: Routledge, 1991.

Jones, Vivien. "The Death of Mary Wollstonecraft." *British Journal for Eighteenth-Century Studies* 20, no. 2 (1997): 187–205.

Jordanova, Ludmilla. *Sexual Visions: Images of Gender in Science and Medicine between the Eighteenth and Twentieth Centuries*. Hemel Hempstead, UK: Harvester/Wheatsheaf; Madison: University Wisconsin Press, 1989.
Kemp, Martin. "'The Mark of Truth': Looking and Learning in Some Anatomical Illustrations from the Renaissance and Eighteenth Century." In *Medicine and the Five Senses*, ed. W. F. Bynum and Roy Porter, 85–121. Cambridge: Cambridge University Press, 1993.
Kipp, Julie. *Romanticism, Maternity, and the Body Politic*. Cambridge: Cambridge University Press, 2007.
Kitson, Peter J. "Sustaining the Romantic and Racial Self: Eating People in the 'South Seas.'" In *Cultures of Taste/Theories of Appetite: Eating Romanticism*, ed. Timothy Morton, 77–96. Houndmills, UK: Palgrave, 2004.
Kristeva, Julia. *Powers of Horror: An Essay in Abjection*. Trans. Leon S. Roudiez. New York: Columbia, 1982.
Kukla, Rebecca. *Mass Hysteria: Medicine, Culture, and Mother's Bodies*. Lanham, MD: Rowman & Littlefield, 2005.
Lajer-Burcharth, Ewa. "The Aesthetics of Male Crisis: The Terror in the Republican Imaginary and in Jean-Louis David's Work from Prison." In *Femininity and Masculinity in Eighteenth-Century Art and Culture*, ed. Gillian Perry and Michael Rossington, 219–243. Manchester: Manchester University Press, 1994.
Lamb, Robert. "The Foundations of Godwinian Impartiality." *Utilitas* 18, no. 2 (2006): 134–153.
Laqueur, Thomas. *Making Sex: Body and Gender from the Greeks to Freud*. Cambridge, MA: Harvard University Press, 1990.
———. "Orgasm, Generation, and the Politics of Reproductive Biology." In *The Making of the Modern Body: Sexuality and Society in the Nineteenth Century*, ed. Thomas Laqueur and Catherine Gallagher, 1–41. Berkeley: University of California Press, 1987.
———. *Solitary Sex: A Cultural History of Masturbation*. New York: Zone Books, 2003.
Lawrence, C. J. "William Buchan: Medicine Laid Open." *Medical History* 19, no. 1 (January 1975): 20–35.
Lefebvre, Henri. *The Production of Space*. Trans. Donald Nicholson-Smith. Oxford: Blackwell, 1991.
Lévi-Strauss, Claude. *The Raw and the Cooked*. 1964. Trans. John and Doreen Weightman. London: Penguin, 1986.
Magubane, Zine. "Which Bodies Matter? Feminism, Postructuralism, Race, and the Curious Theoretical Odyssey of the 'Hottentot Venus.'" In *Gender and Society* 15, no. 6 (December 2001): 816–834.
Mallory, Anne. "Burke, Boredom, and the Theater of Counterrevolution." *PMLA* 118, no. 2 (March 2003): 224–238.
Marshall, Peter. *William Godwin*. New Haven, CT: Yale University Press, 1984.
Maza, Sarah. *Private Lives and Pubic Affairs: The Causes Célèbres of Prerevolutionary France*. Berkeley: University of California Press, 1993.

McCalman, Iain. "The Making of a Libertine Queen: Jeanne de La Motte and Marie-Antoinette." In *Libertine Enlightenment: Sex, Liberty and License in the Eighteenth Century,* ed. Peter Cryle and Lisa O'Connell, 112–144. Houndmills, UK: Palgrave, 2004.

McKeon, Michael. *The Secret History of Domesticity: Public, Private and the Division of Knowledge.* Baltimore: Johns Hopkins University Press, 2005.

McLaren, Dorothy. "Marital Fertility and Lactation, 1570–1720." In *Women in English Society,* ed. Mary Prior, 22–53. London: Methuen, 1985.

Mee, Jonathan. "Libertines and Radicals in the 1790s: The Strange Case of Charles Pigott I." In *Libertine Enlightenment: Sex, Liberty and License in the Eighteenth Century,* ed. Peter Cryle and Lisa O'Connell, 183–203. Houndmills, UK: Palgrave, 2004.

———. "The Political Showman at Home: Reflections on Popular Radicalism and Print Culture in the 1790s." In *Radicalism and Revolution in Britain, 1775–1848: Essays in Honour of Malcom I. Thomis,* ed. Michael T. Davis, 41–55. Houndmills, UK: Palgrave, 2000.

Mellor, Ann. "Sex, Violence, and Slavery: Blake and Wollstonecraft." *Huntington Library Quarterly* 58, nos. 3–4 (1995): 345–370.

Melville, Peter. "'A Friendship of Taste': The Aesthetics of Eating Well in Kant's *Anthropology from a Pragmatic Point of View.*" In *Cultures of Taste/Theories of Appetite: Eating Romanticism,* ed. Timothy Morton, 203–216. Houndmills, UK: Palgrave, 2004.

Mennell, Stephen. *All Manners of Food: Eating and Taste in Britain and France from the Middle Ages to the Present.* Chicago: Illini Books, 1996.

———. "Eating in the Public Sphere in the Nineteenth and Twentieth Centuries." In *Eating Out in Europe: Picnics, Gourmet Dining and Snacks Since the Late Eighteenth Century,* ed. Marc Jacobs and Peter Scholliers, 317–336. Oxford: Berg, 2003.

Micale, Mark. *Approaching Hysteria: Disease and Its Interpretations.* Princeton, NJ: Princeton University Press, 1995.

Monsam, Angela. "Biography as Autopsy in William Godwin's *Memoirs of the Author of 'A Vindication of the Rights of Woman.'*" *Eighteenth-Century Fiction* 21, no. 1 (Fall 2008): 109–130.

Morris, Marilyn. *British Monarchy and the French Revolution.* New Haven, CT: Yale University Press, 1998.

Morton, Timothy. "Joseph Ritson, Percy Shelley and the Making of Romantic Vegetarianism." *Romanticism* 12, no. 1 (2006): 52–61.

———. "Porcine Poetics: Shelley's *Swellfoot the Tyrant.*" In *The Unfamiliar Shelley,* ed. Timothy Webb and Alan Mendel Weinberg, 279–296. Farnham, UK: Ashgate, 2009.

———. *Shelley and the Revolution in Taste: The Body and the Natural World.* Cambridge: Cambridge University Press, 1994.

Myers, Mitzi. "Godwin's Memoirs of Wollstonecraft: The Shaping of the Self and Subject." *Studies in Romanticism* 20 (Fall 1981): 299–316.

Nelson, Craig. *Thomas Paine: Enlightenment, Revolution, and the Birth of Modern Nations*. New York: Viking, 2006.
Neu, James. *A Tear Is an Intellectual Thing: The Meanings of Emotion*. Oxford: Oxford University Press, 2000.
O'Connor, Erin. *Raw Material: Producing Pathology in Victorian Culture*. Durham, NC: Duke University Press, 2000.
Oerlemans, Onno. *Romanticism and the Materiality of Nature*. Toronto: Toronto University Press, 2004.
Pateman, Carole. *The Sexual Contract*. Stanford, CA: Stanford University Press, 1988.
Paulson, Ronald. *Representations of Revolution, 1789–1820*. New Haven, CT: Yale University Press, 1983.
Peace, Mary. "The Economy of Nymphomania: Luxury, Virtue, Sentiment and Desire in Mid-Eighteenth Century Medical Discourse." In *At the Borders of the Human: Beasts, Bodies and Natural Philosophy in the Early Modern Period*, ed. Erica Fudge, Ruth Gilbert, and Susan Wiseman, 239–258. Houndmills, UK: Palgrave, 2002.
Perry, Ruth. "Colonizing the Breast: Sexuality and Maternity in Eighteenth-Century England." *Journal of the History of Sexuality* 2, no. 2 (October 1991): 204–234.
———. *Novel Relations: The Transformation of Kinship in English Literature and Culture, 1748–1818*. Cambridge: Cambridge University Press, 2004.
Poole, Steve. *The Politics of Regicide in England, 1760–1850: Troublesome Subjects*. Manchester: Manchester University Press, 2000.
Porter, Roy. *Bodies Politic: Disease, Death and the Doctors in Britain, 1650–1900*. Ithaca, NY: Cornell, 2001.
———. *Flesh in the Age of Reason*. London: Penguin/Allen Lane, 2003.
Porter, Roy, and George Rousseau. *Gout: The Patrician Malady*. New Haven, CT: Yale University Press, 1998.
Rajan, Tilottama. "Framing the Corpus: Godwin's 'Editing' of Wollstonecraft in 1798." *Studies in Romanticism* 39 (Winter 2000): 511–532.
Richardson, Alan. *British Romanticism and the Science of the Mind*. Cambridge: Cambridge University Press, 2001.
Richardson, Ruth. *Death, Dissection and the Destitute*. 2nd ed. Chicago: University of Chicago Press, 2000.
Rose, Nikolas. "Medicine, History and the Present." In *Reassessing Foucault: Power, Medicine and the Body*, ed. Colin Jones and Roy Porter, 48–72. 1994. Reprint, London: Routledge, 1998.
Rosenberg, Charles. *Explaining Epidemics and Other Studies in the History of Medicine*. Cambridge: Cambridge University Press, 1992.
Rousseau, George. *Nervous Acts: Essays on Literature, Culture and Sensibility*. Houndmills, UK: Palgrave, 2004.
———. "The Pursuit of Homosexuality in the Eighteenth Century: 'Utterly Confused Category' and/or Rich Repository?" In *'Tis Nature's Fault :*

Unauthorized Sexuality During the Enlightenment, ed. Robert Perks Maccubbin, 132–168. Cambridge: Cambridge University Press, 1987.

———. "'A Strange Pathology.'" In *Hysteria beyond Freud*, ed. Sander Gilman et al., 91–221. Berkeley: University of California Press, 1993.

Ruston, Sharon. *Shelley and Vitality*. Houndmills, UK: Palgrave, 2005.

Saint-Amand, Pierre. "Terrorizing Marie Antoinette." *Critical Inquiry* 20 (Spring 1994): 379–400.

Sbiroli, Lynn Salkin. "Generation and Regeneration: Reflections on the Biological and Ideological Role of Women in France (1786–96)." In *Literature and Medicine during the Eighteenth Century*, ed. Marie Mulvey Roberts and Roy Porter, 266–285. London: Routledge, 1993.

Schiebinger, Londa. *Nature's Body: Sexual Politics and the Making of Modern Science*. London: HarperCollins, 1993.

Sedgwick, Eve Kosofsky. "The Character in the Veil: Imagery of the Surface in the Gothic Novel." *PMLA* 96, no.2 (March 1981): 255–270.

Senelick, Laurence. "Mollies or Men of Mode? Sodomy and the Eighteenth-Century London Stage." *Journal of the History of Sexuality* 1 (1990): 33–67.

Sha, Richard. "Scientific Forms of Sexual Knowledge in Romanticism," *Romanticism on the Net* 23 (August 2001). www.erudit.org/revue/ron/2001/v/n23/005993ar.html.

Sheriff, Mary. "The Portrait of the Queen." In *Marie Antoinette: Writings on the Body of the Queen*, ed. Dena Goodman, 45–72. London: Routledge, 2003.

———. "Woman? Hermaphrodite? History Painter? On the Self-Imaging of Elizabeth Vigée-Lebrun." *The Eighteenth Century* 35 (1994): 3–27.

Shildrick, Margrit. *Embodying the Monster: Encounters with the Vulnerable Self*. London: Sage, 2002.

Shuttleton, David. *Small Pox and the Literary Imagination, 1660–1820*. Cambridge: Cambridge University Press, 2007.

Smith, E. A. *George IV*. New Haven, CT: Yale University Press, 1999.

Smith, Virginia. *Clean: A History of Personal Hygiene and Purity*. Oxford: Oxford University Press, 2007.

Smith-Rosenberg, Carroll. *Disorderly Conduct: Visions of Gender in Victorian America*. New York: Knopf, 1985.

Sontag, Susan. *Illness as Metaphor* and *AIDS and Its Metaphors*. London: Penguin, 2002.

Stafford, Barbara Maria. *Body Criticism: Imaging the Unseen in Enlightenment Art and Medicine*. Cambridge, MA: MIT Press, 1991.

Stolberg, Michael. "An Unmanly Vice: Self-Pollution, Anxiety, and the Body in the Eighteenth Century." *Social History of Medicine* 13, no. 1 (2000): 1–22.

Stone, Lawrence. *The Family, Sex and Marriage in England, 1500–1800*. London: Weidenfeld & Nicholson, 1977.

Sussman, George D. *Selling Mothers' Milk: The Wet-Nursing Business in France, 1715–1914*. Urbana: University of Illinois Press, 1982.

Tauchert, Ashley. *Mary Wollstonecraft and the Accent of the Feminine.* Houndmills, UK: Palgrave, 2002.
Thomas, Chantal. *The Wicked Queen: The Origins of the Myth of Marie-Antoinette.* New York: Zone Books, 1999.
Thompson, E. P. *The Romantics: England in a Revolutionary Age.* Woodbridge, Suffolk, UK: Merlin, 1997.
Todd, Janet. *Mary Wollstonecraft: A Revolutionary Life.* London: Weidenfeld & Nicholson, 2000.
Trumbach, Randolph. "Erotic Fantasy and Male Libertinism in Enlightenment England." In *The Invention of Pornography: Obscenity and the Origins of Modernity, 1500–1800,* ed. Lynn Hunt, 253–282. New York: Zone Books, 1993.
——. "Sodomitical Subcultures, Sodomitical Roles, and the Gender Revolution of the Eighteenth Century: The Recent Historiography." In *'Tis Nature's Fault : Unauthorized Sexuality During the Enlightenment,* ed. Robert Perks Maccubbin, 109–121. Cambridge: Cambridge University Press, 1987.
Van Sant, Ann Jessie. *Eighteenth-Century Sensibility and the Novel: The Senses in Social Context.* Cambridge: Cambridge University Press, 1993.
Vickers, Neil. *Coleridge and the Doctors.* Oxford: Oxford University Press, 2004.
Wagner, Corinna. "Domestic Invasions: John Thelwall and the Exploitation of Privacy." In *John Thelwall: Radical Romantic and Acquitted Felon,* ed. Steve Poole, 95–106. London: Pickering & Chatto, 2009.
——, ed. *Gothic Evolutions: Poetry, Tales, Context, Theory.* Peterborough, ON: Broadview, 2013.
——. "Press Scandal and the Struggle for Cultural Authority in the 1790s." *Nineteenth-Century Studies* 22 (2008): 1–14.
Walter, Gérard, ed. *Actes du tribunal révolutionnaire.* Paris: Mercure de France, 1968.
Wennerstrom, Courtney. "Cosmopolitan Bodies and Dissected Sexualities: Anatomical Mis-stories in Ann Radcliffe's *Mysteries of Udolpho.*" *European Romantic Review* 16, no. 2 (April 2005): 193–207.
Wheeler, Roxann. *The Complexion of Race: Categories of Difference in Eighteenth-Century British Culture.* Philadelphia: University of Pennsylvania Press, 2004.
Williams, Raymond. *The Country and the City.* London: Chatto & Windus, 1973.
Wingrove, Elizabeth. *Rousseau's Republican Romance.* Princeton, NJ: Princeton University Press, 2000.
Yalom, Marilyn. *A History of the Breast.* New York: Alfred A. Knopf, 1997.
Youngquist, Paul. *Monstrosities: Bodies and British Romanticism.* Minneapolis: University of Minnesota Press, 2003.

Index

Abernethy, John, 180–81
abjection, 25, 36, 98, 150
abnormality
  birth defects, 37
  Canguilhem on, 31
  categories of, 237
  enlarged clitoris, 32, 34
  nonprocreative sex as, 73
  priapism, 119
  prolapsed uterus, 32
  sexual abstinence as, 156–57, 178
abstinence
  from alcohol, 200
  from meat, 226
  from sex, 154, 155, 156, 179
  from sugar, 176, 222–25
Adams, John, 136–37
addiction
  doctors against brandy, 151–52
  George IV and, 181
  scandal and, 132
  Tom Paine and, 133, 152–54
Address to the People of Great Britain, on the Propriety of Abstaining from West Indian Sugar and Rum (Fox), 222
Admirable Satire on the Death, Dissection, Funeral Procession, and Epitaph, of Mr. Pitt, 82, 85
Adolphus, John, 36
adultery, 37, 44, 120, 126

Advice to Gouty Persons (Kentish), 172
aesthetics
  architecture and, 205
  of anatomy, 94–95
  body and, 193
  clothing and, 138
  gastronomy and, 187, 188, 191, 196, 236
  Kantian, 171, 183–85, 188
Age of Reason (Paine), 163
Aiken, John, 28, 56
alcoholism
  doctors against brandy, 151–52
  George IV and, 181
  scandal and, 132
  Tom Paine and, 133, 152–54
Alcott, William, 270n77
Alderson, John, 141–42, 151
Almanach des gourmands (Grimod), 188–89
Amazon, 64, 70–76
Amazons, A Parisian Society, The, 71–2
American Citizen, 136
American Hall of Fame, 164
American Medical Association, 28
American presidential election (1992), 77
American Revolutionary War (of Independence), 172, 173, 198

Index

Amours de Charlot et Toinette, Les, 25
anarchy, 44, 64, 81, 121, 152, 172
anatomical illustration, 92–98. See also anatomy
Anatomie des parties de la generation de l'homme et de la femme (Figure 3.5), 94–95
anatomy
   Anatomy Act, 12
   comparative anatomy, 20, 31, 209, 228
   Enlightenment developments in, 7, 49, 81
   gender, sexuality, and, 33, 34, 49, 99–101, 118–19, 120
   moral questions surrounding, 12, 103, 112–14, 195, 235–36
   political aspects of, 1, 3
   in political propaganda and satire, 11, 12, 77, 85–86, 91–92, 99, 111
   popular circulation, 8
   racial difference and, 33, 209–10
   reproductive, 39–40, 98
   "School of Flesh and Blood," 92, 95–97
Anatomy of the Human Gravid Uterus, The (Figures 3.6 and 3.7), 94–97
ancien régime, 43, 64, 73, 107, 246n90
ancient world
   Amazons, 70
   dangerous imagination, 39
   early Britons and diet, 198, 216
   Foucault and, 193
   hygiene and, 140, 144, 192–93
   Spartans, 64
   stigma, 146
animals
   animal diet, 226–28
   animal-human hybridity, 133, 150, 209–11
   animalistic instincts, 67, 131, 179, 209
   common people as, 216–18, 221
   George IV as, 211
   hermaphroditic, 31
   Hottentot Venus as, 209–11
   physiology of, 131, 215
Answer to the Jockey Club, 130
Anthropology from a Pragmatic Point of View (Kant), 184–88
anti-Jacobin novels, 7, 71, 110, 122, 139
Anti-Jacobin or Weekly Examiner, 36, 127
Anti-Jacobin Review, 86–87, 104
anti-Paine propaganda, 131, 137, 147–50, 154, 161
anti-revolutionaries, 26, 63, 130, 135–6, 220, 235
Anti-saccharrites; or, John Bull and His Family Leaving Off the Use of Sugar (Figure 6.5) 222–23
antisocial personality disorder, 157
Apacian Morsels (Hummelberger), 189, 196
apathy
   personal ennui, 44, 104–8, 125, 136
   political, 106–7, 176, 235
appetite
   animalistic, 67
   aristocratic, 129, 167, 169, 175
   civilizing of, 189–92, 193
   foreign, 180, 199–202, 208–11, 214, 221–25
   gendered, 115
   George IV's, 186, 202
   medicalization of, 10, 176
   national identities and, 198–201
   sexual, 38, 81, 161
Arbuthnot, John, 107
architectural design, 205, 210–11
Armstrong, John, 140–42, 151, 198
Art of Invigorating and Prolonging Life (Kitchner), 195
Art of Preserving Health: A Poem (Armstrong), 140, 198
artificiality
   culture as, 24, 55–56, 211
   disease and, 114, 168, 175, 194, 211, 212
   foreignness as, 211–12
   in anatomical representation, 97
   in food, 13,
   marriage as, 88

sexual tastes and, 156
Association for Preserving Liberty and Property against Republicans and Levellers, 130, 134, 220
Astruc, John, 17
atavism
  George IV as exhibiting, 183
  Paine as exhibiting, 137, 145, 147, 157–58
  Pigott as exhibiting, 131
atheism, 120, 137, 163
Austrian Woman on the Rampage, The, 21
Authentic Trial at Large of Marie Antoinette, 35
autobiography 5, 92. See also biography
autopsy, 1, 12. See also anatomy

Baartman, Sarah (Hottentot Venus), 209–13, 228, 236
Bachelard, Gaston, 205
bachelorhood, 83–85, 88, 154–55, 158
Baillie, Matthew, 31, 32
Banks, Sir Joseph, 233
barbarism
  personal, 157, 160
  political, 102, 109–10, 164, 220
Barbauld, Anna Letitia, 45, 117
Barker-Benfield, G. J., 119, 122
Barrell, John, 6, 26, 232, 251n20
Barthes, Roland, 204
bathing, 115, 140, 144, 160, 163, 193. See also hygiene
Baudrillard, Jean, 217–18
Belle-alliance, or the female reformers of Blackburn, The (Figure 2.5), 66–67
Beauvilliers, Antoine, 167
Beauvoir, Simone de, 113
Beddoes, Thomas, 122, 174, 176
Beer Street (Hogarth), 200
Bevir, Mark, 10, 161
Bewell, Alan, 171, 200–201, 213, 217, 222
Bichat, Marie François Xavier, 195
Bienville, M. D. T., 22–28

Bignon, Jerome 46
Biographical Anecdotes of the Founders of the French Republic, 70
Biographical Memoirs of the French Revolution (Adolphus), 36
biography, 7
  of Paine, 135–37, 153–54, 156, 159–60, 163
  pathography, 133
  of Sade, 112
  of Wollstonecraft, 91, 92, 114
Biology, 9, 11, 68
  biological determinism, 23, 27–30, 48, 56–58, 77, 101, 114–17, 123–28
  biological dysfunction, 34, 36, 157, 178
  biological transmission, 37–42, 50–51, 142, 213, 217
  biology of incommensurability, 18–20, 39, 47, 76, 116
  of eating, 183, 184, 188
  morality and, 157, 178, 180
  as political determinant, 78
  race and, 209, 211
  related to materialism, 111
  uncertainty of, 23, 33
Bird in the Hand Is Worth Two in the Bush, A, 134
birth. See childbirth
Blackwood's, 100
Blainville, Henri de, 209
Blake, William, 163, 212, 268
Bland, Lucy, 34
Bloody Buoy, The, 37, 220
Boerhaave, Herman, 75
Bold, Henry, 149
Bon Ton, 71–72
Bone to Gnaw for Democrats, A (Cobbett), 220
Bonneville, Nicolas de and Madame, 158
Boothby, Sir Brooke, 134
boredom, 106. See also apathy
botany, 120–21
Botanical Garden (Darwin), 120

Bourdieu, Pierre, 204–5
bourgeois family, 30, 34, 189
Brace, Laura, 52
Braidotti, Rosi, 41
brain, 2, 81, 144
    dualism, 17, 49, 154, 122, 191, 194, 256n118
    John Hunter's views on, 194
    materialist views of, 102–3
    melancholic brain, 123
    mother's brain, 38–39
    origin of sensitivity, 120
brandy, 151–52. See also addiction
Bravo, Bravo! la Reine se penetre de la Patrie (Figure 1.1), 21–22
breast
    as political icon, 53–54, 59–68, 70–72, 77
breast-feeding
    breast sag, 57, 66
    discourse of biological destiny and, 11, 51–60
    Duchess of Devonshire and, 60–63
    fashion and, 56–57
    historical change toward, 50–52
    patriarchal authority over, 58, 60
    physician's advocacy of, 56–58
    politically symbolic, 53, 60, 63–68
    Rousseau and, 53–55
    social concern toward, 59
    wet-nursing, 50, 52, 54, 60
    women's roles, 59–60
Bretonne, Réstif de la, 112–13
Brewer, John, 5–6, 232
bridging concepts, 9–10, 52, 183, 187, 229, 237
Brighton Pavilion, 202–3, 205, 207–8, 211, 213
Brillat-Savarin, Jean-Anthelme, 188, 190, 199
British Critic, 91, 118–19
British Library, 130
Broca, Louis Du, 69, 219
Brown, John, 105–6
Brown, Kathleen, 138, 236
Browne, Sir Thomas, 215
Brunonian medicine, 105–6

Buchan, William, 8, 175, 180, 192
buggery, 75. See also sodomy
Bull, John, 84, 107, 198, 222–23
Burke, Edmund
    on America, 198
    apostrophe to Marie Antoinette, 47
    "drapery of life," 96–97, 99, 121
    First Letter on a Regicide Peace, 36–37, 220
    on hereditary distinction, 174
    political ennui, 106–7
    Reflections, 3–4, 6, 102–3, 106–7, 172
    swinish multitude, 216
    use of cannibal metaphor, 220
Burke, William, 100
"Burking", 100
Bynum, W. F., 7

Cabanis, George, 103
Cadogan, William
    against modern life, 212, 216
    on breastfeeding, 55–56, 57–58
    on gout, 168, 172, 173, 180, 211
Caleb Williams (Godwin), 91
Calhoun, Craig, 232
Campbell, Robert, 157
Cambridge, 129–30
Campan, Jeanne Louise Henriette (Madame Campan), 68
Canguilhem, Georges, 31
cannibal
    as figure of health, 211–12
    as political symbol, 65–66, 73, 218–20
    vegetarianism and, 229
Captain Cook, 220
Cardinal de Rohan, 21
Care of the Self, The (Foucault), 193
Carême, Marie-Antoine, 204
Carlton House, 202, 233, 270n5
Carlyle, Thomas, 103–4, 253
Cartesian dualism, 49, 154, 256n118
Carver, William, 137–39, 154–55
Catechism of Health (Faust), 143, 151
Catholicism, 43

Cavallaro, Dani, 138
Cavendish, Georgiana, Duchess of Devonshire, 60–63, 76
Cavendish, William, Duke of Devonshire, 61
celibacy, 156–57, 178
Chalmers, George (Francis Oldys), 134–36, 148–50, 154, 156, 161, 163
Chambers, Thomas King, 234
Charcot, Jean-Martin, 236
Charon, Louis François, 210
Cheetham, James, 136–40, 147, 152, 154–55, 159–63
Cheyne, George, 167
   on diet, 177, 180, 199–200
   on gout, 168, 175
   on health in the ancient world, 192–93
   on nerves, 122
   on vegetarianism, 226
childbirth. See also maternity and breast-feeding
   birth control, 75
   birth rates, 60
   limited roles and, 50, 58, 67
   puerperal fever, 11, 87, 90–91, 146, 160, 235
   satire on Paine, 150
   satire on Pigott, 131–32
   Wollstonecraft's death in, 90–91, 105, 117, 124–25
chivalry, 74, 86, 106
cholera, 214
chorion, 96
Christie, Thomas, 45–47, 246n6
Citizen Tom Paine (Fast), 163
civic humanism, 226. See also masculinity: republicanisn
Civic Sermons (Barbauld), 45
civilization
   against foreign barbarism, 220–21
   civil liberties and, 225
   civil society and, 1, 5–6, 113
   civility as sign of progress, 121, 131, 137, 145, 162, 164, 196, 212
   civilizing of appetite, 189, 191, 196
   as corrupting, 192–94, 200–201, 211–12, 217–18
   diseases of civilization, 168, 172–73, 175
   mechanisms of civilization, 27, 180, 183, 236
   civilization model of disease, 172–75
Civilizing Process (Elias), 161, 236
Claeys, Gregory, 164
Clark, Anna, 74
class ideologies, 129, 204–5, 171, 237
classical medicine, 140, 144, 192–93
Clayton, William, 143–45, 151
cleanliness. See hygiene
Clinton, Hillary, 77–78
clitoris (enlarged)
   hermaphroditism and, 11, 32, 33
   lesbianism and, 34
   nymphomania and, 23, 29
   reported in African women, 33
clothing, 138–39
Cobbett, William
   as anti-Painite, 158, 162
   as anti-revolutionary, 37, 63, 65, 76, 220
Cody, Lisa Forman, 39
Cohen, Michèle, 250n60
Coleridge, Samuel Taylor, 122, 174
Colley, Linda, 232
colonialism, 173, 198–200, 214, 221, 229
Colwill, Elizabeth, 29, 30, 59
Comments on Corpulency (Wadd), 185
Common Sense (Paine), 133–34, 163, 173
community
   disease and, 143–45, 168, 171, 183, 217
   eating and, 185, 188, 195–96, 200–201, 218
   embodied in architecture, 205
   exclusion from, 146
   luxury and, 186–88
   medical profession as, 33, 192
   motherhood and, 54–55, 63–66
   normative family values and, 3, 45, 54, 236

community *(continued)*
  onanism and, 43, 44
  personal health and, 135, 138, 155, 162, 176, 236
  rationality and, 102–3, 113
  self-interest and, 53, 85, 113, 164
  sensus communis, 12, 185, 186, 196
conception, 39, 41, 131
Condorcet, Nicolas de, 225
Confessions (Rousseau, J.-J.), 158
configuration model of disease, 142–45
conservatism, 3, 5, 108–9, 117, 151, 163, 172, 181
Considerations on Lord Grenville's and Mr. Pitt's Bills (Godwin), 88
Constant, Benjamin, 68
constitution. See also constitutional model of disease
  anatomy and, 112
  constitutional disorders, 227
  English political, 63, 138, 197, 213–14, 225
  female, 12, 32, 48, 51, 56, 124
  foreignness and, 199, 213–14
  French political, 46
  hygiene and health, 143, 159, 167, 264n42
  male, 73, 123
  national identity and, 199–201
  physical and political, 1–6, 9, 82, 152–56, 213, 236, 260n96
constitutional model of disease, 171–75
Constitutional Society, 136
consumption (disease), 42, 123, 132, 146
consumption (food and goods)
  eating and gastronomy, 183, 187, 188, 191, 196, 236
  of foreign foods, 203, 221, 222–25
  George IV and, 181–82
  gout and, 168, 171, 175
  habits of, 12–13, 143, 176, 229
  Kant on, 171, 183–85, 188
  national identity and, 199–201
  of sugar, 222–25

contagion, 12
  clothing and, 138
  contamination and, 142–45, 213–14
  foreign, 4, 140–42, 200, 214–16, 235
  hygiene and, 140–146
  language of, 140
  political, 132, 135, 145
  sexual, 23, 75
  spread of disease, 132, 140
contagious diseases. See disease
contamination model of disease, 142–45, 213–14
Conway, Moncure Daniel, 163
Cook, John, 39–40
Cook's Oracle, The (Kitchiner), 191
Corday, Charlotte, 30
Corpulence; or, Excess of Fat in the Human Body (Chambers), 234
corruption, 104
  breastfeeding and, 56
  eating and, 158, 174, 205, 222, 225
  monstrosity and, 31
  personal life and, 5, 17, 129, 132
cosmopolitanism
  political, 132, 164, 184
  tasteful, 188, 196
Country and the City, The (Williams), 142
Courier, The, 84
Court at Brighton a la Chinese!! (Figure 6.3), 207–8
courtly love, 86
Cow Pock; or, The Wonderful Effects of the New Inoculation!, 150
Craciun, Adriana, 18
Critical Review, 127
Critique of Judgment (Kant), 185
Crooke, Helkiah, 1–2
Crown and Anchor tavern, 130
Cruikshank, George, 66–67, 169, 206–8, 211, 213
Cruikshank, Isaac, 223–24
Cullen, William, 122–123, 192
Cuvier, Georges, 195, 209, 228, 236, 270n77

D'Agoty, Jacques Fabien Gautier, 94–95
D'Israeli, Isaac, 71, 110–11
d'Osmond, Adèle, Comtesse de Boigne, 203
Darby, Robert, 44
Darwin, Erasmus, 120
David, Jean-Louis, 53
Davidson, Arnold, 164
De dissectione partium corporis humani libri tres (Figure 3.4), 93
death
  anatomy, 98, 112
  of Bonaparte, 170
  dirt and, 144–45
  foreign disease and, 214–15
  of French monarchs, 25–26, 41
  of French public women, 30, 69–70
  of George IV, 201, 231
  masturbation and, 42, 56
  Paine's, 159–60
  Pitt's spurious one, 82, 85
  Sadean violence and, 112
  Wollstonecraft's, 86–92, 104–6, 114–24, 235
Deathbed Confession of the Late Countess of Guernsey, 264n29
debauchery, 27, 35, 43, 74, 129, 170, 186–87
decay, 13, 104, 121, 213
décolletage, 56–57
defects, 31–32, 73, 131, 155, 173, 209. See also abnormality
deformity, 75, 152. See also defects; abnormality
degeneration. See also atavism
degenerate bodies, 56, 69, 119
  foreign nations and, 214, 218, 229
  George IV's fork and, 183
  masturbation as, 42–45, 119
  refusal to breastfeed as, 56
  revolution as, 121, 128, 162
Delicate Investigation, 202
Democrat, The (Pye), 71
Dent, William, 81–82
depravity, 5, 37, 54, 65. See also deviance

Deutsch, Helen, 31
deviance
  moral, 126, 143, 148, 156–57
  sexual, 18, 27–30, 41, 111–12, 133–34, 154
  women and, 18, 27–30, 41, 50, 76
diamond necklace affair, 21
Diderot, Denis, 179–80
diet. See dietetics; eating
dietetics, 10, 192–94, 200, 226, 236
Digby, Anne, 243n37
dirt
  contamination, contagion, and, 4, 141–42, 145
  morality and, 142–44
  Paine and, 12, 133–39, 150–164
disability, 156
disaffection, 11, 44, 53, 64, 106. See also apathy
disciplinary boundaries, 7–9
discipline. See Foucault: discipline
Discipline and Punish, (Foucault), 24
disease
  cholera, 214
  civilization model of disease, 172–75
  configuration model of disease, 142–45
  constitutional model of disease, 171–75
  contamination model of disease, 142–45, 213–14
  dysentery, 214
  mange, 217
  mapping of, 213–14
  murrain, 217
  of the womb, 11, 29, 34, 90
  tropical, 214
Dissection, A (Figure 3.2), 81–83
dissection. See also anatomy
  Godwin's textual dissection, 87, 91–92, 102
  of hermaphrodites, 31–33
  medical, 93–101, 128
  Sade and, 112
  of Sarah Baartman, 209
  satire of Pitt, 83–85

dissection *(continued)*
  and sex, 112, 121
Dissertation on the Gout (Cadogan), 172, 211
docile bodies, 9–10
Domestic Medicine (Buchan), 8
domestic virtue
  revolution, moral reform, and, 24, 26, 36, 158
  self-restraint and, 143, 151, 181, 192
  women and, 28, 36, 69
Donald, Diana, 65
Douglas, Mary, 135, 204
Dracula, 145
Dublin University Magazine, 100
Duchess of D—— in the Character of a Mother (Figure 2.2), 61
dysentery, 214

East Indies, 201
eating
  dietetics, 10, 192–94, 200, 226, 236
  foreign foods, 203, 221, 222–25
  gastronomy, 187, 188, 191, 196, 236
  gout and, 168, 171, 175
  immorality and, 176
  Kant on eating, 171, 183–85, 188
  national identity and, 151, 183, 198–201, 226, 229, 230
  obesity, 12–13, 192, 200, 218, 234
  sugar, 222–25
  symbol of utilitarianism, 103
  vegetarianism, 13, 199, 221, 225–29, 270n77
ecology, 142
Eden, Eleanor, 85
Edwards, Daniel, 77–78
Egyptian Hall, Piccadilly Circus, 209
ejaculate, 42, 73
Elements of Medicine (Brown), 105–6
Elements of Morality for the Use of Children (Salzmann), 118–19
Elegie on the Death of the Most Illustrious Prince, The (Lluelyn), 149
Elias, Norbert, 161, 261
Elizabeth, sister of Louis XVI, 35–36

Elliot, Charles Harrington, 147, 156–57
embryology, 30–31
Émile (Rousseau, J-J.), 2, 20, 50, 52, 53–55, 59, 72, 140
emotion
  digestion and, 195, 218
  disordered, 29
  excessive, 110
  indifference, 83, 85, 102–7, 157, 235
  masturbation and, 120
  medicalization of, 111, 122, 236
  nerves and, 39
  sensibility and, 119–26
  women and, 40, 48, 69, 114–16, 123, 125
empiricism, 87, 96, 113
English Malady, The (Cheyne), 122, 200
Englishness. See national identity
Enlightenment
  division of genders, 18–19, 28, 117
  ideas about breastfeeding, 50–63
  materialism, 117–20
  medical, 2, 8, 25
  mind-body connection, 49, 194–95
  moderation and, 151
  rationality, 89, 94, 113–14, 195
  theories of taste, 225
  visuality, 9, 206, 235
ennui. See apathy
epicureanism, 189–95, 216–17
epidemic, 4, 140–42, 200, 214–15, 235
epidemiology, 140, 214, 235
equality
  Kant and, 185
  Paine and, 145, 147
  revolutionary debates about, 63, 69, 72, 89, 132, 158
  of the sexes, 20, 87, 117, 119, 255n99
  Shelley and, 225–26
Essay of Heath and Long Life, An (Cheyne), 167
Essay on Abstinence from Animal Food, as a Moral Duty (Ritson), 226

Essay on the Management, Nursing and Diseases of Children (Moss), 56
Essay on the Nature and Origin of the Contagion of Fevers (Alderson), 141–42
Essay on the True Nature and Due Method of Treating the Gout, An (Cheyne), 168, 175
Essay upon Nursing and the Management of Children from Birth to Three Years of Age (Cadogan), 55
Essays, Moral, Philosophical, and Stomachical, on the Important Science of Good-Living, (Sturgeon), 190
Essays on Physiognomy (Lavater), 37–38
Estates-General, 68, 73
Estienne, Charles, 93–94
etiology
  of disease in general, 31, 41–42
  of gout, 172, 174
  of masturbation, 42
Eton, 129, 130
European Magazine, 91, 127
Evangelicals, 190
Examiner, 233
excitability, 105–7
Explaining Epidemics (Rosenberg), 142
Exposure of the Domestic and Foreign Attempts to Destroy the British Constitution, 63

Falck, Nikolai Detlef, 75
Falk, Gerhard, 146
fame, 30, 136, 156, 164
Fanny Hill (Cleland), 208
fashion, 34, 56–57, 63, 114, 138, 147
Fashion before Ease; or, A Good Constitution Sacrificed, for a Fantastik Form (Figure 4.2), 153
Fast, Howard, 163
fatherhood, 157
Faust, Bernhard, 143, 151–52
Fausto-Sterling, Anne, 209
female-embodied writing, 115–17

Female Jockey Club (Pigott), 63, 129, 180
female penis, 32–33
femme publique, 30
femme-homme, 30
fertility, 44, 53, 60
fetus, 37–40, 93–96, 98
feudalism, 86
fever
  jail, 140–41, 145, 152
  puerperal, 11, 87, 90–91, 146, 160, 235
filth. See dirt; hygiene
Fink, Beatrice, 199
Finke, Leonhard Ludwig, 213
First Letter on a Regicide Peace (Burke), 36–37, 220
fishwives, 66–67, 70
Fissell, Mary, 8
Fitzherbert, Maria, 179
Flim Flams! (D'Israeli), 110–11
Foner, Philip, 164
Foot, Michael, 164
Fordyce, Dr. George, 90
Foreman, Amanda, 60
Foucault, Michel
  biopolitics, 7–8, 171
  deviancy, 9
  discipline, 9–10
  docile bodies, 10, 149
  governmentality, 10, 144, 161–62, 231, 261n108
  on masturbation, 42, 44, 119
  medicopolitical discourse, 7–8
  panopticism, 234
  power, 9–10, 24
  on sexuality, 156
Foul Bodies (Brown), 138–39
Fountain of Regeneration, 53
Fox, Charles James, 60–61, 81–83, 85–86, 179
Fox, Guy, 157–58
Fox, William, 222
French Liberty/British Slavery, 147
French National Convention, 46, 53, 219
Frend, William, 125

302 / Index

Freud, Sigmund, 19, 126, 157
frugality, 176, 191, 222
Fureurs uterines de Marie-Antoinette [Uterine Furors of Marie-Antoinette], 21
Fulford, Tim 86
Full Exposition of the Clintonian Faction, A (Wood), 135

Gall, Franz Joseph, 236
Ganges Delta, 214
gastronomy, 187, 188, 191, 196, 236
  Kant on eating, 171, 183–85, 188
Gatens, Moira, 115–16
Gay, Peter, 43
genealogy, 9, 10, 131, 158, 173, 188
genitals, 19, 30, 32, 81, 83
geographers of taste, 188
geography, 213, 215, 229
George III
  court of, 232
  as Farmer George, 263n25
  as parsimonious, 196
  Royal Marriages Act and, 179–80, 264n29
  satire and, 177–78
  self-restraint and, 176
  sugar and, 222–24
George IV (Prince of Wales, Prince Regent). See also monarchy
  animalistic, 211
  atavistic, 183
  death of, 201, 231
  eating Eastern food, 201–3, 211, 221, 229
  eating turtle, 201
  fear of public opinion, 231–34
  foreign disease and, 213–14
  gout and, 12, 167–71, 216, 221, 230–34
  as host of baccanalian orgies, 202
  as Hottentot Venus, 209, 236
  love of consuming, 181–82
  luxury and, 202–8
  marriage to Caroline, 202, 221
  Oriental architecture and, 203–8, 211

  "Prince of Whales," 233
  satirized as oriental tyrant, 201–2
  secret marriage, 179
  self-interestedness of, 186, 216–18, 226–29
  as solitary eater, 184–85
  two-pronged fork and, 183
  as womanizer, 179, 202, 207, 233
George, Samantha, 120
George the Third (Mangin), 139
Gibbon, Edward, 172
Gigante, Denise, 183, 187–90, 225
Gilbert, Pamela K., 214
Gillray, James. See list of individual illustrations, page ix
Gin Lane (Hogarth), 201
Gladden, Samuel, 218
global spread of disease, 140–42, 200, 214–15, 235
gluttony, 175–76, 189, 190. See also consumption
Godfrey, Richard, 65, 177
Godmiché, La [The royal dildo], 21, 73
Godwin, William
  as anatomist, 12–13, 86, 91–92, 98–103, 106, 111–14, 118–20, 235
  Anti-Jacobin on, 127
  Charles James Fox and, 85–86, 88, 110
  chivalry and, 86, 106, 108, 121
  compared to the Marquis de Sade, 111–13
  compared to *tricoteuses*, 108
  "famous fire cause," 108–10, 254n68
  on impartiality, 86, 91, 108–10
  life of Fénelon, 108–9
  London Corresponding Society, critic of, 88
  Morning Chronicle on, 89
  "new philosophy," 87, 127, 257n131
  opinions on marriage, 86–88, 127
  as rationalist, 12, 71–72, 86, 88–89, 91, 100–21, 161
  Thelwall and, 88–89, 251n20
  William Pitt and, 85–86

Tribune on, 9
Goffman, Erving, 146
gout
   George IV and, 12, 167–71, 216, 221, 230–34
   Louis XVIII and, 167–69
   physicians on, 171–75, 181–83, 192–94, 200, 211
   politics and, 167–75
governmentality, 10, 144, 161–62, 231, 261n108. *See also* Foucault
Gradual Abolition off [sic] *the Slave Trade* (Figure 6.6), 223–24
Graham, Thomas John, 227
Grant, William, 173
Great Windmill Street anatomy school, 99
Green, Thomas, 110
Grenby, Matthew, 87–88
Grimod, Balthazar Laurent de la Reynière, 188–89
Groneman, Carol, 28
Guest, Kristen, 220
guillotine, 37, 106, 108, 152, 219
gynecologist, 28

habeas corpus (suspension of), 5
Habermas, Jürgen, 5, 232
Hacking, Ian, 2
Halberstam, Judith, 164
Hamilton, William, 36
Hamlet (Shakespeare), 131
Hardy, Thomas, 63, 220
Hare, William, 100
Harford, John S, 152–54
Harper's New Monthly Magazine, 198
Hartley, David, 226
Hays, Mary, 117, 125
Heath, William, 168–69, 262n3
Hébert, Jacques René, 35, 42
hereditariness, 38, 132, 172–74, 179, 263n11
hermaphrodites, 11, 19, 28–34, 70
Hertford, Lady, 170, 207
heteronormativity, 30, 161
Hibbert, Christopher, 178, 231, 233
Hippocrates, 37

History of English Thought in the Eighteenth Century (Stephen), 163
History of John Bull, The (Arbuthnot), 107
History of Sexuality (Foucault), 156
Hobbes, Thomas, 149–50, 183, 211, 229
Hogarth, William, 200–201
Hogg, Thomas Jefferson, 217
Home, Everard, 31–32, 244n46
Homer, 193
homoeroticism, 115
homophobia, 74–75
homosexuality, 25, 29, 74–75. *See also* lesbianism
homosociality, 77
homunculous, 131
Hone, William, 205–7
Hottentot apron, 209–10
Hottentot Venus (Baartman, Sarah), 209–13, 228, 236
House of Commons, 12
Howard, Charles, Duke of Norfolk, 4–5
Huish, Robert, 201–2
human ecology, 142
Hume, David, 188, 194
Hummelberger, Gabriel, 189, 196
Humphrey Clinker (Smollett), 201
Hunt, Isaac, 137, 145, 162
Hunt, Leigh and John, 233
Hunt, Lynn, 17, 23
Hunter, James, 1
Hunter, John, 31, 194, 215
Hunter, William, 1, 3, 6, 8, 33–34, 94–97, 112
hybridity
   human-animal, 133, 150, 209–11
   language and genre, 74, 92, 156
hygeia (bodily regimen), 193
Hygeia; or, Essays Moral and Medical (Beddoes), 122–23
hygiene, 236
   ancient ideas of, 140, 144, 192–93
   bathing, 115, 140, 144, 160, 163, 193
   Cheyne on, 192
   contagion and, 140–46

hygiene *(continued)*
  health and, 143, 159, 167, 264n42
  normativity and, 143, 154
  Paine and, 12, 132–61
  sanitation, 7, 12, 144, 214, 237
  self-restraint and, 144, 160
  sensibility and, 138
  Wollstonecraft on, 115
hypochondria, 122–24, 192, 200
hysteria
  about masturbation, 119
  female, 27, 56, 76, 117, 122–24, 242n16
  male, 194
  political, 48, 106
  Wollstonecraft and, 125–26, 236

ideology of incommensurability, 18–20, 39, 47, 76, 116
ideopathology, 217
Imlay, Gilbert, 86, 125, 127
immorality
  anatomy and, 99–100
  excessive eating and, 176, 191, 205
  Godwin, Wollstonecraft, and, 114, 121, 127
  Marie Antoinette and, 18, 30, 35–36
  modernity and, 151, 175
  Pigott and, 129–30
  politicians and, 162
impotence, 25–26, 73, 156, 158
incest
  Marie Antoinette accused of, 17, 21, 35–36, 42
  Princesses Royal and, 180
  Rousseau and, 158
Inchbald, Elizabeth, 127
India, 214, 221
indigenous foods, 188, 198–201, 216, 229
individualism, 4
Indo-Oriental style, 203
Infernal Quixote, The (Lucas), 110
inoculation, 150
Interesting Anecdotes of the Heroic Conduct of Women (Broca), 69, 219

interiority, 6
Introduction to Botany in a Series of Familiar Letters (Wakefield), 120
Isis, 53

Jacobinism, 18, 36, 88, 108, 135, 204, 211
Jeans, Thomas, 175–76
Jenner, Edward, 150
Jockey Club (Pigott), 4, 47, 129–31. See also *Female Jockey Club*
Jones, Henry, 149
Jones, Robert, 203
Jordan, J.S., 150
Jordanova, Ludmilla, 7, 9
Joss and His Folly, The (Figures 6.1 and 6.2), 205–7
journée amoureuse, La, 29
Jukes, Edward, 218
Junius, 202
jury de gustateurs, 188
Justine (Sade), 17, 112

Kant, Immanuel, 183–88, 195–96
Keller, Rose, 112
Kemp, Martin, 94–95
Kentish, Richard, 172
Kenyon, Lloyd, first Baron Kenyon, 126
Kipp, Julie, 52
Kitchner, William, 191
Krafft-Ebing, Richard, 28
Kramnick, Thomas, 164
Kristeva, Julia, 150, 164
Kukla, Rebecca, 52, 55, 58–59

La nouvelle Justine (Sade), 112
L'aristocrate; la democrate (Figure 2.3), 65
L'autrichienne en goguettes, 242n14
Lady's Dispensatory, The, 27
Laqueur, Thomas, 19–20, 42–43
lactation. See breast-feeding
Lady Bessborough, 204
Lajer-Burcharth, Ewa, 73–74
Lamb, Charles, 233–34, 254n68
Lambert, Mary, 154–55

Last Letter of Junius, 202
Laurence, C. J., 192
Lavater, Johann Casper, 38, 235
Le Grand Véfour, 189–90
Le Moniteur Universal, 35
Leake, John, 40, 41
Leake's patent pills, 183
Leclerc, Georges-Louis, Comte de Buffon, 233
Lecture Introductory to the Theory and Practice of Midwifery, A (Leake), 245–81
Lecture on Dirt (Clayton), 143–45, 151
Lectures on Diet and Regimen (Willich), 43–44, 123, 143–44, 146, 151
Lectures on the Lues Venerea (Boerhaave), 75
Lefebvre, Henri, 205
Les curieux en extase (Charon), 210
Les Enfans de Sodome á l'Assemblée Nationale, 73
lesbianism (tribadism), 28–34
lethargy, 106–7. See also ennui
Letters Containing a Sketch of the Politics of France (Williams), 36
Letters on the Elements of Botany Addressed to a Lady (Rousseau, J.-J.), 120
Letters on the Principles of the French Democracy (Hamilton), 36
Letters on the Revolution of France (Christie), 45–47
Letter to a Friend, A (Browne), 215
Letter to a Friend on the Reported Marriage of His Royal Highness, A, (Tooke), 179–80
Letters to Married Women (Smith), 57
Letter to the Prince of Wales, A (Miles), 181, 186
Letters to the Right Honourable Edmund Burke, 26
Letters Written in France (Williams), 45
lettres de cachet, 43, 246n90
Leuwenhoek microscopes, 103
Levee Day, A (Figure 5.2), 169
Lever, Charles, 100

Lévi-Strauss, Claude, 204
Lewes, Sussex, 155
libel (libelles), 5, 17, 130–31, 234
liberty
 Englishness and, 201, 225
 medicine and, 173, 237
 personal, 27, 226
 political, 35–36, 41, 54, 63, 119, 145, 224
liberalism, 116, 132, 163–64, 174, 226, 240
libertinism, 5, 120, 129
Lichtenberg, Georg, 206
Life and Adventures of Job Nott (Price), 220
Life and Character of Mr. Thomas Paine, Put in Metre, 156
Life of Paine (Cheetham), 136–40, 147, 152, 154–55, 159–63
Life of Thomas Pain (Chalmers), 134–36, 148–50, 154, 156, 161, 163
Life of Thomas Paine (Cobbett), 162
Linnaean classification, 31, 120
Linnaeus, Carl, 233, 247n1
literary confession, 5, 7, 11, 112, 158. See also Godwin: *Memoirs*
liver, 2, 227
Lluelyn, Martin, 149
Locke, John, 49, 194
Lombroso, Cesare, 236
London Corresponding Society, 88, 129, 145
London Tradesman (Campbell), 175
Louis Capet, the dauphin, 21, 35–36, 43
Louis XVI (France), 25–27, 72
Louis XVIII (France), 167–69
Love Life of Charlie and Toinette, The, 25
Lucas, Charles, 91, 110
Luddism, 229
luxury
 aristocrats and, 10
 disease and, 27, 120, 141, 168, 175–76, 192–94
 foreign goods and, 180, 202–8, 211, 216, 221–22

luxury (continued)
  George IV and, 202–8
  Kant on, 186–87
  modern moral degeneracy and, 120, 211–12

Macquin, Ange Denis, 190
Making Sex (Laqueur), 19–20
malaria, 214
malformations. See abnormality
Mallory, Anne, 106
Malthusians, 190
man of taste, 12, 122, 171, 184–91, 195–95, 217. See also gastronomy
Manchester Reformation Society, 136
Mandeville, Bernard, 124
Mangin, Edward, 139
Manley, Dr., 159–60
manliness, 4, 86, 163. See also masculinity
maps (medical), 213, 215, 229
Marat, Jean-Paul, 30
Maria lactans (Madonna del latte), 66
Maria; or, The Wrongs of Woman, 115
Marie Antoinette, Queen of France
  accused of incest, 17, 21, 35–36, 42
  Burke on, 4
  depoliticizing of women and, 18, 29–30, 41, 45–49
  hermaphroditism and, 11, 28–34
  Hillary Clinton and, 77–78
  lesbianism and, 28–34
  Louis XVI and, 25–27, 72–73
  Marie Antoinette Syndrome, 77
  nymphomania and, 11, 21–22, 29, 30–31, 35
  onanism and, 11, 33, 35, 41–42
  pornographic pamphlets about, 21–25
  trial of, 18, 35–36, 42
marriage
  courtly love and, 86
  George III and, 178–80
  George IV's, 202, 221
  Godwin's views on, 85–88, 110, 119, 126–27
  heteronormativity and, 27, 30, 34
  loveless, 212
  masturbation and, 42
  Paine's threat to, 151, 154–60
  Pitt and, 85
  "privatized marriage," 157
  public life and, 6,
  Rousseau and, 158
  Royal Marriages Act, 178–80
  toxic, 236
  Wollstonecraft and, 114–15, 119, 126–27
  women's roles and, 47
Marten, John, 42, 44
masculinity
  chivalry and, 86
  emerging modern models of, 76–77, 157, 171, 227
  lesbianism and, 34
  manliness, 4, 86, 163
  moderation and, 227
  politicized women and, 64–65, 71–76
  republicanism and, 18, 54, 59, 64–65, 226
  sodomy and, 73–76
masturbation (onanism), 42–45, 75, 152
  anti-onanists, 43–44
  Foucault on, 42, 44
  Laqueur on, 42–43
  Marie Antoinette and, 11, 33, 35–36, 41
  Pitt and, 84
  Wollstonecraft and, 118–20
materialism, 87, 92, 102–3, 112, 120, 128, 256n118
maternal impression (maternal marking), 37–42, 51
  Paine and, 150
  political angle of, 47, 63,
  in *Tristram Shandy*, 131
maternity. See also breast-feeding; maternal impression
  female-embodiment, 115–17
  lack of maternal feelings, 34–36
  maternal body, 48–49, 58, 92–101
  "nature" of, 11, 27, 76, 101

portraiture of, 66
satire and, 63–68
Maza, Sarah, 17
McCalman, Ian, 18
McKeon, Michael, 6
Mechanical and Critical Enquiry into the Nature of Hermaphrodites, A (Parsons), 19, 33–34
medievalism, 66, 86, 200, 205
Mee, John, 129
melancholy, 44, 105, 125, 192, 200. See also ennui
Melincourt (Peacock), 224–25
Mellor, Anne, 222
Melville, Peter, 185
Memoirs of Emma Courtney (Hays), 125–26
Memoirs of George IV (Huish), 201–2
Memoirs of the Author of the Vindication of the Rights of Woman (Godwin), 11, 86–92, 101–14, 118–21, 127
Memoirs of the Heroic Women of the Revolution (Broca), 69
Mennell, Stephen, 187, 189
mental disorder. See nervous disorder
Méricourt, Théroigne de, 30
methodology, 7, 91–92, 96, 147
Micale, Mark, 242n16
Microcosmographia: The Body of Man (Crooke), 1–2
midwifery, 37, 39, 56, 61
  Satire of Paine, 150
  Wollstonecraft's case, 89, 90
Miles, William Augustus, 181, 186
Mill, James, 103
Mill, John Stuart, 103
Millard, Ann, 100–101
moderation
  in diet, 183, 186, 189–93, 217, 227, 230
  personal and political, 12, 43, 106–7, 251n20
  sexual, 160
Modern Philosophy and Barbarism (Proby), 64, 109–10

modernity, 6, 41, 103, 138, 194
monarchy. See also George IV
  changing political role, 46, 169–70, 229, 233
  Royal Marriages Act, 178–80
  satire of, 177, 203, 222–23
Moniteur universal, 35
Monsam, Angela, 92
monstrosity, 16, 18. See also defects
Montagu, Lady Mary Wortley, 50–52
Monthly Mirror 104–6
mood, 44, 107, 122–24, 195–96. See also apathy
moral philosophy, 52, 59
Morning Chronicle, 89
Morning Post, 83, 130, 233, 251n7
Morris, Marilyn, 177
Morton, Timothy, 65, 216, 228
Moss, William, 56
mulligatawny, 204
Myers, Mitzi, 91–92
Mysteries of Conjugal Love Reveal'd, The, 37–38

Napoleon, 34, 68, 75, 167–70, 204, 244n60
narrative, 9–10, 105, 241n22
  architectural, 205
  gothic, 100,
  mythical, 227
  of foreign exploration, 213–14
  pedagogical, 118
  Sadean, 112
  scandalous, 129, 231, 235
  visual, 94
Narrative of the Incarceration of Count O'Neil, and the Massacre of his Family in France (O'Neil), 74
Nash, John, 203
National Assembly (France), 68, 73, 246n96
national identity, 107
  ancient Britons, 198–200, 216
  drink and, 151
  English physiology and, 107
  food and, 183, 198–201, 226, 229, 230

national identity *(continued)*
  neohumoral theory and, 107
  race and, 200–201, 213–14
Natural Method of Cureing Diseases of the Body (Cheyne), 177–78
neo-Gothic style, 203, 205
neoclassical style, 203
nervous disorders. See also apathy; hysteria
  ennui, 105–6
  gout and, 192
  masturbation and, 42, 48
  melancholy, 44, 105, 125, 192, 200
  sensibility and, 122, 123
  specifically female, 29, 122–24, 128
New Monthly Magazine, 100
New Theory of Generation, The, (Cook), 39–40
Newton, Isaac, 199
New Year's Gift for Mr. Thomas Paine, 135
Nicholas I, Grand Duke of Russia, 204
Nights in Paris (Bretonne), 112–13
Nihell, Elizabeth, 29, 45
Nisbet, William, 194
Normal and the Pathological, The (Canguilhem), 31
normalizing processes. See Foucault; normativity
normativity
  behavior, 13, 236
  cleanliness, 143, 154
  marriage and family, 30, 154–55, 161, 162, 181
  medical, 7
  morality, 135,
  social roles, 58
nostalgia, 151, 194, 216, 228
Nott, John (Theodore Price), 220
Nun, The (Diderot), 180
Nussbaum, Felicity, 31
nutrition, 16. See also dietetics; eating
nymphomania (uterine furor),
  according to Bienville, 22–28
  breastfeeding and, 56
  British physicians on, 17, 27–28
  Marie Antoinette as having, 11, 21–22, 29, 30–31, 35
  treatment of, 27–28
  women and, 17, 30, 56, 70
Nymphomania, or A Dissertation Concerning the Furor Uterinus (Bienville), 22–28

obesity, 12–13, 192, 200, 218, 234
"Observations on the Appeal from the New to the Old Whigs" (Boothby), 134–35
obstetrician, 1, 39, 90–91
O'Connor, Erin, 236
"Ode to Jacobinism," 36
Oedipus Tyrannus; or, Swellfoot the Tyrant (Shelley), 216–219
Oerlemans, Onno, 199
Offrey, Julian de La Mettrie, 195
Ollive, Elizabeth, 155
Onania: Or the Heinous Sin of Self-Pollution (Marten), 42, 44
onanism. See masturbation
O'Neil, Count, 74
one-sex model, 19, 20. See also biology of incommensurability; two-sex model
oophorectomy, 28
Oswald, John, 226

Paine, Thomas
  alcohol and, 133–36, 151–54, 163, 235
  Bonneville family and, 158
  as Cain and Nebuchadnezzar, 146–47
  decision not to have children, 155–58, 235
  doctors and, 156
  historical regicides and, 157
  hygiene and, 12, 133–162
  jail fever, 152
  marriages, 153–58
  political genealogy, 131
  popularity, 134, 137, 160, 163
  sexuality, 129, 133–35, 150, 154–62, 164, 235

stigmata, 146–47
Palais Royale, 190
Paris, Parisians
   cultural life of, 53, 112, 187, 190, 209
   revolutionary, 24, 53, 65, 71–72, 88, 108, 228–29
Paris Commune, 35
Parsons, James, 19, 33–34
Passages from the Diary of a Late Physician, 100
Pateman, Carole, 50
paternalism, 86
pathography, 133, 172
pathology
   eating and, 185, 212, 218, 234
   foreignness and, 214–15
   of indifference, 106
   masturbation as, 36, 119–20
   morality and, 176
   national identity and, 171, 212
   of nervous system, 123
   normal and pathological, 7, 10–13, 31, 75, 101, 128, 237
   political and medical, 174, 217
   satire and, 85
   sexual, 73, 158,
   as tool of scandalmongers, 161–62
   women and, 11, 13, 18, 21, 29, 36, 125
   written on the body, 148, 234
Patriot, The (Hardy), 63
patriotism, 53, 86, 110, 198
Paulson, Ronald, 65, 219
Peacock, Thomas Love, 224–25
penile dysfunction, 25, 42
Peptic Precepts (Kitchner), 195
Perry, Ruth, 52, 58, 157
Persian food, 221
perversion
   anatomy as, 98–100
   George IV as, 203
   obesity as, 218
   scientific, 91, 111–14
   sexual, 18, 24, 74–75, 157, 179
phagic determinism, 199
phallic symbol, 46
phenomenology, 188, 204

Phillips, Richard, 226
phrenology, 148, 235–36
physiognomy, 38, 74, 83
Physiologie du Goût (Brillat-Savarin), 188–90, 199
physiology, 1, 3, 7, 49, 235
   diet and, 176, 196, 228
   emotion as, 120–22
   female, 18, 33, 41, 101, 117
   politics and, 170
Pig's Meat (Spence), 216
Pigott, Charles, 4–6, 129
   on Duchess of Devonshire, 63
   on Duke of Norfolk, 4–6
   on George III, 178
   hygiene of, 131–33
   jail fever, 140
   libertinism of, 129
   on Princesses Royal, 180–81
   on Queen Charlotte, 47–8
   scandalizing of, 130–33
   as Tristram Shandy, 131–32
Pitt, William, the Younger
   announcement of spurious death, 82–85
   as asexual, 84–86
   false announcements of marriage, 85, 251n7
   Godwin and, 88, 110
   "Immaculate Boy," 83
   monarchy and, 263n24
   Regency Crisis and, 179–80
   satirical dissection of, 81–82
   "Signor Pittachio," 84
Plato, 1, 193
Pleasant Draught for Louis, A (Figure 5.1), 168
pleasure, 1, 12
"Poems Concerning the Slave Trade: Sonnet III" (Southey), 222
Poems, Lyrique, Macaronique, Heroique (Bold), 149
poetry, 7, 8, 44, 149
Poignand, physician attending Wollstonecraft, 90
Polignac, Duchess of, 30
polis, 1

Political Affection (Figure 2.1), 61
Political Dictionary (Pigott), 178
political ennui, 105
political iconography, 73
   amazon, 64, 70–76
   breast, 53–54, 59–68, 70–72, 77
   cannibal, 65–66, 73, 218–21, 229
   Marianne as liberty, 53
   pig, 215–29
   sodomite, 73–76
Political Justice (Godwin), 63, 71, 88, 102, 108, 128
pollution, 8, 23, 35, 135. See also contagion; contamination; masturbation
Polwhele, Richard, 12, 117–21, 160
Poovey, Mary, 115
pornography, political, 7, 18, 21–25, 45, 76
porphyria, 48, 179
Porter, Roy, 7, 133, 143, 167, 170–71, 174, 240n17
Post-Mortem Recollections of a Medical Lecturer, 100
postmortem report, 209
power
   female empowerment, 59, 77
   Foucault and, 9–10, 24
   of the imagination, 37
   monarchical, 170, 197
   political, 12, 20, 35, 48, 132, 164, 174, 209
Power/Knowledge (Foucault), 22
pox (syphilis), 75
Practical Treatise on Diet (Nisbet), 194
pregnancy. See reproduction
Presidential Bust of Hillary Rodham Clinton (Figure 2.6), 78
Price, Theodore (John Nott), 220
Priestley, Joseph, 26
Prince Henry Frederick, Duke of Cumberland, 178
Princess Caroline (consort of George IV), 202, 221
Princess Charlotte (daughter of George IV), 208

Princess Marie Louise of Savoy (Princess de Lamballe), 29, 30
Princess Dorothea von Lieven, 203
Principles of Midwifery, or Puerperal Medicine (Aiken), 28
Principles of Surgery (Hunter), 194
Pringle, John, 140
prison fever, 140
Proby, W.C., 64, 109–10
Prometheus, 227
Proteus, 194
psychoanalysis, 157
public and private. See separate spheres ideology
public gaze, 6, 10, 78, 98, 101, 203, 231
public opinion
   emerging as disciplinary mechanism, 6, 24, 26, 126–27, 232
   private life and, 63, 100, 126–27, 232
   revolutionary politics and, 130, 218–219
   taste and, 139, 187
"publicness," 6, 64
puerperal fever, 11, 87, 90–91, 146, 160, 235
Pugin, A.W.N., 205
Purity and Danger (Douglas), 135, 204
Pye, Henry James, 71

Queen Charlotte (consort of George III), 47–48, 176–77, 180, 196, 203, 222–24
Queen Mab (Shelley), 221, 225–26

Rajan, Tilottama, 12
Rambler's Magazine, 61
Ravaillac, François, 157
Reeves, John, 130, 134
Reflections on the Revolution (Burke), 3–4, 6, 102–3, 106–7, 172
Regency style, 203, 209
regeneration, 53, 59–60, 66, 68–69
regional identity, 183–84, 188, 198–200
regulation. See Foucault; self-regulation

reproduction, 7, 30, 39, 44, 235–36
  anatomy and, 92–99
Republic (Plato), 193
"Republican Judge, The" (Cobbett), 33
Republican Refuted, The (Elliot), 156–57
Republican Thomas Paine (Hunt), 137, 145, 162
republicanism, 63, 65, 73, 102, 145, 153, 226
resurrectionists, 99–100
Restorer of Health and Physician of Nature, The, 170
restraint. See self-restraint
Rights of Englishmen: An Antidote to the Poison now Vending by the Transatlantic Republican Thomas Paine (Hunt), 137
Right Hon. Democrat Dissected, A (Figure 3.1), 81–82
Rights of Man (Paine), 64, 136, 139, 150, 156, 163
Ritson, Joseph, 226–228
roast beef, 198–200, 210
Robespierre, 69, 228
Romilly, Samuel, 107
Roland, Marie-Jeanne Phlippon (Madame Roland), 69–70
Roosevelt, Theodore, 163, 261n114
Rose, Nikolas, 7–8
Rosenberg, Charles, 142
Rothschilds, the, 204
Rousseau, George, 7, 42
  on gout, 143, 167, 170–72, 264n42
  on nerves, 124, 240n17, 242n16
  on pathography, 133
Rousseau, Jean-Jacques
  abandonment of his family, 158
  breastfeeding and motherhood, 53–59
  comparative anatomy and, 20
  domesticity and, 20, 54, 59, 69, 76, 114
  gendered sexual difference, 20, 72
  masculinity, 54, 59, 72
  on nature, 2, 20, 52, 53–55, 59, 175, 194, 228

noble savage, 54, 149, 211, 228
  as Paine's progenitor, 158
  sex life, 158
Rowlandson, Thomas, 61, 99–100
Royal College of Surgeons, 19, 244n46
Royal Dildo, The, 21, 73
Royal Marriages Act, 178–80
Royal Medical Society of Edinburgh, 141
Royal Philosophical Society, 31
Ruskin, John, 205
Ruston, Sharon, 240n17, 253n52
Rymsdyk, Jacob van, 94–97, 111

Sade, Marquis de (Donatien Alphonse François)
  Beauvoir's commentary on, 113
  compared with Godwin, 111–14
  experiments on Rose Keller, 112
  on fraternity, 113
  Justine, 17, 112
  La nouvelle Justine, 112
  mother-in-law's claims, 113
  sexual violence and religion, 180
  sexual violence and science, 111–14
Saint-Amand, Pierre, 77
Salic Law, 46
Salkin Sbiroli, Lynn, 68
Salzmann, Christian, 118–19, 255n99
sanitation, 7, 12, 144, 214, 237. See also hygiene
Sartor Resartus (Carlyle), 103
satire. See individual illustrations, listed page ix
scandal, 4–12
  George IV and, 177, 205
  Marie Antoinette, 17–34
  medicalized, 100, 161
  Paine and, 129–39
  politics and, 233, 240
scars, 148–49
Schiebinger, Londa, 52, 209, 247n1
Schwellenberg, Juliane von, 223–24
scopophilia, 210
Secret History of Domesticity (McKeon), 6

Sedgwick, Eve Kosofsky, 146
sedition (seditious words), 1–3, 5, 88, 130, 133, 234
self-abuse. See masturbation
self-interest (selfishness)
  George IV and, 186, 216–18, 226–29
  Godwin and, 81, 85, 88–89, 109, 113
  Hobbesian human nature and, 149–50, 211, 229
  modern culture and, 53, 56, 126, 142
  Paine and, 156
  Sade and, 113
  sex and, 75, 183
self-restraint (self-control), 12, 126
  cleanliness, 144, 160
  dietary restraint, 178, 181, 187–96, 199, 231–34
  Jacobinism and, 87
  masculinity and, 171, 226–29
  masturbation and, 43
  temperance, 160, 199
  women and, 57
self-regulation (self-management). See also discipline
  gastronomy and, 189–96
  governmentality, 144, 161–62
  heteronormativity and, 45
  masculinity and, 171, 226–29
  proper body, 150, 231–36
self-pleasure. See masturbation
semen, 50, 123
semiotics, 204–5
sensibility, 9, 236
  cleanliness and, 138
  diseases of culture and, 191, 240n17
  Duchess of Devonshire and, 63
  eating and, 184–85
  female embodiment and, 114, 119–26
  masculinity and, 227–29
  sensus communis, 12, 185, 186, 196
  sex and, 156–57
separate spheres ideology
  Amazons, homosexuality and, 72–76
  Marie Antoinette and, 20–48

  mothers, breast-feeding and, 58–70
  Wollstonecraft and, 115–25
Sex. See also homosexuality; lesbianism; masturbation
  deviance, 18, 27–30, 41, 111–12, 133–34, 154
  Foucault on, 156
  non-procreative, 73, 155–58, 235
  nymphomania, 22–28
  penile dysfunction, 25, 42
  perversion and anatomy, 98–100
  sexual norms, 13, 154–58, 161–62, 181, 236
  sexual sadism, 111–12
  sexual violence and religion, 180
  sexual violence and science, 111–14
  transparency and, 43, 75, 207
Sha, Richard, 33, 93
shame, 35, 72, 75, 126–27, 161–62, 209
Sharp, Jane, 37
Shelley, Percy Bysshe, 216–22, 225–29
Sheriff, Mary, 30
Shildrick, Margrit, 42, 138, 164
Shuttleton, David, 149–50
Siddons, Sarah, 127
Scientific Magazine and Free-Mason's Repository, The, 104, 127
"Signs of the Times" (Carlyle), 103
Simon, Antoine, 35
sinus pudoris, 209
Sir Thomas More (Southey), 215–16, 222
slavery, 107, 147, 175, 212, 222–25
smallpox, 140, 145–46, 149
Smith, E. A., 232
Smith, Hugh, 57
Smollett, Tobias, 201
Snow, C. P., 7
social contract, 107
social degeneracy. See degeneration
social shame, 126–27
social-constructivist views of gender, 116–17
sodomy, 73–75
soldiers, 21, 71, 76
solipsimus convictorii, 184

Solitary Sex (Laqueur), 42–43
Sontag, Susan, 213
South Sea Islanders, 229
Southey, Robert, 215–16, 222
spatial design, 205
spatial politics, 232
Spence, Thomas, 216
Sphere, Projecting against a Plane, A (figure 3.3), 83–84
Spurzheim, Johann, 235–36
Staël, Germaine de, 68
Stafford, Barbara, 27
Stephen, Leslie, 163
Sterne, Laurence, 131–32
Stevenson, William, 173–76, 181
stigmata, 146–47
Stoker, Bram, 145
Stolberg, Michael, 43
Stomach
  ailments of, 103, 123, 176, 183
  gastronomy and, 190, 191, 194–96
  in political satire, 81–82, 170, 183, 218, 221
Stone, Lawrence, 157
Storer, Horatio, 28
Sturgeon, Lancelot, 190–91
Successful Method of Treating Gout by Blistering (Stevenson), 173
sugar, 176, 222–25
Sure Methods of Improving Health (Graham), 227
susceptibility, 9, 29, 40, 69, 120, 122, 191. See also maternal impression
Sussman, George, 53
Sydenham, Thomas, 167, 215–16
symbiosis, 3, 205, 217, 225
symbolic osmosis, 199
syphilis, 75, 183, 211

Tabella Cibaria: The Bill of Fare (Macquin), 190
taboo, 174. See also Douglas, Mary
Talleyrand, 68, 204
Tatars, 211
Tauchert, Ashley 115–16
taxation, 106, 129, 217

Telegraph, 82
Temperance Enjoying a Frugal Meal (Figure 5.3), 177
Terror, The, 105
Thelwall, John, 26, 88–89, 251–52n20
Thomas, Chantal, 17
Thompson, E. P. 117, 255n95
Thorburn, Grant, 146
Thoughts on Marriage and Criminal Conversation, 126–27
Thoughts on the Probable Influence of the French Revolution on Great-Britain (Romilly), 107
Thousand and One Nights, The, 204
Timaeus (Plato), 193
Tissot, S. A. D., 44
Tom Paine's Nightly Pest (Figure 4.1), 147–48
Tomahawk, 26
Tooke, John Horne, 179–80
Tories, 81, 85, 179, 220
transparency
  anatomical illustration and, 92
  breastfeeding and, 58
  exotic tastes and, 203, 207
  hermaphroditism and, 31,
  political and moral, 6, 23–24, 121, 176, 235
  sexual practices and, 43, 75, 207
  women's bodies and, 27
Treason Trials, 5, 85, 88
Treatise on All the Diseases Incident to Women, A (Astruc), 17
Treatise of the Hypochodriack and Hysterick Diseases (Mandeville), 124
Treatise on Getting and Nursing of Children, 61
Treatise on the Art of Midwifery, A (Nihell), 39
Treatise on the Gout (Sydenham), 167–77
Treatise on the Venereal Disease (Falck), 75
tribadism. See lesbianism
Tribune (Thelwall), 26, 88–89
Tristram Shandy (Sterne), 131–32

"The Triumph of the Whale" (Lamb), 233–34
Two Acts, 5, 85, 88
two-sex model, 19–20. See also biology of incommensurability; one-sex model
typhus, 214

Un petit Soupèr à la Parisiènne: or, A Family of Sans-Culotts Refreshing, after the Fatigues of the Day (Figure 2.4), 64–66
Uncle Sam, 198
The Unsex'd Females (Polwhele), 117–19, 121
Use of Pleasure, The, 193
uterine furore/furor uterinus. See nymphomania
uterine prolapse/prolapsed uterus, 32
utilitarianism
  anatomy and, 101–3
  eating as, 195
  Godwin and, 11–12, 64, 85, 98, 104, 109, 121, 235
  materialism, science, and, 112–14
  Sade and, 112–14

vampirism, 36, 145–47
Van Sant, Ann Jessie, 120
vegetarianism, 13
  Cheyne and, 177–78, 199
  Cuvier and, 270n99
  Ritson and, 226–27
  Shelley and, 221, 225–29
venereal disease, 75, 183, 185, 214
Venette, Nicholas, 37–39
Versailles, 4, 43, 232
Versuch einer allgemeinen medicinisch-praktischen Geographie (Finke), 213
Vickers, Neil, 256n118
"Victim, The," 100
vigor, 4. See also vitality
  male constitution, 73, 123
  mind-body, 154,
  pre-modern bodies, 211, 215
Vindication of the Rights of Men 116

Vindication of the Rights of Woman, 54, 114–116, 118, 120, 125, 128, 129
Vindication of Natural Diet, A (Shelley), 221, 225, 226–27
Visions of the Daughters of Albion (Blake), 212
visuality, politics of, 27, 94–101, 203, 206, 210
vitalism, 102, 194–5
vitality, 6–8, 102. See also vigor
  Englishness and, 107–8
  lack of, 131, 167
  male, 123–24
  masturbation and, 44
  political, 145, 167
vivisection, 112, 133–34
Voltaire, 209
Voluptuary under the Horrors of Digestion, A (Figure 5.4), 176, 182–5
voyeurism, 78, 100, 209–10

Wadd, William, 185
Wakefield, Gilbert, 226
Wakefield, Patricia, 120
Walpole, Horace, 113
Walter, Gérard, 244n61
Warwick, Alexandra, 138
Waterhouse, Benjamin, 136
Wathen, Jonathan, 75
wax anatomical models, 92, 113
well-being, 10
Wells, T. Spencer, 28
Wennerstrom, Courtney, 98, 101
wet nursing, 50, 52, 54, 60. See also breast-feeding
Weymouth, 232
Wheeler, Roxann, 218
Whigs, 4, 60, 81, 83, 129, 179
Whole Works of that Excellent Practical Physician, (Sydenham), 167, 215
Williams, Helen Maria, 36, 45, 117, 125
Williams, Raymond, 142
Willich, A. F. M., 43–44, 123, 143–144, 146, 151

Wilmot, Edward Sloane, 22
Windsor, 231
Wingrove, Elizabeth, 53
Wollstonecraft, Mary, 11–12
  as amazon, 71–72
  botany and, 120–21
  on breast-feeding, 54
  as "concubine," 86
  death in childbirth, 90–91, 105, 117, 124–25
  Fuseli and, 86
  gendered biological difference and, 114–17
  on hygiene, 115
  hysteria and, 125–26, 236
  Imlay and, 86, 125, 127
  as "libertine," 87
  marriage and, 114–15, 119, 126–27
  marriage to Godwin, 110, 124, 126–27
  masturbation and, 118–20
  midwifery and, 89, 90
  overheated emotions, 110–11
  posthumous reputation, 86
  as "prostitute," 87
  puerperal fever, 11, 87, 90–91, 146, 160, 235
  sensibility and, 120–26
  socially shamed, 126–28
  suicide attempts, 86, 125–26
  as translator, 118–19
  womb, 11, 22, 29, 34, 90, 94–98
Wood, John, 135
Wordsworth, William, 121

Yalom, Marilyn, 72
Youngquist, Paul, 20, 98, 101, 240n17

Zimmermann, Johann Georg, 42

www.ingramcontent.com/pod-product-compliance
Lightning Source LLC
Chambersburg PA
CBHW031706230426
43668CB00006B/121